Textbook of Pharmacology for Physiotherapy

Textbook of Pharmacology for Physiotherapy

Padmaja Udaykumar
Professor and Head
Department of Pharmacology
Fr Muller Medical College
Mangalore

JAYPEE BROTHERS
MEDICAL PUBLISHERS (P) LTD
New Delhi

Published by

Jitendar P Vij
Jaypee Brothers Medical Publishers (P) Ltd
EMCA House, 23/23B Ansari Road, Daryaganj, **New Delhi** 110 002,
Phones: +91-11-23272143, 23272703, 23282021, 23245672
Fax: 011-23276490, 23245683 e-mail: jaypee@jaypeebrothers.com
Visit our website: www.jaypeebrothers.com

Branches

- 2/B Akruti Society, Jodhpur Gam Road, Satellite
  Ahmedabad 380 015, Phone: +91-079-30988717, 26926233
  e-mail: jpamdvd@rediffmail.com
- 202 Batavia Chambers, 8 Kumara Krupa Road, Kumara Park East,
  Bangalore 560 001, Phones: +91-80-22285971, 22382956, 30614073
  Tele Fax: +91-80-22281761 e-mail: jaypeemedpubbgl@eth.net
- 282 IIIrd Floor, Khaleel Shirazi Estate, Fountain Plaza Pantheon Road,
  Chennai 600 008, Phones: +91-44-28262665, 28269897
  Fax: +91-44-28262331 e-mail: jpchen@eth.net
- 4-2-1067/1-3, Ist Floor, Balaji Building, Ramkote Cross Road,
  Hyderabad 500 095, Phones: +91-40-55610020, 24758498
  Fax: +91-40-24758499 e-mail: jpmedpub@rediffmail.com
- 1A Indian Mirror Street, Wellington Square,
  Kolkata 700 013, Phones: +91-33-22456075, +91-33-22451926
  Fax: +91-33-22456075 e-mail: jpbcal@cal.vsnl.net.in
- 106 Amit Industrial Estate, 61 Dr SS Rao Road, Near MGM Hospital Parel,
  Mumbai 400 012, Phones: +91-22-24124863, 24104532, 30926896
  Fax: +91-22-24160828 e-mail: jpmedpub@bom7.vsnl.net.in
- "KAMALPUSHPA",38 Reshimbag, Opp.Mohota Science College,
  Umred Road **Nagpur** 440009, Phones: 0712-3945220, 2704275,
  Fax: +91-0712-2704275 e-mail: jpmednagpur@rediffmail.com

Textbook of Pharmacology for Physiotherapy

First Edition : 2004
Reprint : 2006

ISBN 81-8061-278-3

Typeset at JPBMP typesetting unit
Printed at Gopsons Papers Ltd, A-14, Sector 60, Noida

Dedicated

to

Prof. BG Lalitha

Retd. Professor of Zoology

Foreword

Textbook is the most important companion, tool and light of a learning student to lead him, to shape him, enlighten him to perfect himself in the chosen subject of his studies. So it should be reader friendly, descriptive and analytical, to reach those goals, to fit into the mind of the learner. It should also be tailored to the needs of the student to pass his examination, which also is one of the primary goals of a student.

Pharmacology to many, including me, is one of the tough subjects, to learn amongst the medical curriculum. Most of the textbooks in pharmacology have been written, tailored to the needs of a medical student. Dr Padmaja Udaykumar in her own inimitable style has penned this textbook fully looking into the needs of a physiotherapy student. Physiotherapy is one of the most dynamic fields in medicine today to put back the patient to his physical perfection and the student ought to know the pharmacodynamics of the musculoskeletal and neurovascular systems. This book has met all these goals and I find it useful to an orthopaedic and physical medicine postgraduate student as well.

I have known Dr Padmaja for many years. Her tenacity of purpose, vision and enthusiasm has culminated in yet another masterpiece. She is a source of inspiration to the younger generation for academic excellence.

I am sure this textbook will be of immense help to its user and I strongly recommend it, especially to physiotherapy students.

With best wishes

Dr M Shantharam Shetty
Dean and Director-Professor of Orthopaedics
KS Hegde Medical Academy, Mangalore

Preface

Pharmacology is a science that is rapidly growing. Basic knowledge of pharmacology is required for all those who deal with patients. Since there is no standard textbook meant exclusively for physiotherapy students, they are faced with the hardship of having to refer medical pharmacology books. Such volume and depth of pharmacology is unnecessary for physiotherapists and also difficult to çomprehend. Hence this book is written to make pharmacology simple for physiotherapy students. The presentation has been simple so that the students easily understand the subject. Guidelines of the University syllabus has been followed. More importance has been given for topics like analgesics, skeletal muscle relaxants and other musculoskeletal disorders which are emphasized for physiotherapy students. Syllabuses of some universities have recommended topics like 'drugs and exercise', 'vasoconstrictors and vasodilators' for physiotherapy students. They have also been discussed briefly.

I hope this book reduces the burden of students in learning pharmacology.

Padmaja Udaykumar

Acknowledgements

I am extremely grateful to Dr M Shantharam Shetty, Dean and Director-Professor of Orthopaedics, KS Hegde Medical Academy, Mangalore, for writing Foreword to this book.

I am sincerely thankful to the management of Fr Muller Medical College, Director, Fr Baptist Menezes, Administrator—Fr Lawrence D'souza and Dean Dr Sanjeev Rai, for their encouragement and support.

I wish to place on record my sincere thanks to Dr Annappa Kulal for his suggestions. I am thankful to my colleagues Dr Princy Palatty, Dr Prasanna Lakshmi and Dr Vijayalakshmi for their encouragement.

I owe a special note of thanks to my husband Prof Udaykumar K for his constant encouragement and valuable suggestions, which made this work possible.

I also wish to thankfully acknowledge the prompt and meticulous work of M/s Jaypee Brothers Medical Publishers (P) Ltd, New Delhi.

Contents

1

General Pharmacology

- Introduction and sources of drugs
- Routes of drug administration
- Pharmacokinetics
- Pharmacodynamics
- Adverse drug reactions and drug interactions
- Gene therapy

INTRODUCTION AND SOURCES OF DRUGS

Pharmacology is the science that deals with the study of drugs and their interaction with the living systems.

Early man recognised the benefits and toxic effects of many plants and animal products. India's earliest pharmacological writings are from the 'Vedas.' An ancient Indian physician Charaka and then Sushruta and Vagbhata described many herbal preparations included in 'Ayurveda' (meaning the science of life). James Gregory recommended harsh and dangerous remedies like blood-letting, emetics and purgatives to be used until the symptoms of the disease subsided (such remedies often resulted in fatality). This was called 'Allopathy' meaning the other suffering. This word, still being used for the modern system of medicine, is a misnomer. To counter this system, Hannemann introduced the system of Homoeopathy meaning similar suffering in the early 19th century. The principles of this include 'like cures like' and dilution enhances the action of drugs. Thus, several systems of therapeutics were introduced, of which only few survived. The basic reason for failure of many systems is that man's concepts about diseases were incorrect and baseless in those days. By the end of the 17th century the value of experimentation and observation became clear and many physicians applied these to the traditional drugs. Francois Magendie and Claude-Bernard popularised the use of animal experiments to understand the effects of drugs. The development of physiology also helped in the better understanding of pharmacology. The last century has seen a rapid growth of the subject with new concepts and techniques being introduced.

DEFINITIONS

The word pharmacology is derived from Greek word—*Pharmacon* meaning an active principle or drug and *logos* meaning a discourse.

Drug (Drogue—a dry herb in French) is a substance used in the diagnosis, prevention or treatment of a disease. WHO definition—"A Drug is any substance or product that is used or intended to be used to modify or explore physiological systems or pathological states for the benefit of the recipient."

Pharmacodynamics is the study of the effects of the drugs on the body and their mechanisms of action, i.e. what the drug does to the body.

Pharmacokinetics is the study of the absorption, distribution, metabolism and excretion of drugs, i.e. what the body does to the drug (in Greek *Kinesis* = movement).

Therapeutics deals with the use of drugs in the prevention and treatment of disease.

Toxicology deals with the adverse effects of drugs and also the study of poisons, i.e detection, prevention and treatment of poisonings *(Toxicon = poison in Greek).*

Chemotherapy is the use chemicals for the treatment of infections. The term now also includes the use of chemical compounds to treat malignancies.

Pharmacopoeia (In Greek *Pharmacon* = drug; *poeia*=to make) is the official publication containing a list of drugs and medicinal preparations approved for use, their formula and other information needed to prepare a drug; their physical properties, tests for their identity, purity and potency. Each country may follow its own pharmacopoeia to guide its physicians and pharmacists. We thus have the Indian Pharmacopoeia (IP) the British Pharmacopoeia (BP) and the United States Pharmacopoeia (USP). The list is revised at regular periods to delete old useless drugs and to include newly introduced ones.

Pharmacy is the science of identification, compounding and dispensing of drugs. It also includes collection, isolation, purification, synthesis and standardisation of medicinal substances.

SOURCES OF DRUGS

The sources of drugs could be **natural** or **synthetic**.

Natural sources Drugs can be obtained from:

1. *Plants*, e.g. atropine, morphine, quinine, and digoxin.
2. *Animals*, e.g. insulin, heparin, gonadotrophins and antitoxic sera.
3. *Minerals*, e.g. magnesium sulphate, aluminium hydroxide, iron, sulphur and radioactive isotopes.
4. *Microorganisms*—antibacterial agents are obtained from some bacteria and fungi. We thus have penicillin, cephalosporins, tetracyclines and other antibiotics.
5. *Human*—some drugs are obtained from human beings, e.g. immunoglobulins from blood, growth hormone from anterior pituitary and chorionic gonadotrophins from the urine of pregnant women.

Synthetic Most drugs are now synthesized, e.g. quinolones, omeprazole.

Many drugs are obtained by cell cultures, e.g. urokinase from cultured human kidney cells. Some are now produced by recombinant DNA technology, e.g. human insulin, tissue plasminogen activator.

❑ ROUTES OF DRUG ADMINISTRATION

Drugs may be administered by various routes. The choice of the route in a given patient depends on the properties of the drug and the patient's requirements. A knowledge of the advantages and disadvantages of the different routes of administration is essential.

The routes can be broadly divided into:

- Enteral
- Parenteral
- Local.

ENTERAL ROUTE (ORAL INGESTION)

This is the most common, oldest and safest route of drug administration. The large surface area of the gastrointestinal tract, the mixing of its contents and the differences in pH at different parts of the gut facilitate effective absorption of the drugs given orally. However, the acid and enzymes secreted in the gut and the biochemical activity of the bacterial flora of the gut can destroy some drugs before they are absorbed.

Advantages

1. Safest route
2. Most convenient
3. Most economical
4. Drugs can be self-administered
5. Non-invasive route.

Disadvantages

1. Onset of action is slower as absorption needs time.
2. Irritant and unpalatable drugs cannot be administered.
3. Some drugs may not be absorbed due to certain physical characteristics, e.g. streptomycin.
4. Irritation to the gastrointestinal tract may lead to vomiting.
5. There may be irregularities in absorption.
6. Some drugs may be destroyed by gastric juices, e.g. insulin.
7. Cannot be given to unconscious and uncooperative patients.
8. Some drugs may undergo extensive first pass metabolism in the liver.

To overcome some of the disadvantages, irritants are given in capsules, while bitter drugs are given as sugar coated tablets. Sometimes drugs are coated with substances like synthetic resins, gums, sugar, colouring and flavouring agents making them more acceptable.

Enteric Coated Tablets

Some tablets are coated with substances like cellulose-acetate, phthalate, gluten, etc. which are not digested by the gastric acid but get disintegrated in the alkaline juices of the intestine. This will:

1. prevent gastric irritation.
2. avoid destruction of the drug by the stomach.
3. provide higher concentration of the drug in the small intestine.
4. retard the absorption, and thereby prolong the duration of action. But if the coating is inappropriate, the tablet may be expelled without being absorbed at all. Similarly, controlled-release or sustained-release preparations are designed to prolong the rate of absorption and thereby the duration of action of drugs. This is useful for short-acting drugs.

Advantages

- Frequency of administration may be reduced.
- Therapeutic concentration may be maintained specially when nocturnal symptoms are to be treated.

Disadvantages

- There may be 'failure of the preparation' resulting in release of the entire amount of the drug in a short-time leading to toxicity.
- It is more expensive.

Certain precautions are to be taken during oral administration of drugs—capsules and tablets should be swallowed with a glass of water with the patient in upright posture either sitting or standing. This facilitates passage of the tablet into the stomach and its rapid dissolution. It also minimises chances of the drug getting into larynx or behind the epiglottis. Recumbent patient should not be given drugs orally as some drugs may remain in the oesophagus due to the absence of gravitational force facilitating the passage of the drug into the stomach. Such drugs can damage the oesophageal mucosa, e.g. iron salts, tetracyclines.

PARENTERAL ROUTE

Routes of administration other than the enteral (intestinal) route are known as parenteral routes. Here the drugs are directly delivered into tissue fluids or blood.

Advantages

- Action is more rapid and predictable than oral administration.
- These routes can be employed in an unconscious or uncooperative patient.
- Gastric irritants can be given parenterally and therefore irritation to the gastrointestinal tract can be avoided.
- It can be used in patients with vomiting or those unable to swallow.
- Digestion by the gastric and intestinal juices and the first pass metabolism are avoided.

Therefore, in emergencies parenteral routes are very useful routes of drug administration as the action is rapid and predictable and are useful in unconscious patients.

Disadvantages

- Asepsis must be maintained.
- Injections may be painful.
- More expensive, less safe and inconvenient.
- Injury to nerves and other tissues may occur.

Parenteral routes include:

1. Injections
2. Inhalation
3. Transdermal route
4. Transmucosal route.

INJECTIONS

Intradermal

The drug is injected into the layers of the skin raising a bleb, e.g. BCG vaccine, tests for allergy or by multiple punctures of the epidermis through a drop of the drug, e.g. smallpox vaccine. Only a small quantity can be administered by this route and it may be painful.

Subcutaneous (SC) Injection

Here the drug is deposited in the SC tissue, e.g. insulin, heparin. As this tissue is less vascular, absorption is slow and largely uniform making the drug long-acting. It is reliable and patients can be trained for self-administration. Absorption can be enhanced by the addition of the enzyme hyaluronidase.

Disadvantages

- As SC tissue is richly supplied by nerves, irritant drugs can cause severe pain. Hence such drugs cannot be injected.
- In shock, absorption is not dependable because of vasoconstriction.
- Repeated injections at the same site can cause lipoatrophy resulting in erratic absorption.

Hypodermoclysis is the SC administration of large volumes of saline employed in paediatric practice.

Drugs can also be administered subcutaneously as:

1. *Dermojet* In this method, a high velocity jet of drug solution is projected from a fine orifice using a gun. The solution gets deposited in the SC tissue from where it is absorbed. As needle is not required, this method is painless. It is suitable for vaccines.
2. *Pellet implantation* Small pellets packed with drugs are implanted subcutaneously. The drug is slowly released for weeks or months to provide constant blood levels, e.g. testosterone.
3. *Sialistic implants* The drug is packed in sialistic tubes and implanted subcutaneously. The drug gets absorbed over months to provide constant blood levels, e.g. hormones and contraceptives. The empty non-biodegradable implant has to be removed.

Intramuscular (IM)

Aqueous solution of the drug is injected into one of the large skeletal muscles—deltoid, triceps, gluteus or rectus femoris.

As the muscles are vascular, absorption is rapid and quite uniform.Drugs are absorbed faster from the deltoid region than gluteal region especially in women. The volume of injection should not exceed 10 ml. For infants, rectus femoris is used instead of gluteus which is not well-developed till the child starts walking.If the drug is injected as an oily solution, absorption is slow and steady.

Advantages
- Intramuscular route is reliable.
- Absorption is rapid.
- Soluble substances, mild irritants, depot preparations, suspensions and colloids can be injected by this route.

Disadvantages
- Intramuscular injection may be painful and may even result in an abscess.
- Nerve injury should be avoided near a nerve, irritant solutions can damage the nerve if injected.

Intravenous (IV)

Here, the drug is injected into one of the superficial veins so that it directly reaches the circulation and is immediately available for action.

Drugs can be given IV as:

1. A bolus—where an initial large dose is given, e.g. heparin.The drug is dissolved in a suitable amount of the vehicle and injected slowly.
2. Slowly—over 15-20 minutes, e.g. aminophylline.
3. Slow infusion—when constant plasma concentrations are required, e.g. oxytocin in labour or when large volumes have to be given, e.g. dextrose, saline. Generally about one litre of solution is infused over 3 to 4 hours. But the patients condition dictates the rate of infusion.

Advantages
- Most useful route in emergencies as the drug is immediately available for action.
- Provides predictable blood concentrations with 100% bioavailability.

- Large volumes of solutions can be given.
- Irritants can be given by this route as they get quickly diluted in the blood.
- Rapid dose adjustments are possible—if unwanted effects occur, infusion can be stopped; if higher levels are required, infusion rate can be increased—specially for short-acting drugs.

Disadvantages

- Once injected into the vein, the drug cannot be withdrawn.
- Irritation of the veins may cause thrombophlebitis.
- Extravasation of some drugs may cause severe irritation and sloughing.
- Only aqueous solutions can be given IV but not suspensions, oily solutions and depot preparations.
- Self medication is difficult.

Intraperitoneal Peritoneum offers a large surface area for absorption. Fluids are injected intraperitoneally in infants. This route is also used for peritoneal dialysis.

Intrathecal Drugs can be injected into the subarachnoid space for action on the CNS, e.g. spinal anaesthetics. Some antibiotics and corticosteroids are also injected by this route to produce high local concentrations. Strict aseptic precautions are a must.

Drugs are also given extradurally. Morphine can be given epidurally to produce analgesia.

Intra-articular Drugs are injected directly into a joint for the treatment of arthritis and other diseases of the joints. Strict aseptic precautions are required, e.g. hydrocortisone in rheumatoid arthritis.

Intra-arterial Here drug is injected directly into the arteries. It is used only in the treatment of (i) peripheral vascular diseases, (ii) local malignancies and (iii) diagnostic studies like angiograms.

Intramedullary Injection into a bone marrow—now rarely used.

INHALATION

Volatile liquids and gases are given by inhalation, e.g. general anaesthetics. In addition, drugs can be administered as solid particles, i.e. solutions of drugs can be atomised and the fine droplets are inhaled as aerosol, e.g. salbutamol. These inhaled drugs and vapours may act on the pulmonary epithelium and mucous membranes of the respiratory tract and are also absorbed through these membranes.

Advantages
- Almost instantaneous absorption of the drug is achieved because of the large suface area of the lungs.
- In pulmonary diseases, it serves almost as a local route as the drug is delivered at the desired site making it more effective and less harmful.
- First pass metabolism is avoided.
- Blood levels of volatile anaesthetics can be conveniently controlled as their absorption and excretion through the lungs are governed by the laws of gases.

Disadvantage
- Irritant gases may enhance pulmonary secretions-should be avoided.
- This is an important route of entry of certain drugs of abuse.

TRANSDERMAL

Highly lipid soluble drugs can be applied over the skin for slow and prolonged absorption, e.g. nitroglycerine ointment in angina pectoris. Adhesive units, inunction, iontophoresis and jet injection are some forms of transdermal drug delivery.

Adhesive units (transdermal therapeutic systems) are adhesive patches of different sizes and shapes made to suit the area of application. The drug is held in a reservoir between an outer layer and a porous membrane. This membrane is smeared with an adhesive to hold on to the area of application. The drug slowly diffuses through the membrane and percutaneous absorption takes place. The rate of absorption is constant and predictable. Highly potent and short acting drugs are suitable for use in such systems.

Sites of application are chest, abdomen, upper arm, back or mastoid region, e.g. hyoscine, nitroglycerine, fentanyl transdermal patches.

Advantages
- Duration of action is prolonged
- Provides constant plasma drug levels
- Patient compliance is good.

Inunction This route where a drug rubbed into the skin gets absorbed to produce systemic effects is called inunction.

Iontophoresis In this procedure, galvanic current is used for bringing about penetration of lipid insoluble drugs into the deeper tissues where its action is required, e.g. Salicylates.

Jet injection As absorption of drug occurs across the layers of the skin, dermojet may also be considered as a form of transdermal drug administration (description on page 7).

TRANSMUCOSAL

Drugs are absorbed across the mucous membranes. Transmucosal administration includes sublingual, nasal and rectal routes.

Sublingual Here, the tablet or pellet containing the drug is placed under the tongue. It dissolves in the saliva and the drug is absorbed across the sublingual mucosa, e.g. nitroglycerine, nifedipine, buprenorphine.

Advantages
- Absorption is rapid—within minutes the drug reaches the circulation.
- First pass metabolism is avoided.
- After the desired effect is obtained, the drug can be spat out to avoid the unwanted effects.

Disadvantage
Buccal ulceration can occur.

Nasal Drugs can be administered through nasal route either for systemic absorption or for local effects, e.g.
- oxytocin spray is used for systemic absorption.
- for local effect
  - decongestant nasal drops, e.g. oxymetazoline;
  - budesonide nasal spray for allergic rhinitis.

Rectal Rectum has a rich blood supply and drugs can cross the rectal mucosa to be absorbed for systemic effects. Drugs absorbed from the upper part of the rectum are carried by the superior haemorrhoidal vein to the portal circulation (can undergo first pass metabolism), while that absorbed from the lower part of the rectum is carried by the middle and inferior haemorrhoidal veins to the systemic circulation.

Some irritant drugs are given per rectally as *suppositories:*

Advantages

- Gastric irritation is avoided.
- Can be administered by unskilled persons.
- Useful in geriatric patients and others with vomiting and those unable to swallow.

Disadvantages

- Irritation of the rectum can occur.
- Absorption may be irregular and unpredictable.
- Drugs like—indomethacin, chlorpromazine, diazepam and paraldehyde can be given rectally.

Drugs may also be given by this route as **enema**.

Enema is the administration of a drug in a liquid form into the rectum. Enema may be evacuant or retention enema.

Evacuant enema In order to empty the bowel, about 600 ml of soap water is administered per rectally. Water distends and thus stimulates the rectum while soap lubricates. Enema is given prior to surgeries, obstetric procedures and radiological examination of the gut.

Retention enema The drug is administered with about 100 ml of fluids and is retained in the rectum for local action, e.g. prednisolone enema in ulcerative colitis.

TOPICAL

Drugs may be applied on the skin for local action as ointment, cream, gel, powder, paste, etc. Drugs may also be applied on the mucous membrane as in the eyes, ears and nose, as ointment, drops and sprays. Drugs may be administered as **suppository** for rectum, **bougie** for urethra and **pessary** and **douche** for vagina. Pessaries are oval shaped tablets to be placed in the vagina to provide high local concentrations of the drug at the site, e.g. antifungal pessaries in vaginal candidiasis.

Special Drug Delivery Systems

In order to improve drug delivery, to prolong duration of action and thereby improve patient compliance, special drug delivery systems are being tried. Drug targeting, i.e. to deliver drugs at the site where it is required to act is also being aimed at, especially for anticancer drugs. Some such systems are ocusert, progestasert, transdermal adhesive units, prodrugs,osmotic pumps, computerised pumps and methods using monoclonal antibodies and liposomes as carriers.

Ocusert Ocusert systems are thin elliptical units that contain the drug in a reservoir which slowly releases the drug through a membrane by diffusion at a steady rate, e.g. pilocarpine ocusert used in glaucoma is placed under the lid and can deliver pilocarpine for 7 days.

Progestasert is inserted into the uterus where it delivers progesterone constantly for over one year.

Transdermal adhesive units See page 10.

Prodrug is an inactive form of the drug which gets metabolised to the active derivative in the body. A prodrug may overcome some of the disadvantages of the conventional forms of drug administration, e.g. dopamine does not cross the BBB; levodopa, a prodrug crosses the BBB and is then converted to dopamine in the CNS. Prodrugs may also be used to have longer duration of action, e.g. Bacampicillin (a prodrug of ampicillin) is longer acting.

Osmotic pumps are small tablet shaped units consisting of the drug and an osmotic substance placed in two chambers. The osmotic layer swells and pushes the drug slowly out of a small hole. Iron and prazosin are available in this form.

Computerised miniature pumps These are programmed to release drugs at a definite rate either continuously as in case of insulin or intermittently in pulses as in case of GnRH.

Various methods of drug targeting are tried especially for anticancer drugs to reduce toxicity.

Monoclonal antibodies against the tumor specific antigens are used to deliver anticancer drugs to specific tumor cells.

Liposomes are phospholipids suspended in aqueous vehicles to form minute vesicles. Drugs encapsulated in liposomes are taken up mainly by the reticuloendothelial cells of the liver and are also concentrated in malignant tumors. Thus, site-specific delivery of drugs may be possible with the help of liposomes.

❑ PHARMACOKINETICS

Pharmacokinetics is the study of the absorption, distribution, metabolism and excretion of drugs, i.e. the movement of the drugs into, within and out of the body. For a drug to produce its specific response, it should be present in adequate concentrations at the site of action. This depends on various factors apart from the dose. Once the drug is administered, it is absorbed, i.e. enters the blood, is distributed to different parts of the body, reaches the site of action, is metabolised and excreted (Fig. 1.1). All these processes involve passage of the drug molecules across various barriers—like the intestinal epithelium, cell membrane, renal filtering membrane, capillary barrier and so on. To cross these barriers the drug has to cross the cell membrane or pass in-between the epithelial or endothelial cells.

The cell membrane/biological membrane is made up of two layers of phospholipids with intermingled protein molecules (Fig. 1.2). All lipid soluble substances get dissolved in the cell

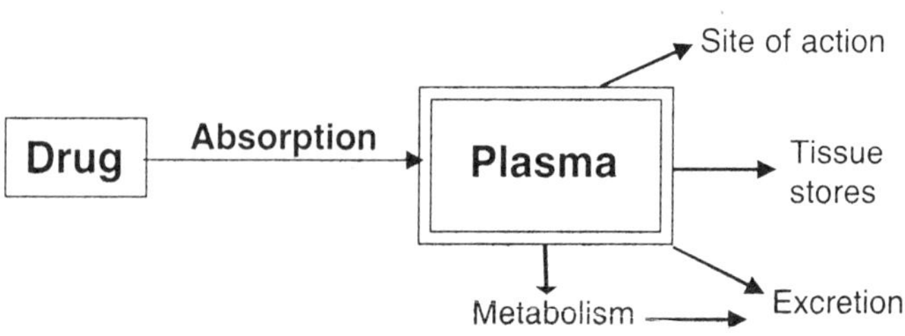

Fig. 1.1: Schematic representation of movement of drug in the body

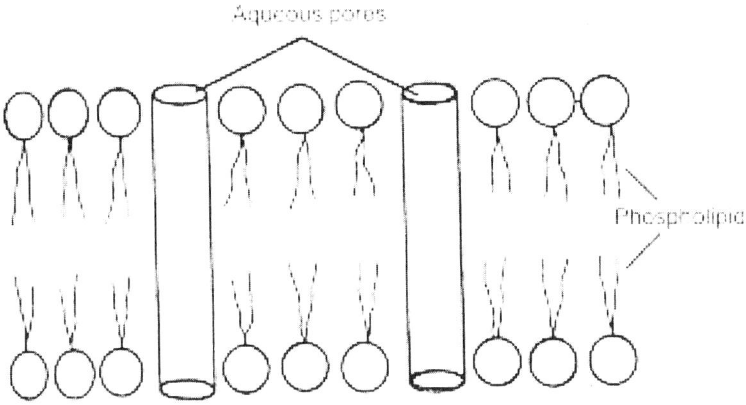

Fig. 1.2: Cell/biological membrane (schematic)

membrane and readily permeate into the cells. The junctions between adjacent epithelial or endothelial cells have pores through which small water-soluble molecules can pass. Movement of some specific substances is regulated by special carrier proteins. The passage of drugs across biological membranes involves processes like passive (filtration, diffusion) and active transport.

Mechanisms of Transport of Drug Across Biological Membranes

Passive transfer	*Carrier-mediated transport*	*Endocytosis*
— Simple diffusion	— Active transport	
— Filtration	— Facilitated diffusion	

Passive Transfer

The drug moves across the membrane without any need for energy either by *simple diffusion* in the direction of its concentration gradient or by *filtration* through aqueous pores in the membrane.

Carrier-mediated Transport

Active transport is the transfer of drugs against a concentration gradient and needs energy. It is carried by a specific carrier protein. Only drugs related to natural metabolites are transported by this process, e.g. levodopa, iron, amino acids.

Facilitated diffusion is a unique form of carrier transport which differs from active transport in that it is not energy dependent and the movement occurs in the direction of the concentration gradient. The carrier facilitates diffusion and is highly specific for the substance, e.g. uptake of glucose by cells, vitamin B_{12} from intestines.

Endocytosis

Endocytosis is the process where small droplets are engulfed by the cell. Some proteins are taken up by this process (like pinocytosis in amoeba).

ABSORPTION

Absorption is defined as the passage of the drug from the site of administration into the circulation. For a drug to reach its site of action, it must pass through various membranes depending on the route of administration. Absorption occurs by one of the processes described above, i.e. passive diffusion or carrier-mediated transport. Thus except for intravenous route, absorption is important for all other routes of administration. Several factors influence the rate and extent of absorption of a drug (Fig. 1.3). They are:

1. **Disintegration and dissolution time** The drug taken orally should break up into individual particles (disintegrate) to be absorbed. It then has to dissolve in the gastrointestinal fluids. In case of drugs given subcutaneously or intramuscularly, the drug molecules have to dissolve in the tissue fluids. Liquids are absorbed faster than solids. Delay in disintegration and dissolution as with poorly water-soluble drugs like aspirin, result in delayed absorption.
2. **Formulation** Pharmaceutical preparations are formulated to produce desired absorption. Inert substances used with drugs as diluents like starch and lactose may sometimes interfere with absorption.
3. **Particle size** Small particle size is important for better absorption of drugs. Drugs like corticosteroids, griseofulvin, digoxin, aspirin and tolbutamide are better

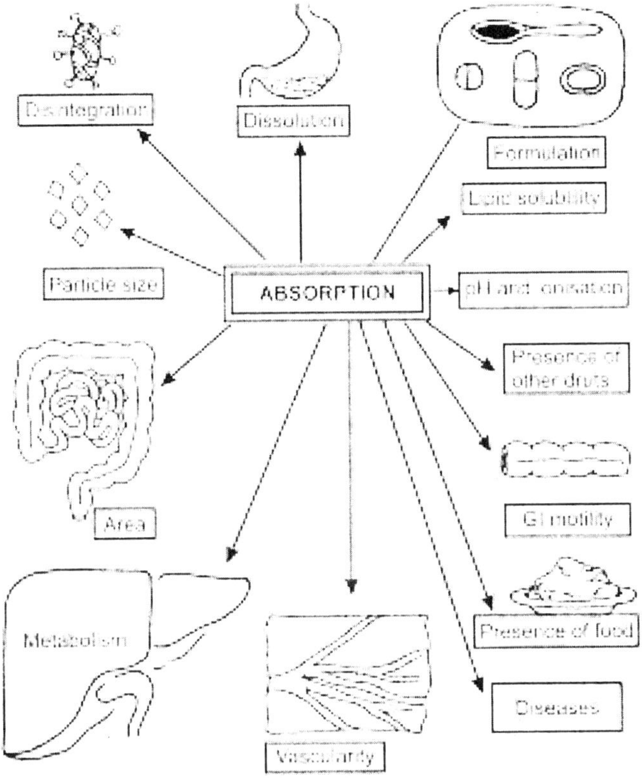

Fig. 1.3: Factors affecting absorption of drugs

absorbed when given as small particles. On the other hand, when a drug has to act on the gut and its absorption is not desired, then particle size should be kept large, e.g. anthelmintics like bephenium hydroxynaphthoate.

4. **Lipid solubility** Lipid soluble drugs are absorbed faster and better by dissolving in the phospholipids of the cell membrane.
5. **pH and ionisation** Ionised drugs are poorly absorbed while unionised drugs are lipid soluble and are well absorbed. Most drugs are weak electrolytes and ionise according to pH. Thus acidic drugs remain unionised in acidic medium of the stomach and are rapidly absorbed,

e.g. aspirin, barbiturates. Basic drugs are unionised when they reach the alkaline medium of intestine from where they are rapidly absorbed, e.g. pethidine, ephedrine.

Strong acids and bases are highly ionised and therefore poorly absorbed, e.g. streptomycin.

6. **Area and vascularity of the absorbing surface** The larger the area of absorbing surface and more the vascularity—better is the absorption. Thus most drugs are absorbed from small intestine.
7. **Gastrointestinal motility**
   Gastric emptying time—if gastric emptying is faster, the passage of the drug to the intestines is quicker and hence absorption is faster.
   Intestinal motility—when highly increased as in diarrhoeas, drug absorption is reduced.
8. **Presence of food** delays gastric emptying, dilutes the drug and delays absorption. Drugs may form complexes with food constituents and such complexes are poorly absorbed, e.g. tetracyclines chelate calcium present in food. Moreover, certain drugs like ampicillin, roxithromycin and rifampicin are well absorbed only on empty stomach.
9. **Metabolism** Some drugs may be degraded in the GI tract, e.g. nitroglycerine, insulin. Such drugs should be given by alternate routes.
10. **Diseases** of the gut like malabsorption and achlorhydria result in reduced absorption of drugs.

First pass metabolism is the metabolism of a drug during its passage from the site of absorption to the systemic circulation. It is also called presystemic metabolism or first pass effect and is an important feature of oral route of administration. Drugs given orally may be metabolised in the gut wall and in the liver before reaching the systemic circulation. The extent of first pass metabolism differs from drug to drug and among individuals, from partial to total inactivation. When it is partial, it can be compensated by giving higher dose of the particular drug, e.g. nitroglycerine, propranolol, salbutamol. But for drugs that undergo extensive first pass metabolism, the route of administration has to be changed, e.g. isoprenaline, hydrocortisone, insulin.

First pass metabolism

- is metabolism of a drug during its first passage through gut wall and liver
- reduces bioavailability
- extent of metabolism depends on the drug and individuals
- consequences— dose has to be increased for some drugs like propranolol
  — route has to be changed for some others like hydrocortisone
- examples: morphine, chlorpromazine, nitroglycerine, verapamil, testosterone, insulin, lignocaine

Bioavailability

Bioavailability is the fraction of the drug that reaches the systemic circulation following administration by any route. Thus for a drug given intravenously, the bioavailability is 100 percent. On IM/SC injection, drugs are almost completely absorbed while by oral route, bioavailability may be low due to incomplete absorption and first pass metabolism. Infact all the factors which influence the absorption of a drug also alter bioavailability.

Bioequivalence

Comparison of bioavailability of different formulations of the same drug is the study of bioequivalence. Often oral formulations containing the same amount of a drug from different manufacturers may result in different plasma concentrations, i.e. there is no bioequivalence. Such differences occur with poorly soluble, slowly absorbed drugs mainly due to differences in the rate of distintegration and dissolution. Variation in bioavailability (nonequivalence) can result in toxicity or therapeutic failure in drugs that have low safety margin like digoxin and drugs that need precise dose adjustment like anticoagulants and corticosteroids. For such drugs, in a given patient, the preparations from a single manufacturer should be used.

DISTRIBUTION

After a drug reaches the systemic circulation, it gets distributed to other tissues. It should cross several barriers before reaching the site of action. Like absorption, distribution also involves the same processes, i.e. filtration, diffusion and specialised transport. Various factors determine the rate and extent of distribution, *viz* lipid solubility, ionisation, blood flow and binding to plasma proteins and cellular proteins. Unionised lipid soluble drugs are widely distributed throughout the body.

Plasma Protein Binding

On reaching the circulation most drugs bind to plasma proteins; acidic drugs bind mainly albumin and basic drugs to alpha-acid glycoprotein. The free or unbound fraction of the drug is the only form available for action, metabolism and excretion while the protein bound form serves as a reservoir. The extent of protein binding varies with each drug, e.g. warfarin is 99% and morphine is 35% protein bound while binding of ethosuximide and lithium is 0%, i.e. they are totally free.

Clinical Significance of Plasma Protein Binding

1. Only free fraction is available for action, metabolism and excretion. When the free drug levels fall, bound drug is released.
2. Protein binding serves as a store (reservoir) of the drug and the drug is released when free drug levels fall.
3. Protein binding prolongs duration of action of the drug.
4. Many drugs may compete for the same binding sites. Thus one drug may displace another from the binding sites resulting in toxicity. For example, indomethacin displaces warfarin from protein binding sites leading to increased warfarin levels.
5. Chronic renal failure and chronic liver disease result in hypoalbuminaemia with reduced protein binding of drugs.

Some highly protein bound drugs

Warfarin	Tolbutamide	Phenytoin
Frusemide	Clofibrate	Sulfonamides
Diazepam	Salicylates	Phenylbutazone
Indomethacin		

Tissue binding Some drugs get bound to certain tissue constituents because of special affinity for them. Tissue binding delays elimination and thus prolongs duration of action of the drug. For example, lipid soluble drugs are bound to adipose tissue. Tissue binding also serves as a reservoir of the drug.

Redistribution When highly lipid soluble drugs are given intravenously or by inhalation, they get rapidly distributed into highly perfused tissues like brain, heart and kidney. But soon they get redistributed into less vascular tissues like the muscle and fat resulting in termination of the action of these drugs. The best example is the intravenous anaesthetic thiopental sodium which induces anaesthesia in 10-20 seconds but the effect stops in 5-15 minutes due to redistribution.

Blood-brain barrier (BBB) The endothelial cells of the brain capillaries lack intercellular pores and instead have tight junctions. Moreover, glial cells envelope the capillaries and together these form the BBB. Only lipid soluble, unionised drugs can cross this BBB. During inflammation of the meninges, the barrier becomes more permeable to drugs, e.g. penicillin readily penetrates during meningitis. The barrier is weak at some areas like CTZ, posterior pituitary and parts of hypothalamus and allows some compounds to diffuse.

Placental barrier Lipid soluble, unionised drugs readily cross the placenta while lipid insoluble drugs cross to a much lesser extent. Thus drugs taken by the mother can cause several unwanted effects in the foetus.

Volume of Distribution (V_d)

Apparent volume of distribution is defined as the volume necessary to accommodate the entire amount of the drug, if the concentration throughout the body were equal to that in plasma. It relates the amount of the drug in the body to the concentration of the drug in plasma. It is calculated as

$$V_d = \frac{\text{Amount of drug in the body}}{\text{Plasma concentration}}$$

For example, if the dose of a drug given is 500 mg and attains a uniform concentration of 10 mg in the body, its $V_d = 50$ litres.

The knowledge of V_d of drugs is clinically important in the treatment of poisoning. Drugs with large V_d like pethidine are not easily removed by haemodialysis.

BIOTRANSFORMATION (Metabolism)

Biotransformation is the process of biochemical alteration of the drug in the body. Body treats most drugs as foreign substances and tries to inactivate and eliminate them by various biochemical reactions. These processes convert the drugs into more polar, water-soluble compounds so that they are easily excreted through the kidneys. Some drugs may be excreted largely unchanged in the urine, e.g. frusemide, atenolol.

Site The most important organ of biotransformation is the liver. But drugs are also metabolised by the kidney, gut mucosa, lungs, blood and skin.

Result of biotransformation Though biotransformation generally inactivates the drug, some drugs may be converted to active or more active metabolites (Table 1.1).

TABLE 1.1: Result of biotransformation

Active drug to inactive metabolite	*Active drug to active metabolite*	*Inactive drug to active metabolite (prodrug)*
e.g. Morphine	e.g. Primidone→ Phenobarbitone	e.g. Levodopa→ Dopamine
Chloramphenicol	Digitoxin→ Digoxin	Prednisone→ Prednisolone
	Diazepam→Oxazepam	Enalapril→Enalaprilat

When the metabolite is active, the duration of action gets prolonged. **Prodrug** is an inactive drug which gets converted into an active form in the body (Table 1.1).

ACTIVE DRUG

↓ *Metabolism*

Inactive drug (Prodrug) → *active metabolite* → **INACTIVATION** ← *active metabolite* ← **Active drug** (Prolongs duration of action)

Enzymes in biotransformation The biotransformation reactions are catalysed by specific enzymes located either in the liver microsomes (microsomal enzymes) or in the cytoplasm and mitochondria of the liver cells and also in the plasma and other tissues (non-microsomal enzymes).

The chemical reactions of biotransformation can take place in two phases (Fig. 1.4).

1. Phase I (Non-synthetic reactions)
2. Phase II (Synthetic reactions).

Phase I reactions convert the drug to a more polar metabolite by oxidation, reduction or hydrolysis. Oxidation reactions are the most important metabolising reactions, mostly catalysed by mono-oxygenases present in the liver. If the metabolite is not sufficiently polar to be excreted, they undergo phase II reactions.

Phase II reactions are conjugation reactions where water-soluble substances present in the body like glucuronic acid, sulfuric acid, glutathione or an amino acid, combine with the drug or its phase I metabolite to form a highly polar compound. This is inactive and gets readily excreted by the kidneys. Large

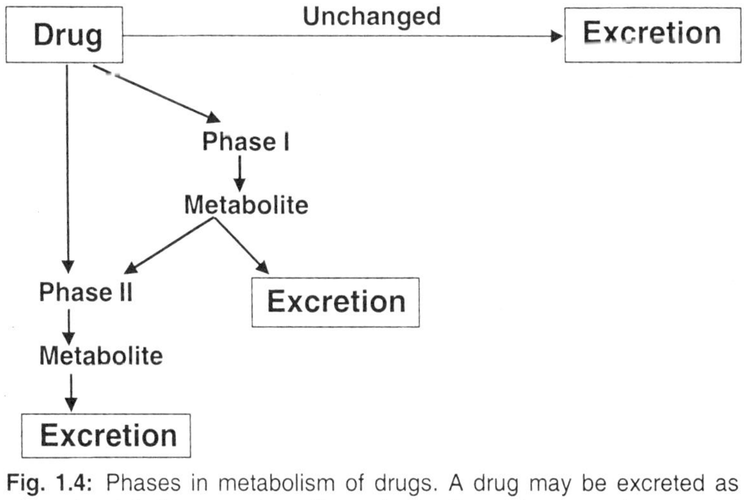

Fig. 1.4: Phases in metabolism of drugs. A drug may be excreted as phase I metabolite or as phase II metabolite. Some drugs may be excreted as such

molecules are excreted through the bile. Thus, phase II reactions invariably inactivate the drug.

Glucuronide conjugation is the most common type of metabolic reaction (Table 1.2).

TABLE 1.2: Important drug biotransformation reactions

Reactions	*Examples of drugs*
Oxidation	Phenytoin, Diazepam, Ibuprofen, Amphetamine, Chlorpromazine, Dapsone
Reduction	Chloramphenicol, Halothane
Hydrolysis	Pethidine, Procaine
Conjugation reactions	
Glucuronide conjugation	Chloramphenicol, Morphine
Acetylation	Sulfonamides, Isoniazid
Methylation	Adrenaline, Histamine
Glutathione conjugation	Paracetamol
Sulfate conjugation	Paracetamol, Steroids

Enzyme Induction

Microsomal enzymes are located in the microsomes of the liver cells. The synthesis of these enzymes can be enhanced by certain drugs and environmental pollutants. This is called *enzyme induction* and this process speeds up the biotransformation of the inducing drug itself and other drugs metabolised by the microsomal enzymes, e.g. phenobarbitone, rifampicin, alcohol, cigarette smoke, DDT, griseofulvin, carbamazepine and phenytoin are some enzyme inducers.

Enzyme induction can result in drug interactions.

Therapeutic application of enzyme induction Neonates are deficient in both microsomal and nonmicrosomal enzymes. Hence their capacity to conjugate bilirubin is low which results in jaundice. Administration of phenobarbitone—an enzyme inducer, helps in rapid clearance of the jaundice in them by enhancing bilirubin conjugation.

Enzyme inhibition Some drugs like cimetidine and ketoconazole inhibit cytochrome P450 enzyme activity. Enzyme inhibition by drugs is also the basis of several drug interactions. Chloramphenicol, Cimetidine, erythromycin, ketoconazole, ciprofloxacin and verapamil are some enzyme inhibitors cimetidine.

EXCRETION

Drugs are excreted from the body after being converted to water-soluble metabolites while some are directly eliminated without metabolism. The major organs of excretion are the kidneys, the intestine, the biliary system and the lungs. Drugs are also excreted in small amounts in the saliva, sweat and milk.

Renal Excretion

Kidney is the most important route of drug excretion. The three processes involved in the elimination of drugs through kidneys are glomerular filtration, active tubular secretion and passive tubular reabsorption.

Glomerular filtration The rate of filtration through the glomerulus depends on GFR, concentration of free drug in the plasma and its molecular weight. Ionised drugs of low molecular weight (< 10,000) are easily filtered through the glomerular membrane.

Active tubular secretion Cells of the proximal tubules actively secrete acids and bases by two transport systems. Thus, acids like penicillin, salicylic acid, probenecid, frusemide; bases like amphetamine and histamine are so excreted. Drugs may compete for the same transport system resulting in prolongation of action of each other, e.g. penicillin and probenecid.

Passive tubular reabsorption Passive diffusion of drug molecules can occur in either direction in the renal tubules depending on the drug concentration, lipid solubility and pH. As highly lipid soluble drugs are largely reabsorbed, their excretion is slow. Acidic drugs get ionised in alkaline urine and are easily excreted while bases are excreted faster in acidic urine. This property is useful in the treatment of poisoning. In poisoning with acidic drugs like salicylates and barbiturates, forced alkaline diuresis (Diuretic + sodium bicarbonate + IV fluids) is employed to hasten drug excretion. Similarly, elimination of basic drugs like quinine and amphetamine is enhanced by forced acid diuresis.

Faecal and Biliary Excretion

Unabsorbed portion of the orally administered drugs are eliminated through the faeces. Liver transfers acids, bases and unionised molecules into bile by specific acid transport processes. Some drugs may get reabsorbed in the lower portion of the gut and are carried back to the liver. Such recycling is called *enterohepatic circulation* and it prolongs the duration of action of the drug; examples are chloramphenicol, tetracycline, oral contraceptives and erythromycin.

Pulmonary Excretion

The lungs are the main route of elimination for gases and volatile liquids viz general anaesthetics and alcohol. This also has legal implications in medicolegal practice.

Other Routes of Excretion

Small amounts of some drugs are eliminated through the sweat and saliva. Excretion in saliva may result in a unique taste of some drugs, e.g. metronidazole and phenytoin. Drugs like iodide, rifampicin and heavy metals are excreted through sweat.

The excretion of drugs in the **milk** is in small amounts and is of no significance to the mother. But, for the suckling infant, it may be sometimes important especially because of the infant's immature metabolic and excretory mechanisms. Though most drugs can be taken by the mother without significant toxicity to the child, there are a few exceptions (Table 1.3).

TABLE 1.3: Example of drugs that could be toxic to the suckling infant when taken by the mother

Sulphasalazine	Doxepin
Theophylline	Amiodarone
Anticancer drugs	Primidone
Salicylates	Ethosuximide
Chloramphenicol	Phenobarbitone
Nalidixic acid	Phenothiazines
Nitrofurantoin	β-blockers

Clearance (CL) is the volume of plasma freed completely of the drug in unit time. It can be calculated by the ratio of the rate of elimination to the plasma concentration.

$$\text{Thus, CL} = \frac{\text{Rate of elimination}}{\text{Plasma concentration}}$$

Clearance is expressed as ml/litre/ unit time.

Clearance is the most important factor determining drug concentration and should be considered when any drug is intended for long-term administration.

Drugs are metabolised/eliminated from the body by:

1. *First-order kinetics* In first order kinetics, a constant *fraction* of the drug is metabolised/eliminated per unit time. Most drugs follow first order kinetics and the rate of metabolism/excretion is dependant on their concentration (exponential) in the body. It also holds good for absorption of drugs.
2. *Zero order kinetics (Saturation kinetics)* Here a constant *amount* of the drug present in the body is metabolised/ eliminated per unit time. The metabolic enzymes get saturated and hence with increase in dose, the plasma drug level increases disproportionately resulting in toxicity.

Some drugs like phenytoin and warfarin are eliminated by both processes, i.e. by first order initially and by zero order at higher concentrations.

Plasma Half-life and Steady State Concentration

Plasma half-life (t½) is the time taken for the plasma concentration of a drug to be reduced to half it's value (Fig. 1.5). Four to five half-lives are required for the complete elimination of a drug. Each drug has its own t½ and is an important pharmacokinetic parameter that guides the dosing regimen. It helps in calculating loading and maintenance doses of a drug. It also indicates the duration of action of a drug.

Biological half-life is the time required for total amount of the drug in the body to be reduced to half.

Biological effect half-life is the time required for the biological effect of the drug to reduce to half. In some drugs like propranolol, the pharmacological effect of the drug may last much

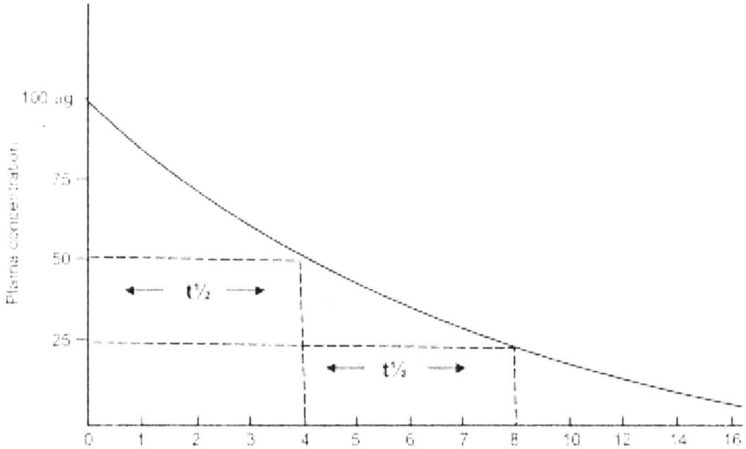

Fig. 1.5: Plasma concentration-time curve following intravenous dose. Plasma t½ = 4 hrs

longer, i.e. even after its plasma levels fall. In such drugs, biological effect half life gives an idea of the duration of action of the drug.

If a drug is administered repeatedly at short intervals before complete elimination, the drug accumulates in the body and reaches a 'state' at which the rate of elimination equals the rate of administration. This is known as the *'Steady-state'* or plateau level (Fig. 1.6). After attaining this level, the plasma concentration fluctuates around an average steady level. It takes 4-5 half-lives for the plasma concentration to reach the plateau level.

DRUG DOSAGE

Depending on the patient's requirements and the characteristics of the drug, drug dosage can be of the following kinds

Fixed dose In case of reasonably safe drugs, a fixed dose of the drug is suitable for most patients, e.g. analgesics like paracetamol—500 mg to 1000 mg 6 hourly is the usual adult dose.

Individualised dose For some drugs especially the ones with low safety margin, the dose has to be 'tailored' to the needs of each patient, e.g. anticonvulsants, antiarrhythmic drugs.

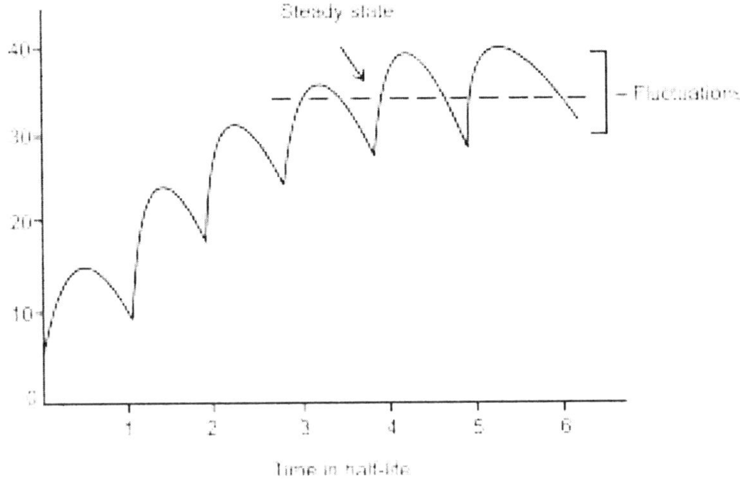

Fig. 1.6: Drug accumulation and attainment of steady state concentration on oral administration

Loading dose In situations when target plasma concentrations have to be attained rapidly, a loading/bolus dose of the drug is given at the beginning of the treatment. A loading dose is a single large dose or a series of quickly repeated doses given to rapidly attain target concentration, e.g. heparin given as 5000 IU bolus dose. Once the target level is reached, a *maintenance dose* is sufficient to 'maintain the drug level' and to balance the elimination.

The disadvantage with the loading dose is that the patient is rapidly exposed to high concentrations of the drug which may result in toxicity.

Therapeutic drug monitoring The response to a drug depends on the plasma concentration attained in the patient. In some situations it may be necessary to monitor treatment by measuring plasma drug concentrations. Such situations are:

1. while using drugs with low safety margin—to avoid therapeutic failure, e.g. digoxin, theophylline, lithium.
2. to reduce the risk of toxicity, e.g. aminoglycosides.
3. to treat poisoning.

METHODS OF PROLONGING DRUG ACTION (Table 1.4)

In several situations it may be desirable to use long-acting drugs. But when such drugs are not available, the duration of action of the available drugs may be prolonged.

TABLE 1.4: Methods of prolonging duration of action of drugs

Processes	*Methods*	*Examples*
ABSORPTION		
Oral	Sustained release preparation, coating with resins, etc.	Iron, deriphylline
Parenteral	1. Reducing solubility — Oily suspension	Procaine + Penicillin Depot progestins
	2. Altering particle size	Insulin zinc suspension as large crystals that are slowly absorbed
	3. Pellet implantation — Sialistic capsules	DOCA Testosterone
	4. Reduction in vascularity of the absorbing surface	Adrenaline + lignocaine (vasoconstrictor)
	5. Combining with protein	Protamine + zinc + insulin
	6. Chemical alteration — Esterification	Estrogen Testosterone
Dermal	Transdermal adhesive patches, Ointments	Scopolamine Nitroglycerine
	Ocuserts (Transmucosal)— used in eye	Pilocarpine
DISTRIBUTION	Choosing more protein bound member of the group	Sulfonamides-like sulfamethoxy-pyridazine
METABOLISM	Inhibiting the metabolising enzyme cholinesterase	Physostigmine prolongs the action of acetylcholine
	By inhibiting enzyme peptidase in renal tubular cells	Cilastatin—prolongs action of imipenem
EXCRETION	Competition for same transport system — for renal tubular secretion	Probenecid prolongs the action of penicillin and ampicillin

The duration of action of drugs can be prolonged by interfering with the pharmacokinetic processes, i.e. by

1. Slowing absorption.
2. Using a more plasma protein bound derivative.
3. Inhibiting metabolism.
4. Delaying excretion.

❑ PHARMACODYNAMICS

Pharmacodynamics is the study of actions of the drugs on the body and their mechanisms of action, i.e. to know what drugs do and how they do it.

Drugs produce their effects by interacting with the physiological systems of the organisms. By such interaction, drugs merely modify the rate of functions of the various systems. But they cannot bring about qualitative changes, i.e. they cannot change the basic functions of any physiological system. Thus drugs act by:

1. Stimulation
2. Depression
3. Irritation
4. Replacement
5. Anti-infective or cytotoxic action
6. Modification of the immune status.

Stimulation is the increase in activity of the specialised cells, e.g. adrenaline stimulates the heart.

Depression is the decrease in activity of the specialised cells, e.g. quinidine depresses the heart; barbiturates depress the central nervous system. Some drugs may stimulate one system and depress another, e.g. morphine depresses the CNS but stimulates the vagus.

Irritation This can occur on all types of tissues in the body and may result in inflammation, corrosion and necrosis of cells.

Replacement Drugs may be used for replacement when there is deficiency of natural substances like hormones, metabolites or nutrients, e.g. insulin in diabetes mellitus, iron in anaemia, vitamin C in scurvy.

Anti-infective and cytotoxic action Drugs may act by specifically destroying infective organisms, e.g. penicillins, or by cytotoxic effect on cancer cells, e.g. anticancer drugs.

Modification of immune status Vaccines and sera act by improving our immunity while immunosuppressants act by depressing immunity, e.g. glucocorticoids.

MECHANISMS OF DRUG ACTION

Most drugs produce their effects by binding to specific target proteins like receptors, enzymes and ion channels. Drugs may act *on* the cell membrane, *inside* or *outside* the cell to produce their effect. Drugs may act by one or more complex mechanisms of action. Some of them are yet to be understood. But the fundamental mechanisms of drug action may be:

- Through receptors
- Through enzymes and pumps
- Through ion channels
- By physical action
- By chemical interaction
- By altering metabolic processes.

1. Through Receptors

Drugs may act by interacting with specific receptors in the body (see below).

2. Through Enzymes and Pumps

Drugs may act by inhibition of various enzymes, thus altering the enzyme-mediated reactions, e.g. allopurinol inhibits the enzyme xanthine oxidase; acetazolamide inhibits carbonic anhydrase.

Membrane pumps like $H^+ K^+$ ATPase, $Na^+ K^+$ ATPase may be inhibited by drugs, e.g. omeprazole, digoxin.

3. Through Ion Channels

Drugs may interfere with the movement of ions across specific channels, e.g. calcium channel blockers, potassium channel openers.

4. Physical Action

The action of a drug could result from its physical properties like:

Adsorption	–	Activated charcoal in poisoning
Mass of the drug	–	Bulk laxatives like psyllium, bran
Osmotic property	–	Osmotic diuretics—Mannitol
	–	Osmotic purgatives—Magnesium sulphate
Radioactivity	–	^{131}I
Radio-opacity	–	Barium sulphate contrast media.

5. Chemical Interaction

Drugs may act by chemical reaction.

Antacids	–	neutralise gastric acids
Oxidising agents	–	like potassium permanganate - germicidal
Chelating agents	–	bind heavy metals making them nontoxic.

6. Altering Metabolic Processes

Drugs like antimicrobials alter the metabolic pathway in the microorganisms resulting in destruction of the microorganism, e.g. sulfonamides interfere with bacterial folic acid synthesis.

Receptor

A receptor is a site on the cell with which an agonist binds to bring about a change, e.g. histamine receptor, α and β adrenergic receptors.

Affinity is the ability of a drug to bind to a receptor.

Intrinsic activity or efficacy is the ability of a drug to produce a response after binding to the receptor.

Agonist An agonist is a substance that binds to the receptor and produces a response. It has affinity and intrinsic activity.

Antagonist An antagonist is a substance that binds to the receptor and prevents the action of agonist on the receptor. It has affinity but no intrinsic activity.

Partial agonist binds to the receptor but has low intrinsic activity.

Ligand is a molecule which binds selectively to a specific receptor.

Last three decades have seen an explosion in our knowledge of the receptors. Various receptors have been identified, isolated and extensively studied.

Site The receptors may be present in the cell membrane, in the cytoplasm or on the nucleus.

Nature of receptors Receptors are proteins.

Synthesis and life-span Receptor proteins are synthesized by the cells. They have a definite life span after which the receptors are degraded by the cell and new receptors are synthesized.

Functions of Receptors

The two functions of receptors are

1. Recognition and binding of the ligand
2. Propagation of the message.

For the above function, the receptor has two functional domains (areas):

i. *A ligand binding domain*—the site to bind the drug molecule
ii. *An effector domain*—which undergoes a change to propagate the message.

Drug-receptor interaction has been considered to be similar to 'lock and key' relationship where the drug specifically fits into the particular receptor (lock) like a key. Interaction of the agonist with the receptor brings about changes in the receptor which in turn conveys the signal to the effector system. The final response is brought about by the effector system through second messengers. The agonist itself is the first messenger. The entire process involves a chain of events triggered by drug receptor interaction.

Receptor Families

Four families types of cell surface receptors are identified. The receptor families are:

1. Ion channels
2. G-protein coupled receptors
3. Enzymatic receptors
4. Transcription factors (receptors that regulate gene transcription).

Receptor Regulation

The number of receptors (density) and their sensitivity can be altered in many situations. Denervation or prolonged deprivation of the agonist or constant action of the antagonist all result in an increase in the number and sensitivity of the receptors. This phenomenon is called **'up regulation.'**

Prolonged use of a β adrenergic antagonist like propranolol results in up regulation of β adrenergic receptors.

On the other hand, continued stimulation of the receptors causes desensitisation and a decrease in the number of receptors—known as **'down regulation'** of the receptors.

Clinical consequences and implications of receptor regulation
After prolonged administration, a receptor antagonist should always be tapered. For example, if propranolol—a β adrenoceptor blocker is suddenly withdrawn after long-term use, it precipitates angina.

Constant use of β adrenergic agonists in bronchial asthma results in reduced therapeutic response due to down regulation of β_2 receptors.

Dose Response Relationship

The clinical response to the increasing dose of the drug is defined by the shape of the dose response curve (DRC). Initially the extent of response increases with increase in dose till the maximum response is reached. The dose response curve has the shape of a rectangular hyperbola (Fig. 1.7). After the maximum effect has been obtained, further increase in doses does not increase the response. If the dose is plotted on a logarithmic scale, the curve becomes sigmoid (Fig. 1.8). The slope of DRC (Fig. 1.9) has clinical significance. A steep slope indicates that a small increase in dose produces a large increase in response, e.g. loop diuretics. Such drugs are more likely to cause toxicity and therefore, individualisation of dose is required. A relatively flat DRC indicates that with an increase in dose, there is little increase in the response, e.g. thiazide diuretics. For such drugs standard doses can be given to most patients.

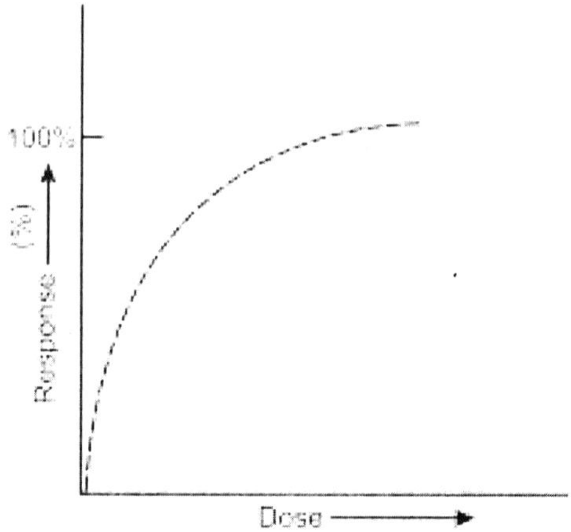

Fig. 1.7: Dose response curve

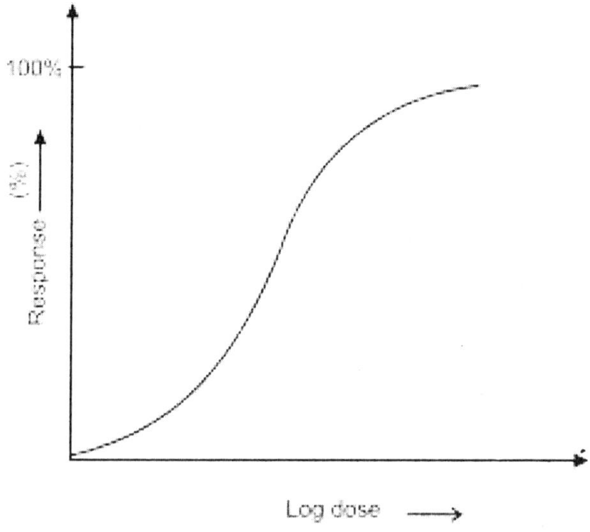

Fig. 1.8: Log dose response curve

Drug Potency and Maximal Efficacy

The amount of drug required to produce a response indicates the **potency**. For example, 1 mg of bumetanide produces the same diuresis as 50 mg of frusemide. Thus, bumetanide is more potent than frusemide. In Figure 1.10, drugs A and B are more

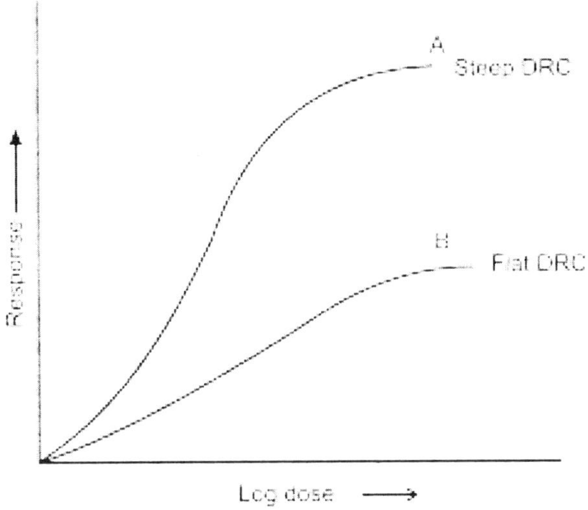

Fig. 1.9: Steep and flat dose response curve

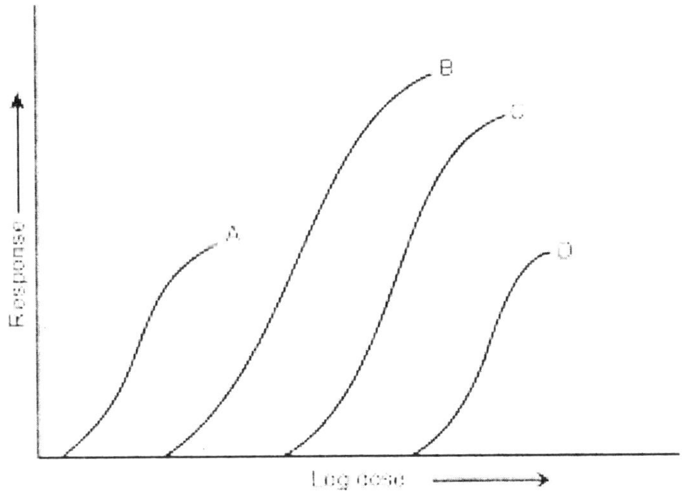

Fig. 1.10: Dose response curves of four drugs showing different potencies and maximal efficacies. Drug A is more potent but less efficacious than B and C. Drug D is less potent and less efficacious than drugs B and C

potent than drugs C and D, drug A being the most potent and drug D—the least potent. Hence higher doses of drugs C and D are to be administered as compared to drugs A and B.

Generally potency is of little clinical significance unless very large doses of the drug needs to be given due to low potency.

Maximal efficacy Efficacy indicates the maximum response that can be produced by a drug, e.g. frusemide produces powerful diuresis, not produced by any dose of amiloride. In Figure 1.10, drugs B and C are more efficacious than drugs A and D. Drug A is more potent but less efficacious than drugs B and C. Such differences in efficacy are of great clinical importance.

Therapeutic index The dose response curves for different actions of a drug could be different. Thus salbutamol may have one DRC for bronchodilation and another for tachycardia. The distance between beneficial effect DRC and unwanted effect DRC indicates the safety margin of the drug (Fig. 1.11).

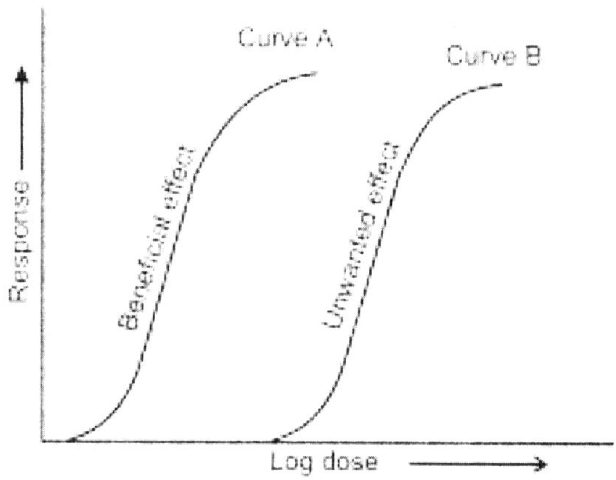

Fig. 1.11: The distance between curves A and B indicates safety margin of the drug. The greater the distance, more selective is the drug

Median lethal dose (LD_{50}) is the dose which is lethal to 50% of animals of the test population.

Median effective dose (ED_{50}) is the dose that produces a desired effect in 50% of the test population.

Therapeutic index (TI) is the ratio of the median lethal dose to the median effective dose.

$$\text{Therapeutic index} = \frac{LD_{50}}{ED_{50}}$$

It gives an idea about the safety of the drug.

- The higher the therapeutic index, the safer is the drug
- TI varies from species to species
- For a drug to be considered reasonably safe, it's TI must be > 1
- Penicillin has a high TI while lithium and digoxin have low TI.

Drug Synergism and Antagonism

When two or more drugs are given concurrently the effect may be additive, synergistic or antagonistic.

Additive Effect

The effect of two or more drugs get added up and the total effect is equal to the sum of their individual actions.

Examples are ephedrine with theophylline in bronchial asthma; nitrous oxide and ether as general anaesthetics.

Synergism

When the action of one drug is enhanced or facilitated by another drug, the combination is **synergistic**. In Greek, *ergon* = work; *syn* = with. Here, the total effect of the combination is greater than the sum of their independent effects. It is often called 'potentiation' or 'supra-additive' effect.

Examples are—acetylcholine + physostigmine
levodopa + carbidopa.

Antagonism

One drug opposing or inhibiting the action of another is antagonism. Based on the mechanisms, antagonism can be

- Chemical antagonism
- Physiological antagonism
- Antagonism at the receptor level
  - — Reversible (Competitive)
  - — Irreversible
- Non-competitive antagonism.

Chemical antagonism Two substances interact chemically to result in inactivation of the effect, e.g. chelating agents inactivate heavy metals like lead and mercury to form inactive complexes;

antacids like aluminium hydroxide neutralize gastric acid.

Physiological antagonism Two drugs act at different sites to produce opposing effects. For example, histamine acts on H_2 receptors to produce bronchospasm and hypotension while adrenaline reverses these effects by acting on adrenergic receptors.

Insulin and glucagon have opposite effects on the blood sugar level.

Antagonism at the receptor level The antagonist inhibits the binding of the agonist to the receptor. Such antagonism may be reversible or irreversible.

Reversible or competitive antagonism The agonist and antagonist compete for the same receptor. By increasing the concentration of the agonist, the antagonism can be overcome. It is thus *reversible antagonism*. Acetylcholine and atropine compete for the muscarinic receptors. The antagonism can be overcome by increasing the concentration of acetylcholine at the receptor. d-tubocurarine and acetylcholine compete for the nicotinic receptors at the neuromuscular junction. The dose response curve shifts to the right (Fig. 1.12) in presence of competitive antagonists.

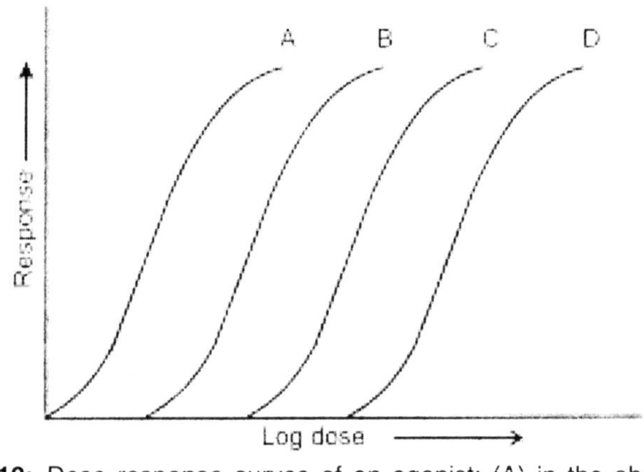

Fig. 1.12: Dose response curves of an agonist: (A) in the absence of competitive antagonist; (B), (C), and (D) in the presence of increasing doses of a competitive antagonist

Irreversible antagonism The antagonist binds so firmly by covalent bonds to the receptor that it dissociates very slowly or not at all. Thus it blocks the action of the agonist and the blockade *cannot* be overcome by increasing the dose of the agonist and hence it is irreversible antagonism, e.g. adrenaline and phenoxybenzamine at alpha adrenergic receptors.

There is progressive flattening of the dose response curve (Fig. 1.13).

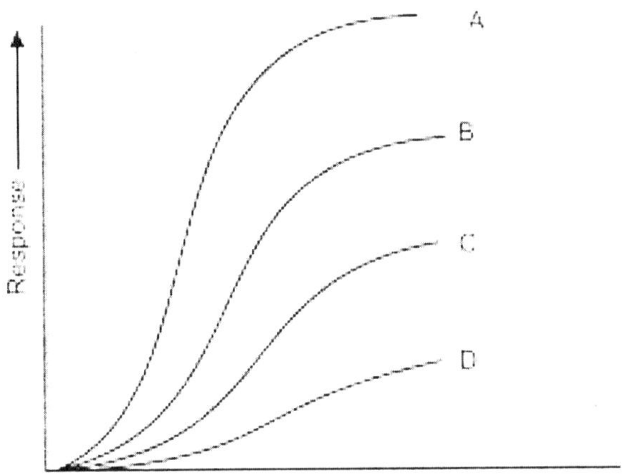

Fig. 1.13: Dose response curves of an agonist: (A) in the absence of antagonist. (B), (C), and (D) in the presence of increasing doses of an irreversible antagonist

Noncompetitive antagonism The antagonist blocks at the level of receptor-effector linkage. There is flattening as well as some rightward shift of the dose response curve (Fig. 1.14). For example, verapamil blocks the cardiac calcium channels and inhibits the entry of Ca^{++} during depolarisation. It thereby antagonises the effect of cardiac stimulants like isoprenaline and adrenaline.

FACTORS THAT MODIFY THE EFFECTS OF DRUGS

The same dose of a drug can produce different degrees of response in different patients and even in the same patient

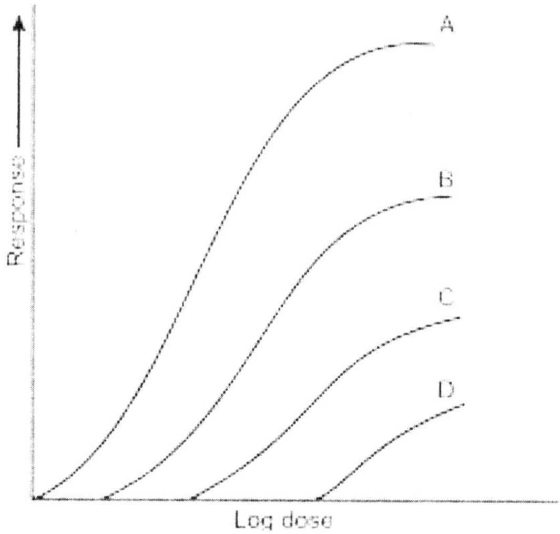

Fig. 1.14: Non-competitive antagonism—there is flattening as well as right ward shift of DRC

under different situations. Various factors modify the response to a drug. They are:

1. Body weight The recommended dose is calculated for medium built persons. For the obese and underweight persons, the dose has to be calculated individually. Though body surface area is a better parameter for more accurate calculation of the dose, it is inconvenient and hence not generally used.

Formula

$$\text{Dose} = \frac{\text{Body weight (kg)}}{70} \times \text{average adult dose}$$

2. Age The pharmacokinetics of many drugs change with age resulting in altered response in extremes of age. In the newborn, the liver and kidneys are not fully mature to handle the drugs, e.g. chloramphenicol can produce grey baby syndrome. The blood-brain barrier is not well-formed and drugs can easily reach the brain. The gastric acidity is low, intestinal motility is slow, skin is delicate and permeable to drugs applied topically. Hence calculation of the appropriate dose, depending on body weight is important to avoid toxicity. Also pharmacodynamic differences could exist, e.g. barbiturates which produce sedation in adults may produce excitation in children.

Formula for calculation of dose for children

Young's formula

$$\text{Child's dose} = \frac{\text{Age (years)}}{\text{Age} + 12} \times \text{Adult dose}$$

In the elderly, the capacity of the liver and kidney to handle the drug is reduced and are more susceptible to adverse effects. Hence lower doses are recommended, e.g. elderly are at a higher risk of ototoxicity and nephrotoxicity by streptomycin.

3. Sex The hormonal effects and smaller body size may influence drug response in women. Special care is necessary while prescribing for pregnant and lactating women and during menstruation.

4. Species and race Response to drugs may vary with species and race. For example, rabbits are resistant to atropine. Then it becomes difficult to extrapolate the results of animal experiments. Blacks need higher doses of atropine to produce mydriasis.

5. Diet and environment Food interferes with the absorption of many drugs. For example, tetracyclines form complexes with calcium present in the food and are poorly absorbed.

Polycyclic hydrocarbons present in cigarette smoke may induce microsomal enzymes resulting in enhanced metabolism of some drugs.

6. Route of administration Occasionally route of administration may modify the pharmacodynamic response, e.g. magnesium sulfate given orally is a purgative. But given IV it causes CNS depression and has anticonvulsant effects. Applied topically (poultice), it reduces local edema. Hypertonic magnesium sulfate retention enema reduces intracranial tension.

7. Genetic factors Variations in an individual's response to drugs could be genetically mediated. **Pharmacogenetics** is concerned with the genetically mediated variations in drug responses. The differences in response is most commonly due to variations in the amount of drug metabolising enzymes since the production of these enzymes are genetically controlled.

Examples

a. ***Acetylation of drugs*** The rate of drug acetylation differs among individuals who may be fast or slow acetylators, e.g. INH, sulfonamides and hydralazine are acetylated. Slow acetylators treated with hydralazine are more likely to develop lupus erythematosus.
b. ***Atypical pseudocholinesterase*** Succinylcholine is metabolised by pseudocholinesterase. Some people inherit atypical pseudocholinesterase and they develop a prolonged apnoea due to succinylcholine.
c. ***G_6PD deficiency*** Primaquine, sulphones and quinolones can cause hemolysis in such people.
d. ***Malignant hyperthermia*** Halothane and succinylcholine can trigger malignant hyperthermia in some genetically predisposed individuals.

8. Dose It is fascinating that the response to a drug may be modified by the dose administered. Generally as the dose is increased, the magnitude of the response also increases proportionately till the 'maximum' is reached. Further increases in doses may with some drugs produce effects opposite to their lower-dose effect, e.g. (i) in myasthenia gravis, neostigmine enhances muscle power in therapeutic doses, but in high doses it causes muscle paralysis, (ii) physiological doses of vitamin D promotes calcification while hypervitaminosis D leads to decalcification.

9. Diseases Presence of certain diseases can influence drug responses, e.g.

- *Malabsorption* Drugs are poorly absorbed.
- *Liver diseases* Rate of drug metabolism is reduced due to dysfunction of hepatocytes. Also protein binding is reduced due to low serum albumin.
- *Cardiac diseases* In CCF, there is edema of the gut mucosa and decreased perfusion of liver and kidneys. These may result in cumulation and toxicity of drugs like propranolol and lignocaine.
- *Renal dysfunction* Drugs mainly excreted through kidneys are likely to accumulate and cause toxicity, e.g. Streptomycin, amphotericin B—Dose of such drugs need to be reduced.

10. Repeated dosing can result in

- cumulation
- tolerance
- tachyphylaxis.

Cumulation Drugs like digoxin which are slowly eliminated may cumulate resulting in toxicity.

Tolerance Tolerance is the requirement of higher doses of a drug to produce a given response. Tolerance may be natural or acquired.

Natural tolerance The species/race shows less sensitivity to the drug, e.g. rabbits show tolerance to atropine; Black race are tolerant to mydriatics.

Acquired tolerance develops on repeated administration of a drug. The patient who was initially responsive becomes tolerant, e.g. barbiturates, opioids, nitrites produce tolerance.

Tolerance may develop to some actions of the drug and not to others, e.g. morphine—tolerance develops to analgesic and euphoric effects of morphine but not to its constipating and miotic effects.

Barbiturates—tolerance develops to sedative but not anti-epileptic effects of barbiturates.

Mechanisms The mechanisms of development of tolerance could be:

Pharmacokinetic Changes in absorption, distribution, metabolism and excretion of drugs may result in reduced concentration of the drug at the site of action and is also known as dispositional tolerance, e.g. barbiturates induce microsomal enzymes and enhance their own metabolism.

Pharmacodynamic Changes in the target tissue, may make it less responsive to the drug. It is also called functional tolerance. It could be due to down regulation of receptors as in opioids or due to compensatory mechanisms of the body, e.g. blunting of response to some antihypertensives due to salt and water retention.

Cross tolerance is the development of tolerance to pharmacologically related drugs, i.e. to drugs belonging to a particular group. Thus chronic alcoholics also show tolerance to barbiturates and general anaesthetics.

Tachyphylaxis is the rapid development of tolerance. When some drugs are administered repeatedly at short intervals, tolerance develops rapidly and is known as tachyphylaxis or acute tolerance, e.g. ephedrine, amphetamine, tyramine and 5-hydroxytryptamine. This is thought to be due to depletion of noradrenaline stores as the above drugs act by displacing noradrenaline from the sympathetic nerve endings. Other mechanisms involved may be slow dissociation of the drug from the receptor thereby blocking the receptor. Thus ephedrine given repeatedly in bronchial asthma may not give the desired response.

11. Psychological factor The doctor patient relationship influences the response to a drug often to a large extent by acting on the patient's psychology. The patients confidence in the doctor may itself be sufficient to relieve a suffering, particularly the psychosomatic disorders. This can be substantiated by the fact that large number of patients respond to placebo. **Placebo** is the inert dosage form with no specific biological activity but only resembles the actual preparation in appearance. *Placebo* = 'I shall be pleasing' (in Latin).

Placebo medicines are used in

1. Clinical trials as a control
2. To benefit or please a patient psychologically when he does not actually require an active drug as in mild psychosomatic disorders and in chronic incurable diseases.

In fact all forms of treatment including physiotherapy and surgery have placebo effect. Substances used as placebo include lactose, some vitamins, minerals and distilled water injections.

12. Presence of other drugs The concurrent use of two or more drugs can influence the response of each other (see Drug Interactions page 51).

❑ ADVERSE DRUG REACTIONS AND DRUG INTERACTIONS

ADVERSE DRUG REACTIONS

All drugs can produce unwanted effects. WHO has defined an adverse drug reaction as "any response to a drug that is noxious and unintended and that occurs at doses used in man for prophylaxis, diagnosis or therapy."

All drugs can cause adverse effects. Some patients are more likely to develop adverse effects to drugs.

1. Side Effects

Side effects are unwanted effects of a drug that are extension of pharmacological effects and are seen with the therapeutic dose of the drug. They are predictable, common and can occur in all people, e.g. hypoglycaemia due to insulin; hypokalaemia following frusemide.

2. Toxic Effects

Toxic effects are seen with higher doses of the drug and can be serious, e.g. morphine causes respiratory depression in overdosage.

3. Intolerance

Drug intolerance is the inability of a person to tolerate a drug and is unpredictable. Patients show exaggerated response to even small doses of the drug, e.g. vestibular dysfunction after a single dose of streptomycin seen in some patients. Intolerance could also be qualitative, e.g. idiosyncrasy and allergic reactions.

Idiosyncrasy is a genetically determined abnormal reaction to a drug, e.g. primaquine and sulfonamides induce haemolysis in patients with G_6PD deficiency; some patients show excitement with barbiturates. In addition, some responses like chloramphenicol-induced agranulocytosis, where no definite genetic background is known, are also included under idiosyncrasy. In some cases the person may be highly sensitive even to low doses of a drug or highly insensitive even to high doses of the drug.

Allergic reactions Allergic reactions to drugs are immunologically-mediated reactions which are not related to the therapeutic effects of the drug. The drug or its metabolite acts as an antigen to induce antibody formation. Subsequent exposure to the drug may result in allergic reactions. The manifestations of allergy are seen mainly on the target organs *viz.* skin, respiratory tract, gastrointestinal tract, blood and blood vessels.

Types of Allergic Reactions and their Mechanisms

Drugs can induce both types of allergic reactions *viz* humoral and cell-mediated immunity. Mechanism involved in type I, II and III are humoral while type IV is by cell-mediated immunity.

Type I (Anaphylactic) reaction The drug induces synthesis of IgE antibodies which are fixed to the mast cells. On subsequent exposure, the antigen-antibody complexes cause degranulation of mast cells releasing the mediators of inflammation like histamine, leukotrienes, prostaglandins and platelet-activating factor. These are responsible for the characteristic signs and symptoms of anaphylaxis like bronchospasm, laryngeal edema and hypotension which could be fatal. Allergy develops within minutes and is called immediate hypersensitivity reaction, e.g. penicillins. Skin tests may predict this type of reactions.

Type II (Cytolytic) reactions The drug binds to a protein and together they act as antigen and induce the formation of antibodies. The antigen antibody complexes activate the complement system resulting in cytolysis causing thrombocytopenia, agranulocytosis and aplastic anaemia.

Type III (Arthus) reactions The antigen binds to circulating antibodies and the complexes are deposited on the vessel wall where it initiates the inflammatory response resulting in vasculitis. Rashes, fever, arthralgia, lymphadenopathy, serum sickness and Steven-Johnson's syndrome are some of the manifestations of arthus type reaction.

Type IV (Delayed hypersensitivity) reactions are mediated by T-lymphocytes and macrophages. The antigen reacts with receptors on T-lymphocytes which produce lymphokines leading to a local allergic reaction, e.g. contact dermatitis.

4. Iatrogenic Diseases (Physician Induced)

These are drug induced diseases. Even after the drug is withdrawn toxic effects can persist, e.g. isoniazid induced hepatitis; chloroquine induced retinopathy.

5. Drug Dependence

Drugs that influence the behaviour and mood are often misused to obtain their pleasurable effects. Repeated use of such drugs result in dependence. Several words like drug abuse, addiction and dependence are used confusingly. Drug Dependence is a state of compulsive use of drugs in spite of the knowledge of risks associated with its use. It is also referred to as drug addiction. Dependence could be 'psychologic' or 'physical' dependence. Psychologic dependence is compulsive drug-seeking behaviour to obtain its pleasurable effects, e.g. cigarette smoking

Physical dependence is said to be present when withdrawal of the drug produces adverse symptoms. The body undergoes physiological changes to adapt itself to the continued presence of the drug in the body. Stopping the drug results in 'withdrawal syndrome.' The symptoms of withdrawal syndrome are disturbing and the person then craves for the drug, e.g. alcohol, opioids and barbiturates.

Mild degree of physical dependence is seen in people who drink too much of coffee.

6. Teratogenicity

Teratogenicity is the ability of a drug to cause foetal abnormalities when administered to the pregnant lady. *Teratos* in Greek means monster. The sedative-thalidomide taken during early pregnancy for relief from morning sickness resulted in thousands of babies being born with phocomelia (seal limbs). This thalidomide disaster (1958-61) opened the eyes of various nations and made it mandatory to impose strict teratogenicity tests before a new drug is approved for use.

Depending on the stage of pregnancy during which the teratogen is administered, it can produce various abnormalities.

i.	Conception to 16 days	—Usually resistant to teratogenic effects. If affected, abortion occurs.
ii.	Period of organogenesis (17 to 55 days of gestation)	—Most vulnerable period; major physical abnormalities occur.
iii.	Foetal period—56 days onwards	—Period of growth and development—hence developmental and functional abnormalities result.

Therefore, in general drugs should be avoided during pregnancy especially in the first trimester. The type of malformation also depends on the drug, e.g. thalidomide causes phocomelia; tetracyclines cause deformed teeth; sodium valproate causes spina bifida.

7. Carcinogenicity and Mutagenicity

Some drugs can cause cancers and genetic abnormalities. For example anticancer drugs can themselves be carcinogenic; other examples are radioactive isotopes and some hormones.

8. Other Adverse Drug Reactions

Drugs can also damage various organ systems.

Organ system affected	Examples
1. Hepatotoxicity	Isoniazid, pyrazinamide, paracetamol, chlorpromazine,6-Mercaptopurine, Halothane, Ethanole, Phenylbutazonl
2. Nephrotoxicity	Analgesics, aminoglycosides, cyclosporine, cisplatin,cephelexin, penicillamine, gold salts
3. Ototoxicity	Aminoglycosides, frusemide
4. Ocular toxicity	Chloroquine, ethambutol
5. Gastrointestinal systems	Opioids, broad spectrum antibiotics
6. Cardiovascular system	Digoxin, doxorubicin
7. Respiratory systems	Aspirin, bleomycin, Busulfan, Amiodarone, Methotrexate
8. Musculoskeletal systems	Corticosteroids, heparin

Contd...

Contd...

	Organ system affected	*Examples*
9.	Behavioural toxicity	Corticosteroids, reserpine
10.	Neurological systems	INH, haloperidol,Ethambutol, Quinine, Doxorubicin vincristine
11.	Dermatological toxicity	Doxycycline, sulfonamides
12.	Electrolyte disturbances	Diuretics, mineralocorticoids
13.	Haematological toxicity	Chloramphenicol, sulfonamides
14.	Endocrine disorders	Methyldopa, oral contraceptives

DRUG INTERACTIONS

Definition Drug interaction is the alteration in the duration or magnitude of the pharmacological effects of one drug by another drug.

When two or more drugs are given concurrently, the response may be greater or lesser than the sum of their individual effects. Such responses may be beneficial or harmful. For example a combination of drugs is used in hypertension—hydralazine + propranolol for their beneficial interaction. But unwanted drug interactions may result in severe toxicity. Such interactions can be avoided by adequate knowledge of their mechanisms and by judicious use of drugs.

Site Drug interaction can occur:

i. *In vitro* in the syringe before administration—mixing of drugs in syringes can cause chemical or physical interactions—such drug combinations are incompatible in solution, e.g. penicillin and gentamicin should never be mixed in the same syringe.
ii. *In vivo,* i.e. in the body after administration.

Pharmacological basis of drug interactions The two major mechanisms of drug interactions include pharmacokinetic and pharmacodynamic mechanisms.

Pharmacokinetic mechanisms Alteration in the extent or duration of response may be produced by influencing absorption, distribution, metabolism or excretion of one drug by another.

Absorption of drugs from the gut may be affected by:

i. Binding—Tetracyclines chelate iron and antacids resulting in reduced absorption
ii. Altering gastric pH
iii. Altering GI motility.

Distribution Competition for plasma protein or tissue binding results in displacement interactions, e.g. warfarin is displaced by phenylbutazone from protein binding sites.

Metabolism Enzyme induction and inhibition of metabolism can both result in drug interactions (see pages 18, 19), e.g. phenytoin, phenobarbitone, carbamazepine and rifampicin are enzyme inducers while chloramphenicol and cimetidine are some enzyme inhibitors.

Excretion When drugs compete for the same renal tubular transport system, they prolong each others duration of action, e.g. penicillin and probenecid.

Pharmacodynamic mechanisms Drugs acting on the same receptors or physiological systems result in additive, synergistic or antagonistic effects. Many clinically important drug interactions have this basis. Atropine opposes the effects of physostigmine; naloxone antagonises morphine; antihypertensive effects of β blockers are reduced by ephedrine or other vasoconstrictors in cold remedies.

❑ GENE THERAPY

Gene therapy is the replacement of defective gene by the insertion of a normal, functional gene. Gene transfer may be done to replace a missing or defective gene or provide extra-copies of a normally expressed gene. Gene therapy is aimed at genetically correcting the defect in the affected part of the body. Unlike all other drugs which only alter the rate of normal cell functions, gene therapy can confer new functions to the cell.

Gene transfer requires the use of vectors to deliver the DNA material, such as:

i. Viral vectors like retroviral vectors and adenoviral vectors.
ii. Liposomes.

Therapeutic applications of gene therapy Gene therapy is at present a developing area. Though originally it was seen as a remedy for inherited single gene defects, gene therapy has now found to be useful in several acquired disorders. The principle applications are in the treatment of cancer, cardiovascular diseases, atherosclerosis, immunodeficiency disorders—particularly AIDS; anaemia, Alzheimer's disease and many infectious diseases.

2

Autonomic Nervous System

- INTRODUCTION TO AUTONOMIC PHARMACOLOGY
- CHOLINERGIC SYSTEM
- ANTICHOLINERGIC DRUGS
- ADRENERGIC SYSTEM
- ADRENERGIC DRUGS (SYMPATHOMIMETICS)
- ADRENERGIC ANTAGONISTS

INTRODUCTION TO AUTONOMIC PHARMACOLOGY

The nervous system is divided (Fig. 2.1) into central and peripheral nervous systems. The peripheral nervous system consists of autonomic and somatic nervous systems.

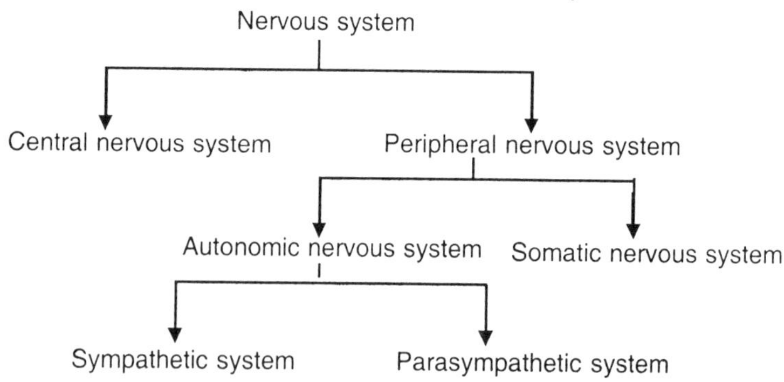

Fig. 2.1: Nervous system

The autonomic nervous system (ANS) (Fig. 2.2) is **not under voluntary control** and therefore was so named by Langley

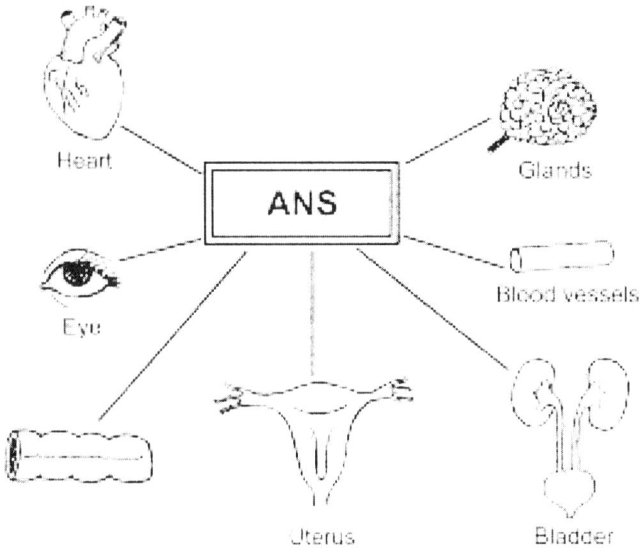

Fig. 2.2: Structures under the control of autonomic nervous system

(*Autos* = self, *nomos* = governing—in Greek). The ANS innervates the heart, the smooth muscles, the glands and the viscera and controls the functions of these organs.

The centres for autonomic reflexes are present in the hypothalamus, medulla and spinal cord. Hypothalamus coordinates the autonomic activity.

The ANS consists of 2 major divisions—the **sympathetic** and the **parasympathetic** (Fig. 2.3). Most of the viscera have both sympathetic and parasympathetic innervation. The two divisions have opposing effects and normally their effects are in a state of equilibrium. The prime function of the sympathetic system is to help the person to adjust to stress and prepare the body for fight or flight reactions, while the parasympathetic mainly participates in tissue building reactions. Man can still survive without sympathetic system but not without parasympathetic.

Autonomic innervation (Fig. 2.4) The autonomic afferents are carried in visceral nerves through nonmyelinated fibres. For

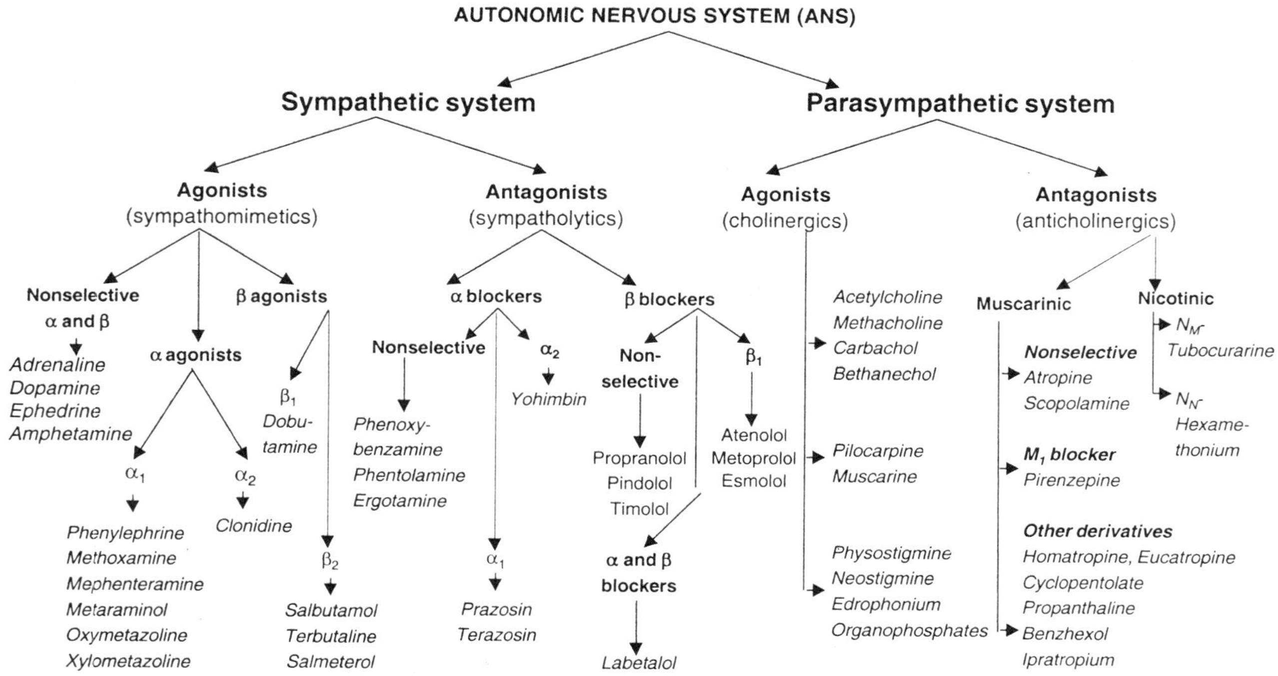

Fig. 2.3: Drugs acting on sympathetic and parasympathetic nervous system

---

Few examples have been given

example, the parasympathetic afferents are carried by the 9th and 10th cranial nerves. The autonomic efferent innervation consists of a myelinated preganglionic fibre which synapses with the axon of a nonmyelinated postganglionic fibre. The postganglionic fibre in turn forms a junction with the receptors of the organs supplied by it. The junction between the pre and postganglionic fibres is called a *ganglion* and that between the postganglionic fibres and the receptors is the *neuroeffector junction*. The travelling of an impulse along the nerve fibre is known as *conduction* while its passage across a synapse is known as *transmission*.

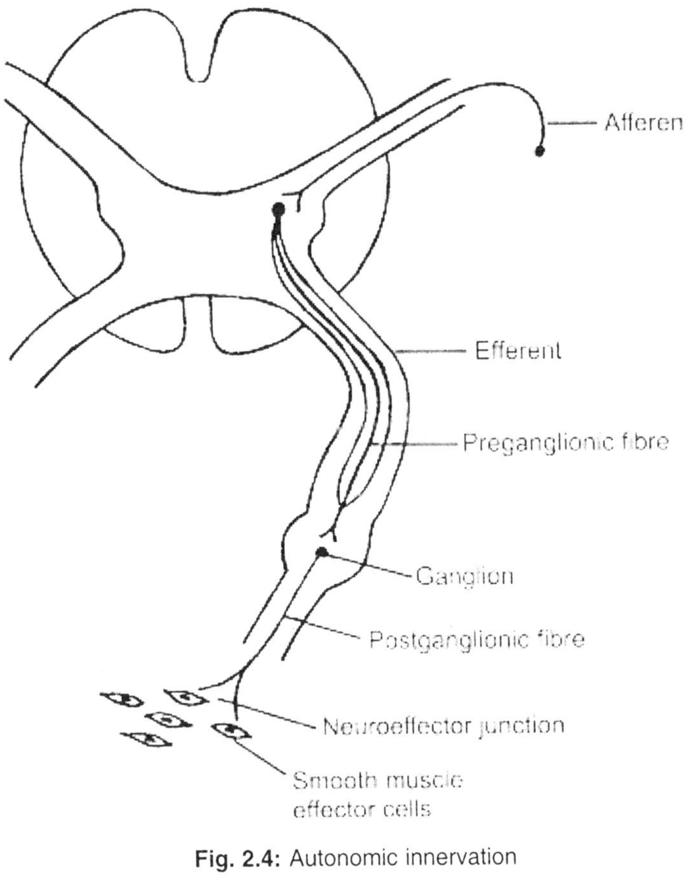

Fig. 2.4: Autonomic innervation

The autonomic efferent is divided into sympathetic and parasympathetic divisions. The parasympathetic afferents are carried through the craniosacral outflow. The sympathetic afferents extend from the first thoracic to second or third lumbar segments (T_1-L_3) of the spinal cord. Adrenal medulla is also considered as sympathetic ganglia and differs from the other sympathetic ganglion in that the principal catecholamine that is released is adrenaline.

Neurotransmitters For the transmission of an impulse across a synapse, a neurohumoral transmitter substance is released into the synaptic cleft. In the ANS, the neurotransmitters released are acetylcholine, noradrenaline, dopamine and in adrenal medulla, it is adrenaline.

❑ CHOLINERGIC SYSTEM

Acetylcholine (ACh) an ester of choline, is an important neurotransmitter of the ANS. The nerves that synthesize, store and release ACh are called *'cholinergic.'*

The **sites** of release of acetylcholine are (Fig. 2.5):

1. Ganglia—All the preganglionic fibres of ANS, i.e. at both the sympathetic and parasympathetic ganglia.
2. The postganglionic parasympathetic nerve endings.
3. Sweat glands—The sympathetic postganglionic nerve endings supplying the sweat glands.
4. Skeletal muscles—somatic nerve endings supplying skeletal muscles.
5. Adrenal medulla.
6. CNS—brain and spinal cord.

Synthesis of ACh Acetylcholine is synthesized from acetyl-CoA and choline, catalysed by the enzyme choline acetyltransferase. This ACh is stored in small oval vesicles in the cholinergic nerve terminals.

Transmission of an impulse When an action potential reaches the presynaptic membrane, ACh is released into the synaptic cleft (Fig. 2.6). This ACh binds to and activates the cholinergic receptor on the postsynaptic membrane leading to the

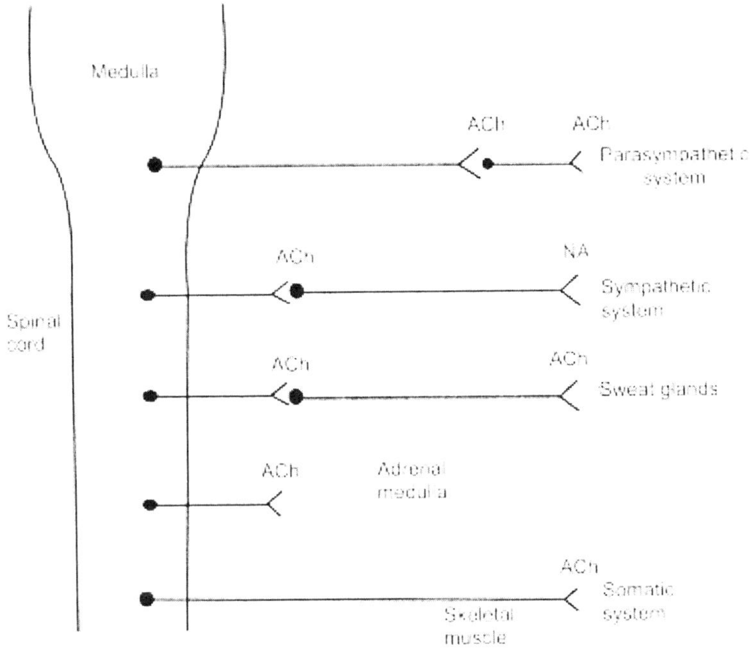

Fig. 2.5: Sites of release of neurotransmitters—acetylcholine and noradrenaline in the peripheral nervous system

depolarisation of this membrane. Thus the impulse is transmitted across the synapse.

ACh released into the synaptic cleft is rapidly destroyed by the acetylcholinesterase (AChE) enzyme. Then the postsynaptic membrane is repolarised.

Cholinesterases Acetylcholine is hydrolysed to choline and acetic acid by the enzymes cholinesterases. Two types of AChE are present:

1. True cholinesterase—at neurons, ganglia and neuromuscular junction.
2. Pseudocholinesterase—in plasma, liver and other organs.

Cholinergic receptors There are two classes of cholinergic receptors—**muscarinic** and **nicotinic**. Muscarinic receptors are

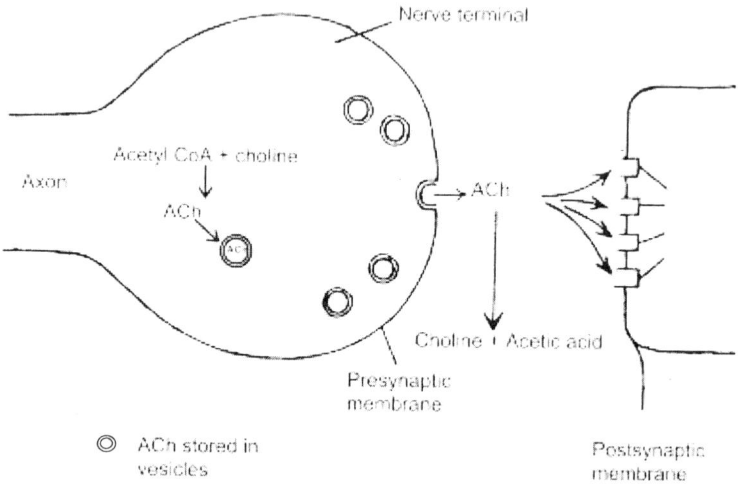

Fig. 2.6: Cholinergic transmission—schematic representation

present in the heart, smooth muscles, glands, eyes and CNS. Five subtypes of muscarinic receptors, M_1-M_5 are recognised (Table 2.1).

TABLE 2.1: Subtypes and location of cholinergic receptors

	Subtypes	*Location*
Muscarinic	M_1	Autonomic ganglia, gastric glands, CNS
	M_2	Heart, nerves, smooth muscles,
	M_3	Glands, smooth muscles
	M_4	CNS
	M_5	CNS
Nicotinic	N_m	Neuromuscular junction
	N_n	Autonomic ganglia Adrenal medulla, CNS

Nicotinic receptors are present in the neuromuscular junction, autonomic ganglia and adrenal medulla. Two subtypes of nicotinic receptors are identified (Table 2.1). N_m receptors are present at the skeletal muscle end plate and N_n receptors at the autonomic ganglia and adrenal medulla.

CHOLINERGIC DRUGS

Cholinergic drugs are chemicals that act at the same site as acetylcholine and thereby mimic its actions. They are therefore called parasympathomimetics or cholinomimetics.

Cholinergic drugs may be classified as:

1. *Esters of choline* Acetylcholine, Methacholine, Carbachol, Bethanechol
2. *Cholinomimetic alkaloids* Pilocarpine, Muscarine
3. *Anticholinesterases*
   Reversible—Neostigmine, Physostigmine
   Irreversible—Organophosphorus compounds.

PHARMACOLOGICAL ACTIONS OF ACETYLCHOLINE

Acetylcholine is taken as the prototype of parasympathomimetic drugs. Acetylcholine produces its actions by binding to muscarinic and nicotinic receptors.

Muscarinic Actions

Muscarinic actions resemble the actions of the alkaloid muscarine found in some mushrooms.

1. Heart The action of ACh is similar to that of vagal stimulation. It reduces the heart rate and force of contraction. In larger doses, AV conduction is depressed.

2. Blood vessels ACh relaxes the vascular smooth muscles and dilates the blood vessels of the skin and mucous membrane. The BP falls due to a fall in total peripheral resistance

3. Smooth muscle ACh increases the tone of all other smooth muscles.

Gastrointestinal tract—tone and peristalsis is enhanced, sphincters are relaxed, resulting in rapid forward propulsion of intestinal contents.

Urinary bladder—detrusor contracts and trigonal sphincter relaxes—promotes voiding of urine.

Bronchial smooth muscle—contracts resulting in bronchospasm.

4. Secretory glands Acetylcholine enhances the secretions of all glands; salivary, lacrimal, nasopharyngeal, tracheobronchial, gastric and intestinal secretions are increased. Sweating is also increased. Enhanced bronchial secretions and bronchospasm result in severe dyspnoea.

5. Eye Acetylcholine brings about constriction of pupil (miosis) by contracting the circular muscles of the iris. It improves drainage of aqueous humor. Ciliary muscle contracts resulting in spasm of accommodation.

Nicotinic Actions

These effects resemble the actions of the alkaloid nicotine.

1. NMJ ACh brings about contraction of skeletal muscles. Large doses cause persistent depolarisation of skeletal muscles resulting in paralysis.

2. Autonomic ganglia ACh stimulates sympathetic and parasympathetic ganglia and the adrenal medulla.

3. CNS ACh is a neurotransmitter at several sites in the CNS.

The important actions of acetylcholine are summarised in Table 2.2.

TABLE 2.2: Actions of acetylcholine

CVS	— ↓ HR ↓ BP
Non-vascular smooth muscle	— contraction, ↑ gut peristalsis, promotes urine voiding, bronchospasm
Glands	— ↑ secretion
Eye	— miosis, spasm of accommodation ↓ IOP
NMJ	— muscle contraction
Ganglia	— stimulation

Uses Acetylcholine is destroyed in the gut when given orally. On intravenous administration, it is rapidly metabolised by pseudocholinesterases in the plasma and by true cholinesterase at the site of action. Therefore it is **not used** therapeutically. Among the choline esters, methacholine is rarely used. Carbachol is used in glaucoma. Bethanechol may be used in some cases of postoperative paralytic ileus and urinary retention.

CHOLINOMIMETIC ALKALOIDS

Pilocarpine is an alkaloid obtained from the leaves of *Pilocarpus microphyllus*. Like ACh it stimulates cholinergic receptors, but its muscarinic actions are prominent.

Its actions on the eye are important—when applied to the eye it causes miosis, spasm of accommodation and a fall in intraocular pressure (IOP). It also increases sweat (diaphoretic) and salivary secretions (sialogogue).

Adverse effects When used as eye drops, burning sensation and painful spasm of accommodation can occur.

Uses

1. Pilocarpine is used in glaucoma (0.5-4% eye drops). Pilocarpine ocusert is available and can deliver pilocarpine constantly for 7 days.

   Glaucoma is an eye disease characterised by increased intraocular pressure. If untreated, irreversible damage can occur, as optic nerve degenerates leading to permanent blindness. Glaucoma is of two types:

   i. Acute congestive/narrow angle glaucoma—In this, iris blocks the drainage of aqueous humour at the canal of Schlemn leading to increased intraocular pressure (Fig. 2.7). It needs immediate treatment.

   ii. Chronic simple/open angle glaucoma—onset is slow; needs long-term treatment. Surgery is the preferred option.

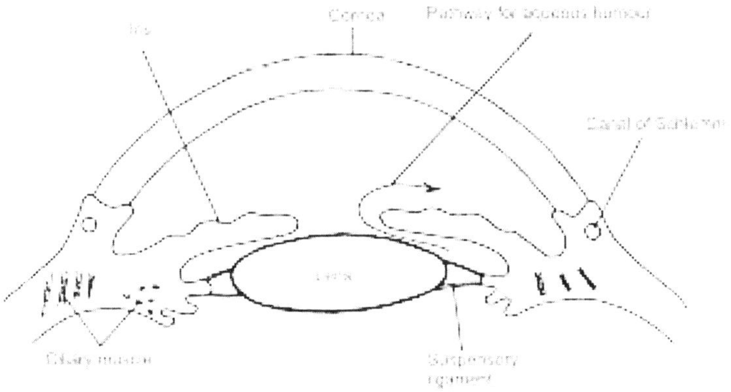

Fig. 2.7: Schematic diagram showing pathway for the drainage of aqueous humour

Durgs used in glaucoma are summarised in Table 2.3.

TABLE 2.3: Drugs used in glaucoma

Drugs	*Routes*	*Mechanisms*
Cholinomimetics		
Pilocarpine, Carbachol	topical	Miosis
Physostigmine, Echothiophate	topical	↑drainage of aqueous humor
Alpha adrenergic agonists		
Adrenaline	topical	↑drainage of aqueous humor
Dipivefrin	topical	
β-blockers		
Timolol	topical	↓ aqueous secretion
Diuretics		
Acetazolamide	oral	↓ aqueous secretion

2. Pilocarpine eye drops are also used alternately with mydriatics like homatropine to break adhesions between the iris and the lens.
3. Pilocarpine can be used to overcome dryness of mouth that is seen following radiation of head and neck.

ANTICHOLINESTERASES

Anticholinesterases (antiChEs) or cholinesterase inhibitors are drugs which inhibit the enzyme cholinesterase. As their structure resembles that of ACh, they bind to AChEs and inactivate them.

Acetylcholine

↓ AChE ←·········AntiChE

Choline + Acetic acid

Thus ACh is not hydrolysed and it accumulates. The actions of these drugs are due to this accumulated ACh. Hence the actions are similar to cholinergic agonists.

Anticholinesterases may be:

1. **Reversible** Physostigmine, Neostigmine, Pyridostigmine, Rivastigmine, Donepezil, Edrophonium.
2. **Irreversible** Organophosphates—Malathion, Sumithion, Toxic nerve gases, Echothiophate.

Physostigmine is an alkaloid obtained from the plant *Physostigma venenosum*. It is a tertiary ammonium compound—hence has better penetration into tissues and also crosses the BBB. It is available as 0.1-1% eye drops. It is used in glaucoma and in atropine poisoning. Its use in glaucoma can cause browache, and on long-term use retinal detachment and cataract.

Neostigmine is a synthetic quaternary ammonium compound—poorly absorbed from the gut; it does not cross the BBB. It is used in myasthenia gravis and post-operative paralytic ileus and atony of urinary bladder.

Edrophonium is rapid and short-acting. It is used in myasthenia gravis, snake bite and in curare poisoning.

Uses of anticholinesterases

1. *As a miotic* Physostigmine causes miosis, spasm of accommodation and a ↓ IOP. It is used:
   a. in glaucoma—can be used with pilocarpine for better effect
   b. alternately with a mydriatic to break adhesions between the iris and the lens.
2. *Myasthenia gravis* Anticholinesterases bring about improvement. Myasthesia gravis is a chronic autoimmune disease characterised by progressive weakness with rapid and easy fatiguability of the skeletal muscles. Antibodies to nicotinic receptors are found, resulting in a decrease in the number of these receptors at NMJ. Edrophonium is used for the diagnosis. Neostigmine (15 mg tab 6 hourly) or pyridostigmine or a combination of these may be given. In addition to its antiChE activity, neostigmine directly stimulates the nicotinic receptors and increases the amount of ACh released during each nerve impulse. AntiChEs enhance ACh levels at NMJ by preventing its destruction. They thus increase the force of contraction and improve muscle power.
3. *Poisoning due to anticholinergic drugs* Physostigmine is used in atropine poisoning and in toxicity due to other drugs with anticholinergic activity like phenothiazines, tricyclic antidepressants and antihistamines.

4. *Curare poisoning* Skeletal muscle paralysis caused by curare can be antagonised by AntiChEs. Edrophonium is preferred for its fast action.
5. *Postoperative paralytic ileus and urinary retention* Neostigmine may be useful.
6. *Cobra bite* Cobra venom, a neurotoxin causes skeletal muscle paralysis. Specific treatment is antivenom. Intravenous edrophonium prevents respiratory paralysis.
7. *Alzheimer's disease* Rivastigmine and danepezil are tried.

Irreversible Anticholinesterases

Organophosphorus compounds are powerful inhibitors of AChE enzyme; binding with the enzyme is permanent—by covalent bonds. Actions are similar to ACh as ACh accumulates in the tissues. Organophosphates are highly lipid soluble and hence are absorbed from all routes including intact skin.

Uses

Glaucoma—echothiophate eye drops are sometimes used in glaucoma.

Organophosphorus Poisoning

As organophosphates are used as agricultural and domestic insecticides, poisoning from them is quite common. Poisoning may be occupational—as while spraying insecticides, accidental or suicidal. Symptoms include muscarinic, nicotinic and central effects; vomiting, abdominal cramps, diarrhoea, miosis, sweating, increased salivary, tracheobronchial and gastric secretions and bronchospasm; hypotension, muscular twitchings, weakness, convulsions and coma. Death is due to respiratory paralysis.

Treatment

1. If poisoning is through skin—remove clothing and wash the skin with soap and water; if consumed by oral route—gastric lavage is given.
2. Maintain BP and patent airway.

3. Drug of choice is atropine (2 mg IV every 10 minutes till pupil dilates).
4. Cholinesterase reactivators—**pralidoxime, obidoxime.** These compounds combine with cholinesterase—organophosphate complex, release the binding and set free AChE enzyme. They should be given within a few hours (< 24 hrs) after poisoning, preferably immediately because the complex undergoes *'ageing'* and then the enzyme cannot be released.

❑ ANTICHOLINERGIC DRUGS

Anticholinergic drugs are agents which block the effects of ACh on cholinergic receptors but conventionally antimuscarinic drugs are referred to as anticholinergic drugs. They are also called cholinergic blocking or parasympatholytic drugs. Drugs that block the nicotinic receptors are ganglion blockers and neuromuscular blockers.

Anticholinergic drugs include atropine and related drugs—atropine is the prototype.

Atropine is obtained from the plant *Atropa belladonna.* Atropine and scopolamine (hyoscine) are the belladonna alkaloids. They compete with acetylcholine for muscarinic receptors and block these receptors—they are muscarinic antagonists.

Actions

The actions of atropine and scopolamine are similar except that atropine is a CNS stimulant while scopolamine is a CNS depressant and causes sedation.

1. CVS—Atropine increases heart rate. In large doses, vasodilation and hypotension occurs.
2. Secretions—Atropine reduces all secretions except milk. Lacrimal, salivary, nasopharyngeal, tracheobronchial and gastric secretions are decreased. Sweating is also reduced.
3. Smooth muscle

   GIT—↓ tone and motility and relieves spasm→may result in constipation.

Biliary tract—smooth muscles are relaxed; biliary spasm is relieved.

Bronchi—atropine causes bronchodilatation.

Urinary bladder—relaxes urinary bladder and may cause urinary retention.

4. Eye—On local instillation, atropine produces mydriasis by blocking the muscarinic receptors in the sphincter pupillae. The ciliary muscle is paralysed resulting in cycloplegia or paralysis of accommodation. Because of mydriasis, the iris may block the drainage of aqueous humor—IOP increases and may precipitate glaucoma in some patients.
5. CNS—In higher doses atropine stimulates the CNS resulting in restlessness, disorientation, hallucinations and delirium. In contrast, scopolamine produces sedation and drowsiness.

Pharmacokinetics Atropine and hyoscine are well-absorbed, cross the BBB and are metabolised in the liver.

Adverse effects are common but not serious and include blurring of vision, dry mouth, dysphagia, dry skin, fever, constipation and urinary retention. Skin rashes may appear. High doses cause palpitation, flushing, restlessness, delirium, hallucinations, psychosis, convulsions and coma. Poisoning is treated with IV physostigmine.

Uses of Belladonna Alkaloids

1. *As antispasmodic* In diarrhoea and dysentry, atropine relieves abdominal pain.

   In renal and biliary colic—atropine is used with morphine (see page 180).

   Nocturnal enuresis in children and in paraplegia atropine reduces urinary frequency.

2. *As mydriatric and cycloplegic*

   Diagnostic for testing error of refraction and fundoscopic examination of the eye.

   Therapeutic To provide rest to the iris in iritis, iridocyclitis and keratitis.

   Mydriatics are used alternately with miotics to break the adhesions between the iris and the lens.

3. *As pre-anaesthetic medication* When administered 30 min before anaesthesia, atropine reduces salivary and respiratory secretions. This will prevent the development of laryngospasm. It also prevents bradycardia during surgery. It's bronchodilator action is of additional value. ***Glycopyrrolate*** an atropine substitute, is most commonly used for this purpose.
4. *In organophosphorus poisoning* Atropine is life saving in OP poisoning and is also useful in mushroom poisoning.
5. *In bronchial asthma, peptic ulcer and parkinsonism* Atropine derivatives are preferred over atropine—see below.
6. *Motion sickness* Hyoscine given 30 minutes before the journey prevents travelling sickness. Transdermal hyoscine patches are available to be applied behind the ear for a prolonged action.
7. Hyoscine can also be used during *labour* to produce sedation and amnesia.

Drug interactions When anticholinergics are given with other drugs that also have anticholinergic property like antihistaminics, phenothiazines, tricyclic antidepressants—side effects get added up.

ATROPINE SUBSTITUTES

Belladonna alkaloids lack selectivity and exert a wide range of effects—producing many side effects. Hence several synthetic and semisynthetic derivatives with selective action were introduced (Table 2.4).

TABLE 2.4: Atropine substitutes

1.	*Derivatives used on the eye*	Homatropine, Eucatropine, Cyclopentolate, Tropicamide
2.	*Antispasmodics*	Atropine methonitrate Propantheline methantheline Oxyphenonium, Glycopyrrolate
3.	*Derivatives used in peptic ulcer*	Pirenzepine, Telenzepine
4.	*Derivatives used in bronchial asthma*	Ipratropium bromide
5.	*Antiparkinsonian drugs*	Benzhexol, Benztropine, Trihexyphenidyl

- Mydriasis and cycloplegia produced by atropine lasts for 7-10 days. The derivatives have a shorter action (6-24 hrs); some can selectively produce either mydriasis or cycloplegia and these can also be used in atropine intolerance.
- Spasmolytics are used in colics, gastritis and peptic ulcer.
- Pirenzepine and telenzapine are selective M_1-blockers—inhibit gastric secretion at doses that do not affect other functions and has been tried in peptic ulcer.
- When used in bronchial asthma, atropine thickens bronchial secretions and interferes with the movement of cilia and thus favours formation of mucous plugs. Ipratropium bromide is a bronchodilator that does not affect mucociliary activity. When given as inhalation, it produces no systemic side effects because of poor absorption. It is used in bronchial asthma and COPD.
- Benztropine, benzhexol and trihexyphenidyl are the derivatives used in drug induced parkinsonism.

❑ ADRENERGIC SYSTEM

The prime function of the adrenergic or sympathetic nervous system is to help the human beings to adjust to stress and prepare the body for fight or flight reactions. When exposed to stress, the heart rate and stroke volume increase with the resultant increase in CO. The blood is shifted from the skin, gut, kidney and glands to the heart, skeletal muscles, brain and lungs, as these organs need more blood during stress. Pupils and bronchi are dilated and sweating is increased. Blood glucose increases by glycogenolysis.

Neurotransmitters of the sympathetic system are noradrenaline (NA, norepinephrine) and dopamine (DA). Adrenaline (epinephrine) is the major hormone secreted by the adrenal medulla.

Synthesis of catecholamines The 3 catecholamines—NA, adrenaline and DA are synthesized from the amino acid tyrosine (Fig. 2.8).

The sympathetic postganglionic nerve fibres that synthesize, store and release NA are called **adrenergic.** Noradrenaline is

Tyrosine
↓ Tyrosine hydroxylase
DOPA
↓ DOPA decarboxylase
Dopamine
↓ DA β-hydroxylase
Noradrenaline
↓ N-methyl transferase
Adrenaline

Fig. 2.8: Biosynthesis of catecholamines

stored in small vesicles in the adrenergic nerve terminals. In response to nerve impulse, NA is released into the synaptic cleft by a process of **exocytosis**. This NA binds to adrenergic receptors located on the postsynaptic membrane to produce the response (Fig 2.9). A small portion of NA is metabolised by the enzyme COMT. But a large portion (nearly 80%) is taken back into the nerve terminals by an active transport process termed **uptake 1**, which is responsible for termination of action of NA. Of this, a fraction is metabolised by MAO and the remaining NA is then transferred to the storage vesicles. Some part of NA released into the synaptic cleft penetrates into the effector cells and is known as **uptake 2**.

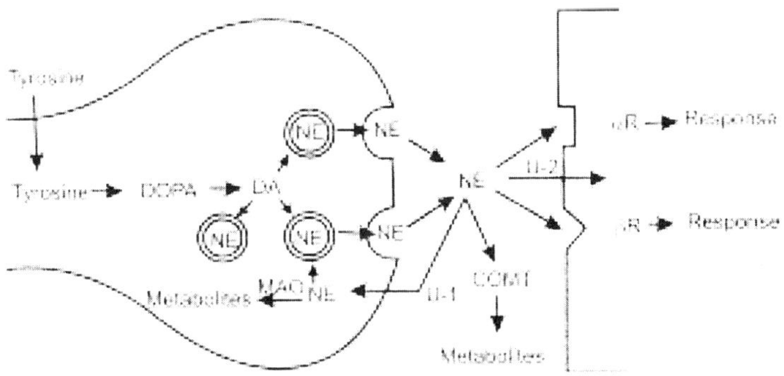

Fig. 2.9: Synthesis, storage, release and metabolism of noradrenaline

Adrenergic receptors Alquist classified adrenergic receptors into 2 types—α and β. With the availability of newer, synthetic, selective drugs, these are further classified into subdivisions. We now know α_1 α_2, β_1, β_2 and β_3 adrenergic receptors.

The stimulation of α receptors mainly produces excitatory effects (exception-GIT); β stimulation causes mainly inhibitory effects (exception- heart). The characteristics of these receptors are given in Table 2.5. α_2 receptors are located on the presynaptic membrane. When the concentration of NA reaches adequate levels, these presynaptic α_2 receptors are stimulated and inhibit the further release of NA. Thus α_2 receptors exert a negative feed back on NA release. α_2 receptors are also present postsynaptically in pancreatic islets, platelets and brain.

TABLE 2.5: Characteristics of adrenergic receptors

Receptor type	*Selective agonist*	*Selective antagonist*	*Location*	*Response*
α_1	Phenylephrine	Prazosin	Vascular smooth muscle	Contraction
			Gut	Relaxation
			Genitourinary smooth muscle	Contraction
			Liver	Glycogenolysis
α_2	Clonidine	Yohimbine	Pancreatic β cells	↓ Insulin release
			Platelets	Aggregation
			Nerve terminals	↓ NE release
β_1	Dobutamine	Metoprolol Atenolol	Heart	↑ Force of contraction, heart rate, AV conduction velocity
β_2	Salbutamol	Butoxamine	Smooth muscle—vascular, bronchial, gut and genitourinary	Relaxation
β_3	—	—	Adipose tissue	Lipolysis

❑ ADRENERGIC DRUGS (Sympathomimetics)

Sympathomimetics are drugs whose actions mimic that of sympathetic stimulation. They may be classified in various ways.

I. *Chemical classification—based on presence/absence of catechol nucleus*

1. *Catecholamines*	Noradrenaline (NA), Adrenaline, Dopamine (DA), Isoprenaline (Synthetic)
2. *Non-catecholamines*	Ephedrine, Amphetamine

II. *Depending on the mode of action*

1. *Directly acting sympathomimetics*	by interacting with adrenergic receptors—NA, Isoprenaline, Dopamine, Adrenaline
2. *Indirectly acting sympathomimetics*	by releasing NA from nerve terminals—Amphetamine, Tyramine
3. *Mixed action amines*	both direct and indirect actions: Ephedrine, Methoxamine

III. *Therapeutic or clinical classification*

1. *Vasopressors*	Noradrenaline, Dopamine, Methoxamine, Metaraminol
2. *Cardiac stimulants*	Adrenaline, Dopamine, Dobutamine, Isoprenaline, Ephedrine
3. *CNS stimulants*	Amphetamine, Ephedrine
4. *Bronchodilators*	Adrenaline, Isoprenaline, Salbutamol, Terbutaline, Salmeterol
5. *Nasal decongestants*	Ephedrine, Pseudoephedrine, Phenylpropanolamine, Phenylephrine, Oxymetazoline, Xylometazoline
6. *Appetite suppressants (anorectics)*	Fenfluramine, Dexfenfluramine
7. *Uterine relaxants*	Salbutamol, Terbutaline, Isoxuprine, Ritodrine

ACTIONS

1. Cardiovascular System

Heart Adrenaline is a powerful cardiac stimulant. Acting through β_1 receptors, it increases the heart rate, force of contraction, cardiac output and conduction velocity. The work done and the resultant O_2 consumption of the heart is increased.

Blood vessels and BP Blood vessels of skin and mucous membrane are constricted (α_1) and that of skeletal muscles are dilated (β_2) by adrenaline.

Moderate doses given IV produce a rapid increase in BP followed by a fall— a biphasic response. The rise in BP is due to α_1 mediated vasoconstriction. Action on β receptors is more persistent and as the action on alpha receptors wears off, the action on β receptors gets unmasked resulting in ↓ BP. Sir Henry Dale demonstrated that when α receptors are blocked (with alpha blockers—ergot alkaloids), adrenaline produces only a fall in BP and this is named after him as **Dale's vasomotor reversal** (or Dale's phenomenon).

Noradrenaline is mainly an alpha agonist and brings about a rise in BP.

Other vascular beds Adrenaline causes renal vasoconstriction resulting in fall in renal blood flow; it also causes pulmonary and mesenteric vasoconstriction.

Cerebral and coronary blood flow is enhanced.

2. Smooth Muscles

Bronchi Adrenaline is a powerful bronchodilator and a weak respiratory stimulant. Pulmonary vasoconstriction relieves bronchial congestion. All these result in an increase in vital capacity.

Uterus Nonpregnant uterus—contracts
Last month of pregnancy—relaxes.

Gut Smooth muscle is relaxed—but weak and transient action.

Splenic capsule Contracts resulting in the release of RBCs into the circulation.

Pilomotor muscles of the hair follicle Contraction.

Bladder Detrusor is relaxed while trigonal sphincter is contracted thereby increasing the holding capacity of the bladder.

3. Eye

Adrenaline causes mydriasis due to contraction of the radial muscles of the iris (α_1); it also reduces intraocular pressure.

4. Metabolic Effects

Adrenaline increases the blood sugar level by enhancing hepatic glycogenolysis. It also inhibits insulin release. It acts on β_3 receptors in the adipocytes to increase the breakdown of triglycerides.

5. Skeletal Muscles

Catecholamines facilitate neuromuscular transmission by action on both α and β receptors—they enhance the amount of ACh released.

Pharmacokinetics As catecholamines are rapidly inactivated in the gut and the liver they are not given orally. Adrenaline and NA are metabolised by COMT and MAO.

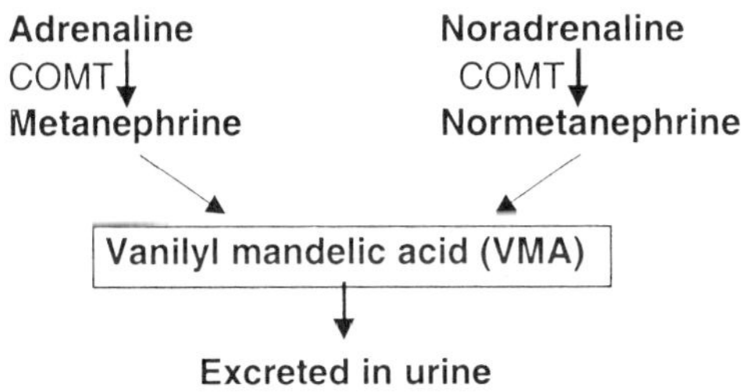

Adverse reactions Anxiety, palpitation, weakness, tremors, pallor, dizziness, restlessness and throbbing headache may follow adrenaline/NA administration. In patients with ischaemic heart disease, both adrenaline and NA can precipitate anginal pain. Rapid IV injection can cause sudden sharp rise in BP which may precipitate, arrthythmias, subarachnoid haemorrhage or hemiplegia.

Preparations Adrenaline 1:1000, 1: 10,000 and 1:1,00,000 solutions are available for injection. Adrenaline is given SC/IM; intracardiac in emergencies. Adrenaline aerosol for inhalation and 2% ophthalmic solution are also available.

Uses of adrenaline

1. **Anaphylactic shock** Adrenaline is the drug of choice (0.3-0.5 ml of 1:1000 solution). It promptly reverses hypotension, laryngeal oedema and bronchospasm and is life saving in anaphylactic shock. IM route is preferred as absorption by SC route is not reliable in shock.
2. **Cardiac arrest** Sudden cardiac arrest due to drowning, electrocution, etc. are treated with intracardiac adrenaline.
3. **Control of haemorrhage** Adrenaline in 1: 10,000 to 1 : 20,000 concentration is used as a topical hemostatic to control bleeding. Bleeding stops due to vasoconstriction. Adrenaline packs are used.
4. **With local anaesthetics** (see page 148) Injected with LA, adrenaline produces vasoconstriction and reduces the rate of absorption of LA. By this it prolongs the action and reduces systemic toxicity of LA. 1: 10,000 to 1: 2,00,000 adrenaline is used.
5. **Acute bronchial asthma** SC/inhalation adrenaline produces bronchodilation (see page 180).
6. **Glaucoma** Adrenaline ↓ IOP and can be used in glaucoma.

Noradrenaline Can be used in shock to increase BP—but it is very rarely used.

Isoprenaline (Isoproterenol, Isopropylarterenol) is a synthetic catecholamine with predominantly β receptor stimulant action and negligible α actions. It has cardiac stimulant and smooth muscle relaxant properties. Due to vasodilation BP falls; it is a potent bronchodilator. Adverse effects include palpitation, angina, headache and flushing.

Isoprenaline is used in heart block and shock for its cardiac stimulant actions. It can be used in bronchial asthma (page 180).

Dopamine is the precursor of NA. It acts on the dopaminergic and adrenergic receptors. It is a central neurotransmitter. Low doses stimulate vascular D_1 receptors in renal, mesenteric and coronary beds causing vasodilatation in these vessels. Higher doses cause cardiac stimulation through β_1 receptors and in high doses α_1 receptors are activated resulting in vasoconstriction and ↑ BP.

Adverse effects Nausea, vomiting, palpitation, angina, sudden ↑ in BP may occur.

Uses DA is used in the treatment of shock—cardiogenic, hypovolaemic and septic shock. It is specially useful when there is renal dysfunction and low cardiac output.

Dobutamine a derivative of dopamine, is a relatively selective β_1 agonist. Though it also activates α receptors, in therapeutic doses the only dominant action is an increase in the force of contraction of the heart without a significant increase in the heart rate. Thus, it is used in patients with CCF or acute myocardial infarction or following cardiac surgery when there may be pump failure.

Non-catecholamines are devoid of catechol nucleus, they act both by direct stimulation of adrenergic receptors and indirectly by releasing NA. In contrast to catecholamines, they are effective orally, relatively resistant to MAO and therefore are longer-acting; they cross the blood-brain barrier and have CNS effects.

Ephedrine is an alkaloid obtained from the plants of the genus *Ephedra*. It acts by direct stimulation of α and β receptors and indirectly through release of NA. Repeated administration at short intervals result in tachyphylaxis. Ephedrine ↑ BP by peripheral vasoconstriction and by increasing the cardiac output. Like adrenaline it relaxes smooth muscles; it is a CNS stimulant and produces insomnia, restlessness, anxiety, tremors and increased mental activity.

Adverse effects include stomach upset, sleeplessness, tremors and difficulty in micturition.

Uses

1. **Bronchial asthma** Ephedrine is useful in mild, chronic bronchial asthma (see page 240) but it is not preferred.
2. **Nasal decongestion** Nasal drops of ephedrine are used. Pseudoephedrine—an isomer of ephedrine is used orally for decongestion.
3. **Mydriasis** Ephedrine eye drops are used to produce mydriasis without cycloplegia.

4. **Hypotension** For prevention and treatment of hypotension during spinal anaesthesia—IM ephedrine is used.
5. **Narcolepsy** is a condition with an irresistible desire and tendency to sleep. As ephedrine is a CNS stimulant, it is useful in narcolepsy.
6. **Nocturnal enuresis (Bed wetting)** in children may be treated with ephedrine as it increases the holding capacity of the bladder. Drugs should be used only when non-pharmacological measures have failed.

Amphetamine is a synthetic compound with actions similar to ephedrine, tachyphylaxis can occur on repeated use. Amphetamine is a potent CNS stimulant; it produces increased mental and physical activity, alertness, increased concentration and attention span, elation, euphoria and increased capacity to work. It also increases initiative and self confidence, postpones fatigue and improves physical performance (temporarily) as seen in athletes. All these properties make amphetamine a drug of dependence and abuse. Higher doses produce confusion, delirium and hallucinations. The effects may be reversed with overdosage.

Respiration Amphetamine stimulates respiration—analeptic.

Depression of appetite Acting on the feeding centre in the hypothalamus, amphetamine reduces hunger and suppresses appetite.

Amphetamine also has weak anticonvulsant property.

Adverse effects include restlessness, tremors, insomnia, palpitation, anxiety, confusion and hallucinations. Prolonged use may precipitate psychosis.

High doses cause angina, delirium, arrhythmias, hypertension, acute psychosis, coma and death due to convulsions.

Dependence Amphetamine causes psychologic dependence.

Uses

1. *Attention deficit hyperactivity disorder (ADHD)* in children is characterised by decreased ability to concentrate and hold attention, aggressive behaviour and hyperactivity; Amphetamine increases attention span in such children and improves performance in school.

2. *Narcolepsy* Amphetamine is preferred over ephedrine.
3. *Obesity* Though appetite is suppressed, due to risk of dependence and other side effects, amphetamine should not be used for this purpose.
4. *Epilepsy* Amphetamine can be used as an adjuvant and to counter the sedation due to antiepileptics.

VASOPRESSORS

These are α_1 agonists and include metaraminol, mephenteramine, phenylephrine and methoxamine. They increase the BP by increasing total peripheral resistance (TPR) or cardiac output (CO) or both. They are given parenterally with constant monitoring of BP. Tachyphylaxis may develop.

Uses Vasopressors are used to raise the BP in hypotension as seen in cardiogenic or neurogenic shock and during spinal anaesthesia.

Metaraminol is an alpha stimulant and also acts indirectly by NA release. CO is increased. It is also a nasal decongestant.

Mephenteramine acts on both α and β receptors to ↑ TPR, ↑ CO and thereby raises BP. It is orally effective. Pressor effect is accompanied by bradycardia.

Phenylephrine is a selective α_1 stimulant; it is also a nasal decongestant. Reflex bradycardia is prominent. It produces mydriasis without cycloplegia.

Methoxamine has actions similar to phenylephrine.

NASAL DECONGESTANTS are α agonists which relieve congestion due to vasoconstriction.

They may be used:

1. *Orally* Ephedrine, Pseudoephedrine
2. *Topically* Oxymetazoline, Xylometazoline, Naphazoline, Phenylephrine, Mephenteramine, Metaraminol

- Irritation and after congestion are disadvantages
- On prolonged use nasal decongestants may cause atrophy of the mucosa due to intense vasoconstriction.

Uses Rhinitis in upper respiratory infection, allergic and vasomotor rhinitis, sinusitis and blocked eustachian tubes—nasal decongestants afford symptomatic relief.

SELECTIVE β_2 STIMULANTS include orciprenaline, salbutamol, terbutaline and salmeterol. These are smooth muscle relaxants which produce bronchodilatation, vasodilation and uterine relaxation without significant cardiac stimulation. They can be given by inhalation and are used in:

i. Bronchial asthma (see chapter 8)
ii. As uterine relaxants to delay premature labour.

Side effects include muscle tremors, palpitation and arrhythmias.

Isoxuprine is a selective β receptor stimulant used as uterine relaxant in premature labour, threatened abortion and dysmenorrhoea.

ANORECTIC AGENTS (ANOREXIANTS)

Though amphetamine suppresses appetite, it is not recommended for the treatment of obesity due to its central stimulant effects. Many amphetamine-like drugs which suppress appetite but lack significant CNS stimulant effects are now available. They are fenfluramine, dexfenfluramine, mazindol, phenylpropanolamine and others. *Adverse effects* include risk of abuse, drowsiness and depression because of which they are only used for short periods as adjuncts to other measures.

❑ ADRENERGIC ANTAGONISTS

Adrenergic blockers bind to the adrenergic receptors and prevent the action of adrenergic drugs. They may block alpha or beta receptors or both.

ALPHA ADRENERGIC BLOCKING AGENTS

Alpha receptor antagonists block the adrenergic responses mediated through alpha adrenergic receptors. Some of them have selectivity for α_1 or α_2 receptors.

Actions

The important effects of α receptor stimulation are α_1 mediated vasoconstriction and α_2-(presynaptic) receptor mediated inhibition of NA release. The result of blockade of these alpha receptors by α-antagonists is hypotension with tachycardia. This effect is due to:

i. α_1-blockade—inhibits vasoconstriction--leading to vasodilation and thereby ↓ BP. This fall in BP is opposed by the baroreceptor reflexes which tend to ↑ heart rate and cardiac output.
ii. α_2-blockade—enhances release of NA which stimulates β receptors (α are already blocked) β_1 stimulation in heart results in tachycardia and ↑ cardiac output.

Selective α_1-blockade—results in hypotension without significant tachycardia.

Selective α_2-blockade—↑ NA release resulting in hypertension.

α-blockade also results in miosis and nasal stuffiness. α-blockade in the bladder and prostate leads to decreased resistance to the flow of urine.

Adverse effects of α-blockers—postural hypotension, palpitation, nasal stuffiness, miosis and impaired ejaculation which may result in impotence.

Classification

1. *Non-selective*

a. *Non-competitive blocker*	Phenoxybenzamine
b. *Competitive blockers*	Ergot alkaloids (ergotamine), Tolazoline, Phentolamine, Chlorpromazine

2. *Selective*

a. *α_1-blockers*	Prazosin, Terazosin
b. *α_2-blocker*	Yohimbine

Phenoxybenzamine binds covalently to alpha receptors causing irreversible blockade. Given IV, blood pressure gradually falls and is associated with tachycardia. The action lasts for 3-4 days.

Ergot alkaloids Ergotamine, ergotoxine and their derivatives are competitive α antagonists and the blockade is of short duration.

Phentolamine and tolazoline are imidazoline derivatives. They are competitive α-blockers. In addition they also block 5-HT receptors, stimulate gut motility and ↑ gastric secretion. Hence they can cause vomiting and diarrhoea in addition to the effects of α-blockade.

Prazosin is a potent, highly selective, α_1-blocker with 1000 times greater affinity for α_1 receptors. Arterioles are dilated more than veins resulting in hypotension. There is no significant tachycardia (as α_2 receptors are spared there is no ↑ in NA release).

It is orally effective and is metabolised in the liver.

Adverse effects First dose phenomenon—1 hour after the initial dose, marked postural hypotension occurs which may lead to fainting. To avoid this, prazosin should be started with a low dose and taken at bed time.

Terazosin is longer-acting and can be given once daily.

Yohimbine is a relatively selective α_2-blocker which increases BP and heart rate due to ↑ NA release. It causes congestion of genitals for which it is used to treat psychogenic impotence. It is also claimed to be an aphrodisiac though the effect is only psychological.

Uses of α-blockers

1. *Hypertension* Selective α_1-blockers like prazosin are used in the treatment of hypertension (page 130). Phenoxybenzamine or phentolamine can be used in hypertensive crisis.
2. *Pheochromocytoma* is an adrenal medullary tumor which secretes large amounts of catecholamines resulting in hypertension. The tumor has to be removed surgically. Phenoxybenzamine and phentolamine are used for the preoperative management of the patient and during the operation. Inoperable cases are put on long-term treatment with phenoxybenzamine.

3. *Peripheral vascular diseases* Like Raynaud's phenomenon may be benefited by α-blockers which afford symptomatic relief.
4. *Congestive cardiac failure* Because of its vasodilator action, prazosin is useful in CCF. But ACE inhibitors are preferred.
5. *Benign prostatic hypertrophy (BPH)* Blockade of α_1 receptors in the bladder, prostate and urethra reduce resistance to urine outflow. Prazosin is useful in patients who cannot be operated upon.

BETA ADRENERGIC BLOCKING AGENTS

β-blockers are drugs that block the actions of catecholamines mediated through the β receptors.

Classification

1. *Non-selective*: Propranolol, Nadolol, Timolol, Sotalol
2. *Cardioselective (β_1)* Metoprolol, Atenolol, Acebutolol, Esmolol
3. *Partial agonists* Pindolol, Oxprenolol
4. *With additional alpha blocking property* Labetalol.

Pharmacological Actions

1. *CVS* β-blockers decrease heart rate, force of contraction and cardiac output. Blood pressure falls. The effect is more pronounced in presence of increased sympathetic tone than in a normal situation.
   AV conduction is delayed. Myocardial oxygen requirement is reduced due to reduced cardiac work.
   High doses produce membrane-stabilising activity like quinidine, causing direct depression of the heart.
2. *Exercise* β-blockers prevent the increase in heart rate and force of contraction which are brought about by exercise. β-blockers may also reduce the work capacity. These effects are less prominent with β_1 selective agents. This is because blockade of β_2 receptors prevents the increase in blood flow to the skeletal muscles during exercise. β-blocker improve exercise tolerance in patients with angina.
3. *Respiratory tract* Blockade of β_2 receptors in the bronchial smooth muscle causes increase in airway resistance—may precipitate acute attacks in asthmatics.

4. *Eye* Many β-blockers reduce intraocular pressure by decreased secretion of aqueous humour.
5. *Metabolic* β-antagonists block lipolysis and glycogenolysis induced by sympathetic stimulation. Plasma triglycerides may increase and HDL levels decrease in some patients.

Pharmacokinetics

Though well absorbed on oral administration, some β-blockers like propranolol undergo extensive first pass metabolism. Most of them have short t½ and are metabolised in the liver.

Adverse Reactions

1. **Bradycardia** is common.
2. **CCF** In patients with impaired cardiac function, sympathetic activity supports the heart. β-blockade eliminates this and may result in CCF.
3. **Cold extremities** especially in patients with peripheral vascular disease may occur.
4. β-blockers can precipitate **acute asthmatic attacks** and is contraindicated in asthmatics.
5. **CNS** Sedation, depression and rarely hallucinations can follow the use of β-blockers.
6. **Metabolic effects** Weakness, ↓ exercise capacity may be seen due to its metabolic effects.
7. Abrupt withdrawal of β-blockers after prolonged use can cause **rebound hypertension** and precipitate anginal attacks. This is due to up-regulation of β receptors. Hence β-blockers should be gradually withdrawn over many weeks.

Some important drug interactions

1. Propanol + insulin—when diabetics on insulin also receive propranolol:
   i. β-blockade masks tachycardia which is the first warning signal of hypoglycaemia.
   ii. β-blockade delays the recovery from hypoglycaemia by preventing glycogenolysis induced by sympathetic

stimulation. This may be avoided by using a β_1-selective blocker.

2. Propranolol + verapamil—since both cause myocardiac depression, profound depression may result. Hence the combination should be avoided.

Cardioselective β-blockers e.g. Atenolol, Metoprolol, Esmolol.

These drugs:

- Selectively block β_1 receptors, β_2-blockade is weak
- Bronchospasm is less/negligible
- Inhibition of glycogenolysis is lower—hence safer in diabetics
- Exercise performance impaired to a lesser degree
- Reduced chances of peripheral vascular disease.
- Atenolol is long-acting—given once daily.
- Esmolol is very short-acting and can be given intravenously in emergencies.
- Osmolol

Partial agonists—Pindolol, Oxprenolol.

These have intrinsic sympathomimetic activity due to their partial β-agonistic property. As a result, bradycardia and myocardiac depression are less marked. They are therefore preferred in patients with low cardiac reserve or those who are likely to have severe bradycardia.

Uses of β-blockers

1. **Hypertension** β-blockers are useful in the treatment of mild to moderate hypertension. A β-blocker can be used alone or with other antihypertensives (page 129).
2. **Angina pectoris** β-blockers are useful in the prophylaxis of exertional angina. Both the severity and frequency are reduced (page 124).
3. **Cardiac arrhythmias** β-blockers are useful in the treatment of both ventricular and supraventricular arrhythmias. (page 119).
4. **Myocardial infarction** IV β-blockers in acute MI may limit the size of the infarct.

   In patients who have recovered from MI, long-term treatment with β-blockers prolongs survival.

5. **Obstructive cardiomyopathy** β-blockers are found to be beneficial.
6. **Pheochromocytoma** Propranolol is given with α-blockers before surgery to control hypertension.
7. **Thyrotoxicosis** Propranolol controls palpitation, tremors and affords symptomatic relief in thyrotoxicosis.
8. **Glaucoma** Timolol is used topically in open angle glaucoma.
9. **Prophylaxis of migraine** Propranolol reduces frequency and severity of migraine headache; used for prophylaxis.
10. **Anxiety** Propranolol prevents the acute panic symptoms seen in public speaking, examination and other such anxiety-provoking situations. Performance in musicians can be improved. Tremors, tachycardia and other symptoms of sympathetic overactivity are alleviated.

Alpha and Beta-adrenergic Blockers

Labetalol Blocks both α_1 and β (β_1 and β_2) receptors. It is a competitive antagonist. Heart rate, contractility, AV conduction and BP fall. Blood flow to the limbs increases.

Side effects include postural hypotension, GI disturbances and other effects of alpha and β-blockade.

Uses Labetalol is used in hypertensive emergencies and pheochromocytoma. **Carvedilol** and **medroxalol** also block both alpha and beta receptors.

3

Musculoskeletal System

- Skeletal muscle relaxants
- Drugs used in the treatment of local muscle spasm
- Drugs used in the other musculoskeletal diseases
- Drugs used in disorder of bone, agents used in osteoporosis
- Drugs and exercise

SKELETAL MUSCLE RELAXANTS

Skeletal muscle relaxants (SMR) are drugs that reduce the muscle tone either by acting peripherally at the neuromuscular junction (neuromuscular blockers) or centrally in the cerebrospinal axis or directly on the contractile mechanism. They reduce the spasticity in a variety of neurological conditions and are also useful in surgeries.

CLASSIFICATION

1. **Drugs acting peripherally at the NMJ**
   Competitive blockers—d-Tubocurarine, Pancuronium, Alcuronium, Rocuronium, Atracurium
   Non-depolarising agents Mivacurium, Doxacurium, Pipecurium, Vecuronium, Rapacuronium, Gallamine
   Depolarising blockers—Succinylcholine, Decamethonium
2. **Drugs acting centrally**—Diazepam, Baclofen, Mephenesin, Tizanidine
3. **Drugs acting directly on the muscle**—Dantrolene

PERIPHERALLY ACTING SKELETAL MUSCLE RELAXANTS

Neuromuscular Blockers (NMB)

Competitive Blockers

Curare was used by the South American Indians as arrow poison for hunting wild animals because curare paralysed the animals. On extensive research, the active principle from curare, **tubocurarine** was identified. d-tubocurarine (d-Tc) is the dextrorotatory quarternery ammonium alkaloid obtained from the plant *Chondrodendron tomentosum* and plants of the Strychnos species (l-tubocurarine is less potent). Several synthetic agents have been developed. All these are quarternary ammonium compounds, because of which they are not well absorbed and are quickly excreted.

Mechanism of action Non-depolarising blockers bind to nicotinic receptors on the motor end plate and block the actions of acetylcholine by competitive blockade (Fig. 3.1). These compounds slowly dissociate from the receptors and transmission is gradually restored. Thus, their action is reversible.

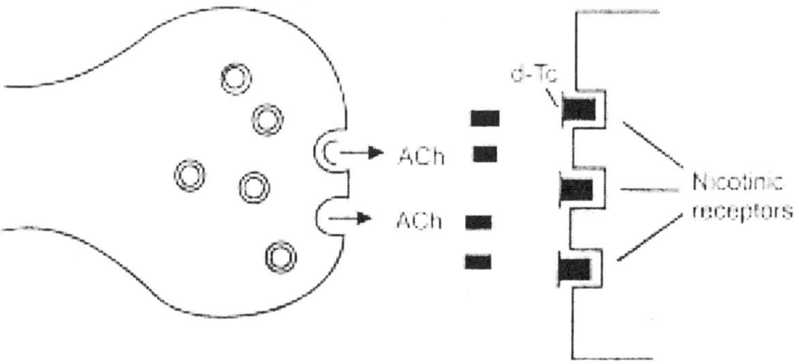

Fig. 3.1: d-Tc molecules bind to nicotinic receptors and prevent the binding of ACh on these receptors

Pharmacological actions

Skeletal muscle On parenteral administration, tubocurarine initially causes muscular weakness followed by flaccid paralysis. Small muscles of the eyes and fingers are the first to be affected, followed by those of the limbs, neck and trunk. Later the intercostal muscles and finally the diaphragm are paralysed and respiration stops. Consciousness is not affected throughout. Recovery occurs in the reverse order, i.e. the diaphragm is the first to recover. The effect lasts for 30-60 minutes (Table 3.1).

TABLE 3.1: Duration of action of competitive neuromuscular blockers

Drug	*Duration (min)*
Tubocurarine	35-60
Gallamine	35-60
Pancuronium	35-80
Doxacurium	90-120
Atracurium	20-35
Vecuronium	20-35
Mivacurium	12-18
Pipecuronium	80-100
Rapacuronium	15-30
Rocuronium	30-60

Autonomic ganglia In high doses tubocurarine can block autonomic ganglia and adrenal medulla resulting in hypotension.

Histamine release Tubocurarine can cause histamine release the mast cells from leading to bronchospasm, increased salivary, tracheobronchial and gastric secretions and this also contributes to hypotension.

Pharmacokinetics d-Tc is a quarternary ammonium compound—hence not absorbed orally. It is given either IM or IV.

Adverse reactions

1. Respiratory paralysis and prolonged apnoea. It should be treated with artificial ventilation. Neostigmine reverses the skeletal muscle paralysis.
2. Hypotension due to ganglion blockade and histamine release.
3. Flushing and bronchospasm due to histamine release by d-Tc; this is not seen with newer agents.

Synthetic Competitive Blockers

Pancuronium, atracurium, vecuronium, gallamine, doxacurium, mivacurium, pepecuronium, rapacuronium, rocuronium (Table 3.1) are synthetic competitive blocks. Tubocurarine, doxacurium and gallamine have a slow onset (about 5 minutes) but long duration of action; pancuronium, vecuronium, atracurium and mivacurium have intermediate onset (2-4 minutes) while rapacuronium and rocuronium have fast onset of action (1-2 minutes). The synthetic compounds have the following advantages over tubocurarine.

- Less/no histamine release.
- Do not block autonomic ganglia hence cause less hypotension
- Spontaneous recovery takes place with most of these drugs.
- Some are more potent than tubocurarine.
- Atracurium can be safely used in patients with renal impairment because it is degraded by plasma esterases and does not depend on kidney for elimination.
- The newer agents rapacuronium and rocuronium have a rapid onset of action. Hence they can be used as alternative to succinylcholine (SCh) for muscle relaxation before endotracheal intubation.
- Rocuronium does not cause hypotension, tachycardia and is fast acting.

Tubocurarine causes histamine release, ganglion blockade (resulting in hypotension) and its muscle relaxant effect needs to be reversed with drugs. Hence tubocurarine is not used now. The synthetic compounds are preferred.

Depolarising Blockers

Succinylcholine (SCh, Suxamethonium) is a quaternary ammonium compound with the structure resembling two molecules of acetylcholine joined together.

Mechanism of action The neuromuscular effects of SCh are like those of ACh. SCh reacts with nicotinic receptors and depolarises the skeletal muscle membrane. But, unlike ACh, it is destroyed very slowly by pseudocholinesterase. Thus continued presence of the drug causes persistent depolarisation resulting in flaccid paralysis. This is phase I block. In high doses

SCh produces a dual block—initial depolarising block followed by non-depolarising block. The membrane gets slowly repolarised but cannot be depolarised again. The mechanism of this phase II block is not clearly known.

Pharmacological actions

Skeletal muscle on intravenous administration onset of action is very rapid—within 1 minute. Initial transient muscular fasciculations and twitchings, mostly in the chest and abdominal regions are followed by skeletal muscle paralysis. The fasciculations are maximum in 2 minutes and subside in 5 minutes. It is due to stimulation of the muscle fibres by a discharge of action potentials in them. SCh is a short-acting muscle relaxant and the effect lasts for 5-10 minutes. Hence it has to be given continuously as an infusion for longer effect.

CVS Initially hypotension and bradycardia may result from stimulation of the nicotinic receptors in vagal ganglia. This is followed by tachycardia and hypertension due to stimulation of sympathetic ganglia. Higher doses can cause cardiac arrhythmias. SCh can also cause histamine release if injected rapidly.

Other effects SCh can cause hyperkalemia as it triggers the release of K^+ from the cells by increasing the permeability to cations. It can also cause a transient increase in intraocular pressure.

Pharmacokinetics SCh is rapidly hydrolysed by pseudocholinesterase—hence it is short-acting (about 5 minutes). Some people (1 in 2000) have an abnormal pseudocholinesterase, a hereditary defect; SCh does not get metabolised and even the usual dose results in prolonged apnoea and paralysis which may last for several hours. Artificial ventilation and fresh blood transfusion are needed.

Adverse reactions Postoperative muscle pain is a common adverse effect of SCh. It may be due to the damage to muscle fibres that occurs during initial fasciculations.

Hyperkalemia: This may result in cardiac arrest in patients with burns and nerve injuries.

Cardiac arrhythmias: SCh can cause cardiac arrhythmias.

Malignant hyperthermia: It is a rare genetically determined condition where there is a sudden increase in body temperature and severe muscle spasm due to release of intracellular Ca^{++} from the sarcoplasmic reticulum. Certain drugs like halothane, isoflurane and succinylcholine can trigger this process which can be fatal. Combination of halothane and SCh is the most common triggering factor. Intravenous dantrolene is life-saving in malignant hyperthermia. Oxygen inhalation and immediate cooling of the body also help.

Drug interactions

1. General anaesthetics augment the action of SMRs.
2. Anticholinesterases like neostigmine—reverse the action of competitive blockers.
3. Aminoglycosides and calcium channel blockers potentiate the action of SMRs.

Uses of Peripherally Acting Skeletal Muscle Relaxants

Inappropriate use of peripherally acting SMRs can be fatal. Hence they should be given only by qualified anaesthetists or adequately trained doctors.

1. *Adjuvant to anaesthesia* Adequate muscle relaxation is essential during surgeries. Skeletal muscle relaxants are used as adjuvants to general anaesthesia. Short-acting SMRs like succinylcholine is used during endotracheal intubation. SMRs are also useful in laryngoscopy, bronchoscopy, oesophagoscopy and in orthopaedic procedures like reduction of fractures and dislocations.
2. *In electroconvulsive therapy* SMRs protect the patient from convulsions and trauma during ECT.
3. *In spastic disorders* SMRs are used to overcome the spasm of tetanus, athetosis and status epilepticus.

CENTRALLY ACTING MUSCLE RELAXANTS

These drugs act on higher centres and cause muscle relaxation without loss of consciousness. They also have sedative properties.

Mechanism of Action

Centrally acting muscle relaxants depress the spinal polysynaptic reflexes. These reflexes maintain the muscle tone. By depressing these spinal reflexes, centrally acting SMRs reduce the muscle tone.

Diazepam has useful antispastic activity. It can be used in relieving muscle spasm of almost any origin including local muscle trauma (see page 155).

Baclofen is an analog of the inhibitory neurotransmitter GABA. It is a GABA agonist—it depresses the monosynaptic and polysynaptic reflexes in the spinal cord. It relieves painful spasms including flexor and extensor spasms and may also improve bladder and bowel functions in patients with spinal lesions. Normal tendon reflexes and voluntary muscle power are not affected. Baclofen is generally given orally.

Side effects are drowsiness, weakness and ataxia. Baclofen should be gradually withdrawn after prolonged use.

Mephenesin is not preferred due to its side effects. A number of related drugs like *carisoprodol, methocarbamol, chlorzoxazone* are used in acute muscle spasm caused by local trauma. All of them also cause sedation.

Tizanidine is a congener of clonidine. It is a central α_2 agonist like clonidine. It increases presynaptic inhibition of motor neurons and reduces muscle spasms. Adverse effects include drowsiness, weakness, hypotension and dry mouth. Tizanidine is used in the treatment of spasticity due to stroke, multiple sclerosis and amyotropic lateral sclerosis.

Other centrally acting spasmolytic agents include riluzole, gabapentin and progabide. Riluzole has both presynaptic and postsynaptic effects. It inhibits glutamate release in the CNS. It is well tolerated with minor adverse effects like nausea and diarrhoea. It is used to reduce spasticity in AML.

Uses of Centrally Acting Muscle Relaxants

1. *Musculoskeletal disorders* like muscle strains, sprains, myalgias, cervical root syndromes, herniated disc syndromes, low backache, dislocations, arthritis, fibrositis and bursitis all cause painful muscle spasms. Muscle relaxants are used with analgesics in these.
2. *Spastic neurological disorders* like cerebral palsy, multiple sclerosis, poliomyelitis, hemiplegia and quadriplegia are treated with diazepam or baclofen.
3. *Tetanus* Diazepam is given IV.
4. *ECT* Diazepam is given along with peripherally acting SMRs.
5. *Orthopaedic procedures* like fracture reduction may be done after administering diazepam.

Directly Acting Muscle Relaxants

Dantrolene directly affects the skeletal muscle contractile mechanism. It inhibits the muscle contraction by preventing the calcium release from the sarcoplasmic reticulum.

Adverse effects include drowsiness, dizziness, fatigue, muscle weakness, diarrhoea and rarely hepatotoxicity. Liver function tests should be done to look for hepatotoxicity.

Uses

Dantrolene is used in spastic disorders and malignant hyperthermia (page 92). Dantrolene prevents the release of Ca^{++} from the sarcoplasmic reticulum and relieves muscle spasm in malignant hyperthermia.

❑ DRUGS USED IN THE TREATMENT OF LOCAL MUSCLE SPASM

Several agents are used for the treatment of local muscle spasms which may result from injury or strain. Cyclobenzaprine, metaxalone, carisoprodol, chlorzoxazone, meprobamate, and methocarbamol are some of them. They have the following common features:

- All these drugs act by depressing spinal polysynaptic reflexes.
- Common adverse reactions include drowsiness and dizziness.
- Cyclobenzaprine has anticholinergic effects and can therefore cause dryness of mouth, drowsiness and dizziness.
- Many of them are available in combination with NSAIDs.
- NSAIDs are equally or more effective in relieving muscle spasms.

Botulinum toxin is produced by the anaerobic bacterium Clostridium botulinum. The toxin inhibits the release of acetylcholine at the cholinergic synapses resulting in flaccid paralysis of skeletal muscles.

Botulinum toxin is useful (local injection) in the treatment of dystonias, including sports or writers cramps muscle spasms, tremors, cerebral palsy and in rigidity seen in extrapyramidal disorders. It is commonly used to relieve blepharospasm Botilinum toxin is also gaining popularity in cosmetic therapy to remove facial lines by local injection.

❑ DRUGS USED IN OTHER MUSCULOSKELETAL DISEASES

Osteomalacia Vitamin D deficiency results in osteomalacia. Vitamin D is used for the prevention and treatment of osteomalacia.

Paget's disease—NSAIDs, calcitonin and bisphosphonates are used. Analgesics reduce pain while calcitonin and bisphosphonates reduce bone resorption.

Osteoarthritis—NSAIDs and glucocorticoids are used.

DRUGS USED IN SPASTICITY

Spasticity is due to hypertonic contraction of the skeletal muscles. Spastically is seen in cerebral palsy, stroke and multiple sclerosis. Drugs used in spasticity include baclofen, diazepam and dantrolene.

OTHER MUSCULAR DISORDERS

Some muscular disorders like congenital myotonia, Lambert-Eaton syndrome, McCardle syndrome and tetany are due to impaired neuromuscular transmission.

Congenital myotonia is characterized by violent muscle spasm, which results from irritability of the muscle fiber membrane. Membrane stabilizing agents like phenytoin and quinine are found to be useful in this condition.

Lambert-Eaton syndrome is characterized by muscular weakness and easy fatiguability. It is associated with some cancers like lung cancer. Physical exercise and calcium are found to be useful in improving muscle power.

McCardle syndrome in some people, glycogen cannot be converted to glucose in the muscle due to an enzyme deficiency. Hence after some exercise such persons develop severe muscle weakness, stiffness and pain. It can be treated with large doses of glucose or by adrenaline injection, which releases glucose from the liver.

Tetany Hypocalcaemia results in tetany and increased neuromuscular excitabitability. Calcium salts, should be given orally or in more severe cases intravenously.

❑ DRUGS USED IN THE DISORDERS OF BONE, AGENTS USED IN OSTEOPOROSIS

Disorders of bone include:
- Osteoporosis
- Osteomalacia and rickets
- Paget's disease

Drugs used in disorders of bone are
- *Bisphosphonates*
  - — Alendronate etidronate
  - — Pamidronate residronate
- *Raloxifene* (selective estrogen receptor modulator)

AGENTS USED IN THE PREVENTION AND TREATMENT OF OSTEOPOROSIS

Drugs may be used either to prevent bone resorption or promote bone formation or a combination of both in the prevention and treatment of osteoporosis. These agents reduce the risk of fractures in patients with osteoporosis.

Drugs that prevent bone resorption are

- Calcium (↑BMD)
- Vitamin D (↑absorption of calcium)
- Estrogens (prevents osteoporosis)
- Raloxifene—a SERM (↑BMD)
- Calcitonin (prevents bone resorption, ↑BMD*)
- Bisphosphonates (↓bone resorption, ↑BMD*)

*BMD (Bone mineral density)

Drugs that promote bone formation

- Fluoride (in small doses ↑osteoblastic activity →↑bone mass — but generally not preferred)
- Testosterone (in hypogonadal men)
- Anabolic steroids (in postmenopausal women)
- PTH analogs are being tried.

❑ DRUGS AND EXERCISE

Effect of Exercise on the Cardiorespiratory Function

During exercise, oxygen consumption of the skeletal muscle increases. Hence it requires more oxygen supply. In order to meet this increased demand, various changes take place in the cardiovascular and respiratory system. The heart rate, force of contraction and thereby the cardiac out put increase; the respiratory rate, depth and thereby tidal volume increase. The blood vessels of skeletal muscles are dilated which increases blood supply as well as washes away the metabolites formed.

Drugs that Influence Exercise

Drugs like amphetamines, anabolic steroids, methylxanthines and cocaine improve exercise performance while β-blockers decrease exercise tolerance.

Amphetamine improves both mental and physical performance (see page 78). It improves alertness and performance even in highly tiring conditions. It postpones fatigue and brings about a significant improvement in athletic performance in sportsmen. Amphetamines are banned in sports. Amphetamine is a drug of dependence.

Cocaine Like amphetamine, cocaine is a psychomotor stimulant. It produces euphoria and increased motor activity. It inhibits the uptake of catecholamines in the nerve terminals resulting in increased sympathetic activity. Cocaine is a drug of dependance and its long-term use results in various adverse effects.

Anabolic steroids are androgens with selective anabolic effects and lesser degree of androgenic effects. Anabolic steroids improve muscle strength. They are misused by athletes and are now banned in them. But androgens can cause various side effects if used over a long-time including reduced sperm production and decreased fertility. Some cause gynaecomastia, hepatotoxicity, increase serum cholesterol and psychological disorders. Androgens cause virilization in women.

Bronchodilators *Methylxanthines*, (see page 239) The main compounds are theophylline and caffeine. They are present in coffee, tea and cocoa. Methylxanthines are CNS stimulants. They reduce fatigue, improve alertness and physical performance. They are mild psychomotor stimulants. They also bring about bronchodilation and cardiac stimulation which add to their beneficial effects on exercise.

β-adrenergic agonists Adrenaline and selective β_2-agonists like salbutamol, terbutaline and salmeterol are bronchodilators. Though their bronchodilator effect may help better oxygenation during respiration, these drugs cause skeletal muscle tremors. The exact mechanism is not known but they may act through β-receptors to increase the discharge of muscle spindles. *Clenbuterol* is a β_2-agonist used by sportsmen for its anabolic effects.

Drugs that Decrease Exercise Tolerance

β-adrenergic blockers prevent the exercise induced increase in heart rate and force of contraction. β-blockers reduce the work capacity and impair exercise performance. The increase in blood flow to the skeletal muscle during exercise is reduced by β_2 blockade. They also prevent the rise in blood glucose level brought about by catecholamines. They may also increase airway resistance. By all these effects, β-blockers reduce exercise tolerance.

4

Drugs Acting on the Kidney

- DIURETICS
- ANTIDIURETICS

DIURETICS AND ANTIDIURETIC DRUGS

Kidney, the excretory organ of our body serves the important functions of excretion of waste products, regulation of fluid volume and electrolyte content of the extracellular fluid.

PHYSIOLOGY OF URINE FORMATION

Normally about 180 litres of fluid is filtered everyday, of which 99% gets reabsorbed and about 1.5 litres of urine is formed. For simplification, the nephron can be divided into four sites (Fig. 4.1).

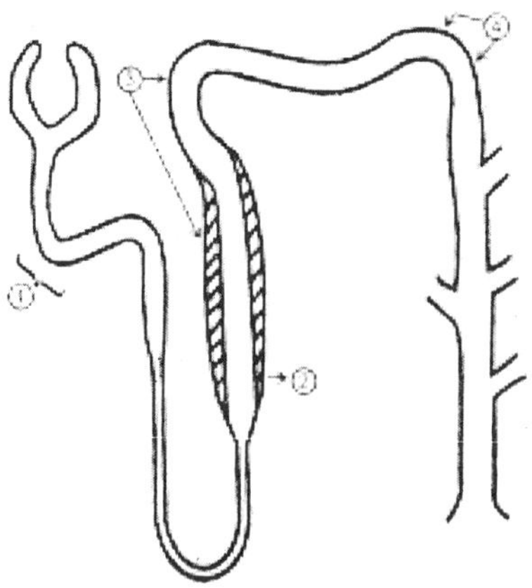

Fig. 4.1: Simplified diagram of a nephron showing sites of action of diuretics (1) Proximal tubule—osmotic diuretics, mannitol, (2) Ascending limb of Henle's loop—loop diuretics, (3) Early distal tubule—thiazides, (4) Distal tubule and collecting duct—K^+ sparing diuretics

Proximal tubule Sodium bicarbonate, sodium chloride, amino acids and glucose are reabsorbed in the proximal tubule along with water by specific transport mechanisms. Osmotic diuretics act here.

Henle's loop In the thin descending limb of the loop of Henle, water is reabsorbed by osmotic forces. Hence osmotic diuretics are acting here too. The thick ascending limb actively reabsorbs sodium chloride from the lumen (but is impermeable to water) by $Na^+/K^+/2Cl^-$ co-transporter. 'Loop diuretics' selectively block this transporter.

Distal convoluted tubule In the early distal tubule, sodium chloride is reabsorbed by an electrically neutral Na^+ and Cl^- transporter. This transporter is blocked by thiazide diuretics.

Collecting tubule In the late distal tubule and collecting duct, $NaCl^-$ is actively reabsorbed, in exchange for K^+ and H^+ to maintain the ionic balance-regulated by aldosterone. Absorption of water is under the control of antidiuretic hormone (ADH).

❑ DIURETICS

Diuretic is an agent which increases urine and solute excretion.

CLASSIFICATION

1. **High efficacy diuretics** *(Loop diuretics)* — Furosemide, Bumetanide, Piretanide, Ethacrynic acid, Torsemide
2. **Moderate efficacy diuretics**
   - *Thiazides* — Benzothiadiazines like Chlorothiazide, Hydrochlorothiazide, Polythiazide, Bendroflumethiazide
   - *Thiazide related agents* — Chlorthalidone, Clopamide, Indapamide, Metolazone, Xipamide
3. **Low efficacy diuretics**
   - *Potassium sparing diuretics* — Triamterene, Amiloride, Spironolactone

Carbonic anhydrase inhibitors	Acetazolamide
Osmotic diuretics	Mannitol, Urea, Glycerol
Methylxanthines	Theophylline

High efficacy or Loop Diuretics

Loop diuretics act by inhibiting $NaCl^-$ reabsorption in the thick ascending limb of the Henle's loop. They inhibit the Na^+, K^+, $2Cl^-$, co-transport mechanism. As a large amount of $NaCl^-$ is absorbed in this segment, they are highly efficacious. Diuretic response increases with dose and higher doses can cause dehydration (high ceiling of effect).

Loop diuretics also enhance the excretion of K^+, Ca^{++} and Mg^{++} (But Ca^{++} is reabsorbed in the distal tubule—hence no hypocalcaemia). They increase reabsorption of uric acid in the proximal tubule. They also alter renal haemodynamics to reduce fluid and electrolyte reabsorption in the proximal tubule.

Frusemide (Furosemide) is a sulfonamide derivative. It is the most popular loop diuretic. Given intravenously it acts in 2-5 minutes, while following oral use, it takes 20-40 minutes; duration of action is 3-6 hours.

IV furosemide relieves pulmonary congestion and reduces left ventricular filling pressure by causing venodilation in congestive heart failure and pulmonary edema.

Pharmacokinetics Furosemide is rapidly absorbed orally, highly bound to plasma proteins and excreted by kidneys.

Bumetanide is a sulfonamide like frusemide but is 40 times more potent. Bioavailability is 80% and is better tolerated.

Ethacrynic acid is more likely to cause adverse effects and hence is not commonly used.

Adverse Effects of Loop Diuretics

1. *Hypokalaemia and metabolic alkalosis* is dose dependent and can be corrected by K^+ replacement and correction of hypovolaemia.
2. *Ototoxicity* Loop diuretics cause hearing loss by a toxic effect on the hair cells in the internal ear—more common with ethacrynic acid. It is dose-related and generally reversible. Concurrent use of other ototoxic drugs should be avoided.

3. *Hyperuricaemia* may precipitate acute attacks of gout.
4. *Hypocalcaemia and hypomagnesaemia* After prolonged use this may result in osteoporosis.
5. *Hyponatraemia, dehydration and hypovolaemia* should be treated with saline infusion.
6. *Hyperglycaemia and hyperlipidaemia* are mild in therapeutic doses.
7. *GIT disturbances* like nausea, vomiting and diarrhoea are common with ethacrynic acid.
8. *Allergic reactions* like skin rashes are more common with sulfonamide derivatives.

Uses

1. *Oedema* Frusemide is highly effective for the relief of oedema of all origins like cardiac, hepatic and renal oedema.
   - Acute pulmonary oedema is relieved by IV frusemide due to its immediate vasodilator effect and then by diuretic action.
   - In cerebral oedema, frusemide is used as an alternative to osmotic diuretics.
2. *Forced diuresis* In poisoning due to drugs like barbiturates and salicylates, frusemide is used with IV fluids.
3. *Hypertension* with renal impairment may be treated with loop diuretics.
4. *Hypercalcaemia and hyperkalaemia* Loop diuretics enhance the excretion of Ca^{++} and K^+. But Na^+ and Cl^- should be replaced to avoid hyponatraemia and hypochloraemia.

Thiazides and Thiazide-like Diuretics

Chlorothiazide was the first thiazide to be synthesized. All thiazides have a sulfonamide group.

Actions

This group of drugs block Na^+/Cl^- co-transport in the early distal tubule (site 3). They also inhibit carbonic anhydrase activity. Thiazides also enhance excretion of Mg^+ and K^+ (in the distal segments, Na^+ in the lumen is exchanged for K^+ which is then excreted). But they inhibit urinary excretion of Ca^{++} and uric acid.

Pharmacokinetics

Thiazides are well-absorbed orally and are rapid acting. Duration varies from 6-48 hr (see Table 4.1). They are excreted by the kidney.

Adverse Effects

Hypokalaemia, metabolic alkalosis, hyperuricaemia, hypovolaemia, dehydration, hyponatraemia, hypercalcaemia, and hyperlipidaemia are similar to that seen with loop diuretics. Hyperglycaemia induced by thiazides may precipitate diabetes mellitus probably by inhibition of insulin secretion. It is more common when long-acting thiazides are used for a long time. Weakness, fatigue and allergic reactions like rashes and photosensitivity can be seen.

Uses

1. *Hypertension* Thiazides are the first line drugs (see page 127).
2. *Congestive heart failure* Thiazides are the first line drugs in the management of oedema due to mild to moderate CHF.
3. *Oedema* Thiazides may be tried in hepatic or renal oedema.
4. *Renal stones* Hypercalciuria with renal stones can be treated with thiazides which reduce calcium excretion.
5. *Diabetes insipidus* Thiazides reduce plasma volume and GFR and benefit such patients.

Potassium Sparing Diuretics

Spironolactone is an aldosterone antagonist. It binds aldosterone receptors on distal tubule and collecting duct and competitively inhibits the action of aldosterone (aldosterone promotes Na^+ reabsorption and K^+ secretion). As major amount of Na^+ is already reabsorbed in the proximal parts, spironolactone has low efficacy. Spironolactone also reduces K^+ loss due to other diuretics.

It enhances the excretion of calcium by a direct action on the renal tubules.

Adverse effects include gynaecomastia, drowsiness, hyperkalaemia especially in renal insufficiency; metabolic acidosis and skin rashes.

Amiloride and triamterene are directly acting agents which enhance Na^+ excretion and reduce K^+ loss by acting on ion channels in the distal tubule and collecting duct. They block the Na^+ transport through ion-channels in the luminal membrane. Since K^+ secretion is dependent on Na^+ entry, these drugs reduce K^+ excretion.

Adverse effects are gastrointestinal disturbances, hyperkalaemia and metabolic acidosis.

Uses of potassium sparing diuretics

1. *With thiazides and loop diuretics* to prevent potassium loss.
2. *Oedema* In cirrhosis and renal oedema where aldosterone levels may be high.
3. *Hypertension* Along with thiazides to avoid hypokalaemia and for additive effect.
4. *Primary or secondary aldosteronism* Spironolactone is used.

Drug Interactions with Diuretics

1. Frusemide and ethacrynic acid are highly protein bound and may compete with drugs like warfarin and clofibrate for protein binding sites.
2. Other ototoxic drugs like aminoglycosides should not be used with loop diuretics to avoid enhanced toxicity.
3. Hypokalaemia induced by diuretics enhance digitalis toxicity.
4. NSAIDs blunt the effect of diuretics as they cause salt and water retention to avoid enhanced toxicity.
5. Diuretics enhance lithium toxicity by reducing renal excretion of lithium.
6. Other drugs that cause hyperkalaemia (ACE inhibitors) and oral K^+ supplements should be avoided with K^+ sparing diuretics because, together they can cause severe hyperkalaemia.

Carbonic Anhydrase Inhibitors

Carbonic anhydrase is an enzyme that catalyses the formation of carbonic acid which spontaneously ionises to H^+ and HCO_3^-. This HCO_3^- combines with Na^+ and is reabsorbed.

$$H_2O + CO_2 \rightleftharpoons H_2CO_3$$

$$H_2CO_3 \rightleftharpoons H^+ + HCO_3^-$$

Carbonic anhydrase is present in the nephron, eyes, gastric mucosa, pancreas and other sites.

Acetazolamide, inhibits the enzyme a carbonic anhydrase and enhances the excretion of sodium, potassium, bicarbonate and water. The loss of bicarbonate leads to metabolic acidosis.

Other Actions

1. *Eye* Bicarbonate and sodium ions are required for the production of aqueous humour. Carbonic anhydrase inhibition results in decreased formation of aqueous humour and thereby reduces intraocular pressure.
2. *Brain* Bicarbonate is secreted into CSF and carbonic anhydrase inhibition reduces the formation of CSF.

Adverse Effects

1. Metabolic acidosis, renal stones, hypokalaemia, drowsiness and allergic reactions can occur.

Uses

1. Glaucoma—(see page 64)
2. To alkalinize the urine—as required in overdosage of acidic drugs.
3. Metabolic alkalosis—acetazolamide enhances HCO^-_3 excretion.
4. Mountain sickness—In mountain climbers who rapidly ascend great heights, severe pulmonary oedema or cerebral oedema may occur. Acetazolamide may help by reducing CSF formation.
5. Epilepsy—acetazolamide is used as an adjuvant as it increases the seizure threshold.

Osmotic Diuretics

Mannitol is a pharmacologically inert substance. When given IV (orally not absorbed), mannitol gets filtered by the glomerulus but not reabsorbed. It causes water to be retained in the kidney by osmotic effect resulting in water diuresis. There is also some loss of Na^+.

Adverse effects are dehydration, ECF volume expansion, headache and allergic reactions.

Uses

1. To maintain urine volume in conditions like shock.
2. To reduce intracranial and intraocular pressure—following head injury and glaucoma respectively.

Glycerol is effective orally—reduces intraocular and intracranial pressure.

Methylxanthines like theophylline have mild diuretic effect.

TABLE 4.1: Dose and duration of action of commonly used diuretics

Diuretic	*Daily dose (mg)*	*Duration (hrs)*	*Brand name*
Furosemide	20-80 mg	3-6	LASIX
Bumetanide	0.5-2 mg	3-6	BUMET
Hydrochlorothiazide	25-100	8-12	ESIDREX
Polythiazide	1-3	24-48	NEPHRIL
Chlorthalidone	50-100	48-72	HYTHALTON
Xipamide	20-60	24-36	XIPAMID
Metolazone	5-10	18-24	ZAROXYLIN
Spironolactone	50-100	6-12	ALDACTONE
Triamterene	50-100	4-6	DYTIDE (with benzthiazide)
Amiloride	5-10	20-24	LASIRIDE (with frusemide)

❑ ANTIDIURETICS

Antidiuretics are drugs that reduce urine volume. These include

1. Antidiuretic hormone (Vasopressin)
2. Thiazide diuretics
3. Miscellaneous
   — Chlorpropamide
   — Carbamazepine.

Antidiuretic hormone (ADH) is secreted by the anterior pituitary along with oxytocin. It is synthesized in the supraoptic and paraventricular nuclei of the hypothalamus, transported along the hypothalamo-hypophyseal tract to the posterior pituitary and it is stored there. ADH is released in response to two stimuli—dehydration and rise in plasma osmolarity.

Actions

ADH acts on vasopressin receptors and enhances water reabsorption, causes vasoconstriction and raises BP. It also acts on other smooth muscles to increase peristalsis in the gut and contracts the uterus.

It is given parenterally as injection or as intranasal spray.

Adverse Effects

When used intranasally ADH can cause nasal irritation, allergy, rhinitis and atrophy of the nasal mucosa. Other effects include nausea, abdominal cramps and backache (due to contractions of the uterus).

Uses

1. Diabetes insipidus of pituitary origin.
2. Bleeding oesophageal varices—ADH constricts mesenteric blood vessels and may help.
3. Before abdominal radiography—expels gases from the bowel.
4. Haemophilia—may release factor VIII.

Thiazides Paradoxically thiazides reduce urine volume in diabetes insipidus of both pituitary and renal origin by an unknown mechanism.

Chlorpropamide an oral hypoglycaemic, sensitizes the kidney to ADH action.

Carbamazepine an antiepileptic, stimulates ADH secretion.

5

Cardiovascular System

- Cardiac glycosides and treatment of cardiac failure
- Antiarrhythmic drugs
- Drugs used in the treatment of angina pectoris
- Antihypertensive drugs
- Pharmacotherapy of shock
- Plasma expanders

CARDIAC GLYCOSIDES AND TREATMENT OF CARDIAC FAILURE

The cardiac muscle is a specialised tissue with unique properties like excitability, contractility and automaticity. The myocardium has two types of cells—the contracting cells and the conducting cells. The contracting cells participate in the pumping action of the heart. Parts of the conducting tissue have the characteristic property of automaticity. **Automaticity** is the ability of the cell to generate electrical impulses spontaneously. SA node, AV node and His-Purkinje system comprise the conducting tissue of the heart. Normally the SA node acts as the pace maker. **Excitability** is the ability of the cell to undergo depolarization in response to a stimulus. **Contractility** is the ability of the myocardium to adequately contract and pump the blood out of the heart.

Cardiac action potential When a stimulus reaches the cardiac cell, specific ions move into and out of the cell eliciting an action potential. Such movement of ions across the cardiac cell may be divided into phases (Fig. 5.1).

Phase 0 is rapid depolarisation of the cell membrane during which there is fast entry of sodium ions into the cell through the sodium channels. This is followed by repolarisation.

Phase 1 is a short, initial, rapid repolarisation due to efflux of potassium ions.

Phase 2 is a prolonged plateau phase due to slow entry of calcium ions into the cell through the calcium channels. Cardiac cell differs from other cells in having this phase of action potential.

Phase 3 is a second period of rapid repolarisation with potassium ions moving out of the cell.

Phase 4 is the resting phase during which potassium ions return into the cell while sodium and calcium ions move out of it and the resting membrane potential is restored.

During phases 1 and 2, the cell does not depolarise in response to another impulse, i.e. it is in absolute refractory period. But during phases 3 and 4, the cell is in relative refractory period and may depolarise in response to a powerful impulse.

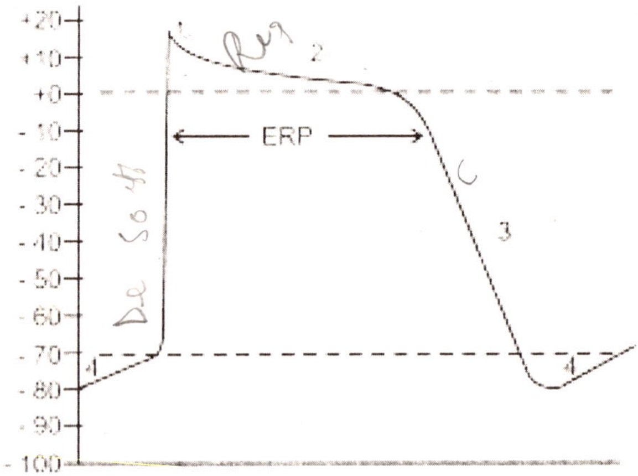

Fig. 5.1: Cardiac action potential phases 0-4: Phase 0—indicates rapid depolarisation, Phases 1-3—indicate repolarisation, Phase 4—gradual depolarisation during diastole

The cardiac output is determined by heart rate and stroke volume. The stroke volume in turn depends on the preload, afterload and contractility. **Preload** is the load on the heart due to the volume of blood reaching the left ventricle. It depends on the venous return. **Afterload** is the resistance to the left ventricular ejection, i.e. the total peripheral resistance.

Congestive cardiac failure (CCF) is one of the common causes of morbidity and mortality. In congestive cardiac failure, the heart is unable to provide adequate blood supply to meet the body's oxygen demand. The pumping ability of the heart is reduced and the cardiac output decreases. The ventricles are not completely emptied resulting in increased venous pressure in the pulmonary and systemic circulation. This causes pulmonary oedema, dyspnoea, liver enlargement and peripheral oedema. As a compensatory mechanism, there is stimulation of the sympathetic system and renin angiotensin system which help in maintaining the cardiac output. The myocardium also undergoes structural alterations like ventricular hypertrophy and remodelling to adapt itself to the stressful situation. These compensatory changes maintain the cardiac output for sometime.

Low output failure could result from ischaemic heart disease, hypertension, valvular and congenital heart diseases. High output failure results from anaemia, thyrotoxicosis, beriberi and certain congenital heart diseases.

The drugs used in CCF include **diuretics, vasodilators** and **cardiac glycosides**. The pharmacology of cardiac glycosides has been discussed first, followed by the role of other drugs in CCF.

CARDIAC GLYCOSIDES

Cardiac glycosides are obtained from the plants of the foxglove family. William Withering, an English physician first described the clinical effects of digitalis in CCF in 1785.

Source Digitoxin is obtained from the leaves of *Digitalis purpurea*. From the leaves of *Digitalis lanata*, digitoxin and digoxin are derived and the seeds of *Strophanthus gratus* contain ouabain. They are all called cardiac glycosides but digoxin is the most commonly used of them because of its favourable pharmacokinetic properties. The word digitalis is used to mean cardiac glycosides.

Chemistry The glycosides consist of an aglycon attached to sugars. The aglycon has pharmacodynamic activity while sugars influence pharmacokinetic properties.

Pharmacological actions

1. **Cardiac actions** Digoxin is a cardiotonic drug.

Positive ionotropic effect Cardiac glycoside increase the force of contraction of the heart—the stroke volume increases and thereby the cardiac output. The systole is shortened and the diastole is prolonged which allows more rest to the heart. The ventricles are more completely emptied because of more forceful contractions.

The *heart rate* is reduced due to:

a. increased vagal tone
b. decreased sympathetic overactivity due to improved circulation
c. by a direct action on SA and AV nodes.

The effects on *electrophysiological properties* of the heart varies with dose and in different parts of the heart. Digitalis shortens ventricular refractory period, depresses AV conduction and enhances automaticity of the ventricles and the Purkinje cells. Digitalis also produces the characteristic ECG changes.

Blood pressure No significant effects in CCF patients. Pulse pressure may increase.

Coronary circulation improves due to increased cardiac output and prolonged diastole during which the coronaries get filled better.

2. **Extracardiac actions**
   - *Kidney*—Diuresis occurs which relieves oedema in CCF patients.
   - *CNS*—High doses stimulate CTZ resulting in nausea and vomiting.

Mechanism of action Cardiac glycosides inhibit the enzyme Na^+/K^+ ATPase—also called 'sodium pump' present on the cardiac myocytes. This results in an increase in intracellular

Na^+ and Ca^{++}. Thus more calcium is available for contraction, resulting in increased force and velocity of contraction.

Pharmacokinetics Digoxin is well-absorbed (Table 5.1). Presence of food in the stomach delays absorption. Bioavailability varies with different manufacturers and because the safety margin is low, in any given patient, the preparations from the same manufacturer should be used. Glycosides are cumulative drugs.

Adverse effects Cardiac glycosides have a low safety margin and adverse effects are common.

TABLE 5.1: Pharmacokinetic properties of digoxin and digitoxin

Properties	*Digoxin*	*Digitoxin*
Absorption	40-60%	90-100%
Plasma protein binding	25%	95%
Onset of action	15-30 min	30-120 min
t½	24-48 hr	5-7 days
Route of elimination	Renal excretion	Hepatic metabolism
Time for digitalization (without loading dose)	5-7 days	25-30 days
Daily dose (slow loading or maintenance)	0.125-0.5 mg	0.05-0.2 mg
Rapid digitalising dose	0.5-0.75 mg every 8 hours 3 doses	0.2-0.4 mg every 12 hours 3 doses

Extracardiac Anorexia, nausea, vomiting and diarrhoea are the first symptoms to appear. Weakness, confusion, hallucinations, blurred vision and gynaecomastia can occur.

Cardiac toxicity Arrhythmias of any type including extrasystoles, bradycardia, pulses bigeminy and AV block (ventricular tachycardia and fibrillation) can be caused by cardiac glycosides. Hypokalaemia enhances digitalis toxicity.

Treatment of toxicity

- Stop digitalis
- Oral or parenteral K^+ supplements are given
- Ventricular arrhythmias are treated with IV phenytoin
- Bradycardia is treated with atropine and supraventricular arrhythmias with propranolol
- Antidigoxin immunotherapy is now available.

TABLE 5.2: Drug interactions

Drugs that enhance digoxin toxicity
- Diuretics (due to hypokalaemia), calcium
- Quinidine, verapamil, methyldopa—↑digoxin levels

Drugs that reduce digoxin levels
- Antacids, neomycin, metoclopramide—↓ absorption
- Rifampicin, phenobarbitone—hasten metabolism due to enzyme induction

TABLE 5.3: Precautions and contraindications to digitalis therapy

- Hypokalaemia—enhances toxicity
- MI, thyrotoxicosis patients—more prone to arrhythmias
- Acid base imbalance-prone to toxicity

Uses

1. Congestive cardiac failure (see below)
2. Cardiac arrhythmias
   - Atrial fibrillation and atrial flutter—digoxin reduces the ventricular rate
   - Paroxysmal supraventricular tachycardia (PSVT)—digoxin is an alternative to verapamil.

Other Positive-inotropic Drugs

Phosphodiesterase inhibitors *Amrinone (inamrinone) and milrinone* inhibit the enzyme phosphodiesterase (which degrades cAMP) resulting in ↑cAMP levels. They increase force of contraction and also cause vasodilatation. But because of the adverse effects and increased mortality seen with the use of these drugs, they are generally not preferred.

DRUGS USED IN CONGESTIVE CARDIAC FAILURE

In congestive cardiac failure, the heart is unable to provide adequate blood supply to meet the demand. The aim of treatment is to reduce morbidity and mortality by restoring cardiac output and relieving congestion.

The drugs used in CCF include:

1. Diuretics—frusemide
2. Vasodilators—hydralazine, nitrates, ACE inhibitors, sodium nitroprusside, prozosin, calcium channel blockers

3. Positive inotropic agents
   — Digitalis
   — Beta adrenergic agonists
   — Phosphodiesterase (PDE) inhibitors

1. **Diuretics** High ceiling diuretics like frusemide are used. They increase salt and water excretion and reduce blood volume. By this they *reduce preload* and venous pressure, improve cardiac performance and relieve oedema.

2. **Vasodilators** reduce the mortality in patients with cardiac failure. Vasodilators may be arteriolar or venular dilators or both.

- Arteriolar dilators (↓after load)—hydralazine relaxes arterial smooth muscles, thus reducing peripheral vascular resistance (↓afterload). As a result, the work load on the heart is reduced.
- Venodilators (↓preload)—nitrates-reduce the venous return to the heart (↓preload) thus reducing the stretching of the ventricular walls and myocardial oxygen requirements.
- Both arteriolar and venular dilators—ACE inhibitors, sodium nitroprusside, prazosin, calcium channel blockers - these reduce both preload and afterload.

  Organic Nitrates: Nitroglycerine and isosorbide dinitrate are good vasodilators with a rapid and short action. They can be used for short periods to decrease the ventricular filling pressure in acute heart failure. Nitroglycerine can be used IV in acute CCF. Nitrates may be given in combination with hydralazine.

Angiotensin converting enzyme inhibitors (ACE-I)(page 132). ACE-I like Captopril, Enalapril, Lisinopril and Ramipril act by

i. *reduction of afterload* Angiotensin II is a powerful vasoconstrictor present in the plasma in high concentrations in cardiac failure. ACE-inhibitors prevent the conversion of angiotensin I to angiotensin II and thereby reduce the afterload.
ii. *reduction of preload* Aldosterone causes salt and water retention and increases plasma volume. ACE-I prevent the formation of aldosterone (by reducing Ang-II) and thereby reduce the preload.

iii. *reversing compensatory changes* Angiotensin II formed locally in the myocardium is responsible for various undesirable compensatory changes like ventricular hypertrophy and ventricular remodelling seen in CCF. ACE-I reverse these changes.

ACE inhibitors are the most preferred drugs in chronic congestive cardiac failure.

3. Positive inotropic agents

Digitalis Mild to moderate cases of low output failure are treated with diuretics and vasodilators (ACE-inhibitors preferred). When patients are not controlled by these, they may be put on digoxin. Digoxin improves cardiac performance in the dilated, failing heart. If there is associated atrial fibrillation, digoxin is the preferred drug in such patients.

❑ ANTIARRHYTHMIC DRUGS

An arrhythmia is an abnormality of the rate, rhythm or site of origin of the cardiac impulse or an abnormality in the impulse conduction. Cardiac arrhythmias may be due to abnormal generation or conduction of impulses. Factors like hypoxia, electrolyte disturbances, trauma, drugs and autonomic influences can cause arrhythmias (Table 5.4).

CLASSIFICATION

Vaughan Williams classified antiarrhythmics as follows:

Class I. **Sodium channel blockers**

A. Prolong repolarization
   — Quinidine, Procainamide, Disopyramide
B. Shorten repolarization
   — Lignocaine, Mexiletine, Phenytoin
C. Little effect on repolarization
   — Encainide, Flecainide

Class II. **β-adrenergic blockers**
(reduce sympathetic tone)
— Propranolol, Acebutolol, Esmolol, etc.

Class III. **K^+ channel blockers**
(Prolong repolarization)
— Amiodarone, Sotalol, Dofetilide, Ibutilide

Class IV. **Ca^{++} channel blockers**
(Prolong conduction and refractoriness specially in SA and AV nodes).
— Verapamil, Diltiazem

Sodium Channel Blockers

Class I A drugs

Prevent inward sodium movement by blocking Na^+ channels, depress phase-0 depolarization and prolong repolarization.

Quinidine is the D-isomer of quinine obtained from the cinchona bark. By blocking Na^+ channels, it depresses all cardiac properties—automaticity, excitability, conduction velocity and prolongs repolarization: quinidine thus has membrane—stabilizing activity, i.e. it inhibits the propagation of the action potential.

Quinidine also has vagolytic and α-blocking properties. It is also a skeletal muscle relaxant.

Pharmacokinetics Given orally quinidine is rapidly absorbed, 90% bound to plasma proteins, metabolised in the liver and excreted in the urine.

Adverse effects Quinidine is not well-tolerated due to adverse effects and may need to be stopped. Quinidine itself can cause arrhythmias and heart block. Hence treatment should be monitored. Hypotension, nausea, vomiting, diarrhoea, hypersensitivity and idiosyncratic reactions can occur. Higher doses can cause cinchonism like quinine.

Procainamide a derivative of the local anaesthetic procaine has the advantages over quinidine that it has weak anticholinergic properties and is not an α-blocker. It is better tolerated than quinidine.

Disopyramide has significant anticholinergic properties.

Uses Class I A drugs are useful in almost all types of arrhythmias. They are used in atrial fibrillation and atrial flutter and in ventricular arrhythmias. Because of the adverse effects, quinidine is not preferred in arrhythmias but it can be used in malaria in place of quinine.

Class I B Drugs

Class I B drugs block the sodium channels and also shorten repolarization.

Lignocaine suppresses the electrical activity of the arrhythmogenic tissues while the normal tissues are not much affected. It is a local anaesthetic. Given orally lignocaine undergoes high first pass metabolism and has a short t½—hence used parenterally. It may cause drowsiness, hypotension, blurred vision, confusion and convulsions. Lignocaine is used in the treatment of ventricular arrhythmias, especially that caused by acute myocardial infarction or open heart surgery.

Phenytoin is an antiepileptic also useful in ventricular arrhythmias and digitalis induced arrhythmias.

Mexiletine can be used orally; causes dose related neurologic adverse effects including tremors and blurred vision. Nausea is common. It is used as an alternative to lignocaine in ventricular arrhythmias.

Class I C Drugs

Class I C drugs are the most potent sodium channel blockers. Because of the risk of cardiac arrest, sudden death and other adverse effects, they are not commonly used. They may be used in severe ventricular arrhythmias.

Class II Drugs

β-blockers like propranolol exert antiarrhythmic effect due to blockade of cardiac β receptors (in high doses has membrane stabilising activity). They depress myocardial contractility, automaticity and conduction velocity.

Propranolol is used in the treatment of supraventricular arrhythmias especially those associated with exercise, emotion or hyperthyroidism.

TABLE 5.4: Choice of drugs in cardiac arrhythmias

Arrhythmia	*Cause*	*Treatment*
Sinus tachycardia	↑ sympathetic tone, fever, thyrotoxicosis	• Treat the cause • If severe—propranolol
Atrial extrasystoles	Excess caffeine, nicotine, alcohol	• Treat the cause • Reassurance • If severe—propranolol/ disopyramide
Atrial flutter/fibrillation	Rheumatic heart disease, cardiomyopathy, hypertension	• Cardioversion • Proponolol/quinidine/ disopyramide/digitalis
PSVT		• Vagal manouvers like carotid massage • Verapamil/adenosine • β-blockers
Ventricular ectopics	Normal heart—benign; also in cardiomyopathy, ischaemic, digitalis induced	• β-blockers • Lignocaine
Ventricular tachycardia	Organic heart disease and ventricular dysfunction, drug-induced	• Cardioversion • Lignocaine
Ventricular fibrillation	Acute MI, organic heart disease, surgical trauma, drug-induced	• Cardioversion • Lignocaine • Class I A drugs for prevention
Digitalis induced tachyarrhythmias	Digitalis toxicity	• Phenytoin • Potassium • Lignocaine
Sinus bradycardia		• Atropine

Esmolol given intravenously is rapid and short-acting and can be used to treat arrhythmias during surgeries and other emergencies.

Sotalol a β-blocker also prolongs the action potential duration and is often preferred when a β-blocker is needed.

Class III Drugs

These drugs prolong the action potential duration and refractory period by blocking the potassium channels.

Amiodarone is a powerful antiarrhythmic. In addition to prolonging action potential duration, it also blocks β adrenergic receptors and sodium channels.

Amiodarone can cause various adverse effects like heart block, cardiac failure, hypotension, hypothyroidism, pulmonary fibrosis and hepatotoxicity. It is used only in resistant cases of chronic ventricular arrhythmias and to prevent recurrence of atrial fibrillation and flutter.

Bretylium is an adrenergic neurone blocker used in resistant ventricular arrhythmias.

Class IV Drugs

Calcium channel blockers inhibit the inward movement of calcium resulting in reduced contractility, automaticity and AV nodal conduction. Verapamil and diltiazem have prominent cardiac effects.

Verapamil is used to terminate paroxysmal supraventricular tachycardia (PSVT). It is also used to control ventricular rate in atrial flutter or fibrillation.

Miscellaneous

Adenosine is a purine nucleotide having rapid and short antiarrhythmic action. Given IV it suppresses automaticity, AV conduction and dilates the coronaries. Adenosine is the drug of choice for acute termination of paroxysmal supraventricular tachycardias (PSVT).

Adverse effects are nausea, dyspnoea, flushing and headache but are of short duration.

❑ DRUGS USED IN THE TREATMENT OF ANGINA PECTORIS

Angina pectoris is the symptom of ischaemic heart disease (IHD) characterised by sudden, severe, substernal discomfort or pain which may radiate to the left shoulder and along the flexor surface of the left arm. Myocardial oxygen consumption is mainly determined by preload (venous return and stretching of the heart), afterload (peripheral arterial resistance) and heart rate. When the oxygen supply to the myocardium is insufficient for its needs, myocardial ischaemia develops. Pain is due to accumulation of metabolites in the cardiac muscle. Two forms of angina are:

1. *Classical angina (stable angina, angina of effort)* Pain is induced by exercise or emotion, both of which increase myocardial oxygen demand. As there is narrowing of the coronary arteries due to atherosclerosis, they cannot dilate to increase the blood supply during exercise. Hence there is imbalance between oxygen supply and demand.
2. *Variant or Prinzmetal's angina* occurs at rest and is caused by spasm of the coronary artery.

Drugs are used to improve the balance between oxygen supply and demand either by increasing oxygen supply to the myocardium (coronary dilation) or by reducing the oxygen demand (reducing preload/afterload/heart rate or all of these).

ANTIANGINAL DRUGS

1. **Nitrates**—Nitroglycerine, Isosorbide dinitrate, Isosorbide mononitrate, Penta erythritol tetranitrate.
2. **Calcium channel blockers**—Verapamil, Diltiazem, Amlodipine.
3. **β-blockers**—Propranolol, Atenolol, etc.
4. **Potassium channel openers** —Nicorandil
5. **Miscellaneous**—Aspirin

Nitrates

Nitrates are vasodilators (mainly venodilators). They are converted to nitric oxide which leads to relaxation of the vascular smooth muscles. Venodilation reduces venous return to the heart thereby reducing preload. Arteriolar dilation reduces vascular resistance thus decreasing afterload. As both preload and afterload are reduced, work load of the heart is decreased thereby reducing oxygen requirement of the heart.

In variant angina, nitrates relieve vasospasm due to coronary vasodilation.

Nitrates also cause dilation of blood vessels in the skin—resulting in flushing; dilatation of the meningeal vessels result in headache.

Bronchial smooth muscles are also relaxed.

Adverse effects Headache is common; flushing, sweating, palpitation, weakness, postural hypotension and rashes can occur. Tolerance to vascular effects develops on repeated long term use.

Uses

1. *Angina* Sublingual nitroglycerine is the drug of choice for acute anginal attacks. It relieves pain in 3 minutes. If the pain is not relieved, the dose may be repeated (up to 3 tablets in 15 minutes).

   Orally nitrates are also used for the prophylaxis of angina. Nitroglycerine ointment may be applied over the chest.
2. *Cardiac failure* Nitrates are useful due to their vasodilator property.
3. *Myocardial infarction* IV nitroglycerine is used by many physicians.

TABLE 5.5: Some nitrates used in angina pectoris

Drug	*Dose and route*	*Duration of action*
Nitroglycerine (GTN) (ANGISED)	0.5 mg SL	15-40 min
	5 mg oral	4-8 hr
	2% Skin ointment applied 1-2 inches on the precardial region	4-6 hr
Isosorbide dinitrate (SORBITRATE)	5-10 mg SL	20-40 min
	10-20 mg oral	2-3 hr
Isosorbide mononitrate (ISMO)	10-20 mg oral	6-8 hr

4. *Cyanide poisoning* Nitrates convert haemoglobin to methemoglobin which binds to cyanide, forming cyanmethaemoglobin. It thus protects the important enzymes from binding to cyanide. Amyl nitrite is preferred. Early treatment is very important.

Calcium Channel Blockers

The depolarisation of cardiac and vascular smooth muscle cells depend on the entry of extracellular calcium into the cell through calcium channels. This calcium triggers the release of intracellular calcium from the sarcoplasmic reticulum. All these calcium ions cause contraction. Calcium channel blockers (CCB) inhibit the entry of Ca^{++} by blocking the Ca^{++} channels. This results in the following actions:

1. *Smooth muscle relaxation* Arteriolar dilatation reducing peripheral vascular resistance, leading to a fall in BP. Reflex tachycardia may occur with some.
2. *Heart* CCBs depress myocardial contractility, reduce heart rate, cardiac work and myocardial O_2 consumption.
3. *Coronary circulation* Coronary vasodilation occurs, increasing coronary blood flow. Hence CCBs are useful in variant angina.

   CCBs include:

   Dihydropyridines

   Nifedipine, Nimodipine, Nicardipine, Amlodipine, Felodipine, Isradipine, Nitrendipine, Nisoldipine

   Others

   Verapamil, Diltiazem

Verapamil has prominent myocardiac depressant actions. AV conduction is depressed and usually bradycardia is seen. Hence it should not be combined with β-blockers. Fall in BP is mild as the vasodilator effect of verapamil is less potent.

Adverse effects include constipation, bradycardia, heart block and hypotension. It may precipitate CCF in patients with diseased heart.

Nifedipine a dihydropyridine, is a potent vasodilator and causes a significant fall in BP and evokes reflex tachycardia.

Myocardiac depressant effect is weak. It can be given sublingually.

Adverse effects are headache, flushing, palpitation, dizziness, fatigue, hypotension, leg cramps and ankle oedema.

Other CCBs like amlodipine, felodipine, nitrendipine and nicardipine are similar to nifedipine with some pharmacokinetic variations. They have higher vascular selectivity. Nimodipine selectively relaxes cerebral vasculature. Diltiazem has less potent vasodilator effects but is a myocardiac depressant.

Pharmacokinetics CCBs are well-absorbed but undergo extensive first pass metabolism. They are all highly plasma protein bound and are metabolized in the liver.

Uses of CCBs

1. *Angina Pectoris* CCBs are used in both types of angina. Nifedipine can be combined with β-blockers like propranolol.
2. *Hypertension* Verapamil, nifedipine, amlodipine and diltiazem can be used. Nifedipine is used sublingually in hypertensive crisis.
3. *Arrhythmias* Verapamil is the drug of choice in PSVT.
4. *Peripheral vascular disease* Nifedipine is useful in Raynaud's disease due to its vasodilator effects.

β-blockers

β-blockers reduce the frequency and severity of attacks of exertional angina and are useful in the prevention of angina. Exercise, emotion and similar situations increase sympathetic activity leading to increased heart-rate, force of contraction and BP, thereby increasing O_2 consumption by the heart. β-blockers prevent angina by blocking all these actions. They are used for the long-term prophylaxis of classical angina and may be combined with nitrates. β-blockers should always be tapered after prolonged use. They are *not* useful in variant angina.

Potassium Channel Openers

Nicorandil is an arterial and venous dilator. Opening of the K^+ channels results in hyperpolarization and therefore relaxation of the vascular smooth muscles. Adverse effects are headache, flushing, dizziness and hypotension.

Miscellaneous

Aspirin Low dose aspirin is given for a long period for its antiplatelet aggregatory property. It has been shown to prevent myocardial infarction in patients with angina.

Pharmacotherapy of Angina

Acute attack Sublingual nitroglycerine is the drug of choice. If the pain does not subside in 5 minutes, repeat the dose. After the relief of pain, the tablet should be discarded.

Acute prophylaxis Sublingual nitroglycerine given 15 minutes before an exertion (e.g. walking uphill) can prevent the attack. The prophylactic effect lasts for 30 minutes.

Chronic prophylaxis Long-acting nitrates or β-blockers (preferred) or calcium channel blockers can be used. All are given orally.

If one drug is not effective, a combination of drugs may be used.

Combinations of Drugs in Angina

1. Nitrates + β-blockers—very effective in exertional angina. Reflex tachycardia due to nitrates is countered by β-blockers. Ventricular dilatation due to β-blockers is opposed by nitrates.
2. Nifedipine + β-blockers. The antianginal effects are additive. Reflex tachycardia due to nifedipine is countered by β-blockers.
3. Nitrates + CCBs—nitrates decrease preload, CCBs reduce afterload and the combination reduces cardiac work load.
4. CCBs + β-blockers + Nitrates—if the angina is not controlled by 2 drug combinations, 3 drugs can be used. Nitrates reduce preload, CCBs reduce afterload while β-blockers decrease heart rate. This combination is useful in severe angina.

Unstable angina includes:

— patients with exertional angina developing angina at rest

— severe, prolonged anginal attacks without ECG evidence of MI

— angina developing after myocardial infarction.

Such patients with unstable angina are at a high risk of developing MI or sudden death and need hospitalisation and rigorous treatment for its prevention.

Drugs used in unstable angina Aspirin, heparin and IV nitroglycerine may be used in unstable angina. Long-term administration of β-blockers like atenolol or CCB like verapamil is beneficial.

Drugs used in myocardial infarction Rupture of an atheromatus plaque in the coronary artery results in the formation of a thrombus which blocks the artery leading to acute myocardial infarction.

Drugs used are IV opioid analgesics like morphine/pethidine to relieve pain and anxiety, thrombolytics like streptokinase to dissolve the thrombus and aspirin for its antiplatelet aggregatory effect.

Atenolol, ACE inhibitors and O_2 inhalation also help.

❑ ANTIHYPERTENSIVE DRUGS

Hypertension is an elevation of systolic and/or diastolic BP above 140/90 mm of Hg. It is a common cardiovascular condition. Hypertension may be *primary* (essential) hypertension—where the cause is not known or *secondary*—when it is secondary to other conditions like renal, endocrine or vascular disorders.

Based on the degree of severity, hypertension can be graded as:

- Mild—diastole up to 104
- Moderate—105-114
- Severe— more than 115.

Blood pressure is determined by cardiac output (CO) and total peripheral vascular resistance (PVR). Blood pressure is controlled by baroreceptor reflexes acting through autonomic nervous system along with the renin-angiotensin-aldosterone system.

Prolonged hypertension damages the blood vessels of the heart, brain and the kidneys and may result in several complications like stroke, coronary artery disease or renal failure. Hence hypertension needs to be treated.

Antihypertensives act by influencing the BP regulatory systems *viz* the autonomic system, renin-angiotensin system, calcium channels or sodium and water balance (plasma volume).

CLASSIFICATION

1. **Diuretics**
   - *Thiazides* Hydrochlorothiazide, Chlorthalidone, etc.
   - *Loop diuretics* Frusemide
   - *K^+ Sparing diuretics* Spironolactone, Amiloride, Triamterene.
2. **Sympatholytics**
   - *Centrally acting drugs* Clonidine, Methyldopa
   - *Ganglion blockers* Trimethaphan
   - *Adrenergic neuron blockers* Guanithidine, Reserpine
   - *Adrenergic receptor blockers:*
     — β-blockers Propranolol, Atenolol, etc.
     — α-blockers Prazosin
   - *Mixed α and β blockers* Labetalol.
3. **Vasodilators**
   - *Arteriolar dilators* Hydralazine, Minoxidil, Diazoxide
   - *Arteriolar and venular dilators* Sodium nitroprusside
4. **Ca^{++} channel blockers** Verapamil, Nifedipine, etc.
5. **Angiotensin converting enzyme inhibitors** Captopril, Enalapril, Lisinopril, Ramipril.
6. **Angiotensin II receptor antagonist** Losartan, candesartam, valsartan.

Diuretics (see Chapter 3) The antihypertensive effect of diuretics is mild—BP falls by 15-20 mm Hg over 2-4 weeks. Diuretics act as antihypertensives as follows.

Diuretics enhance the excretion of sodium and water resulting in

1. ↓ Plasma volume → ↓ cardiac output → ↓ BP
2. ↓ Body sodium → relaxation of vascular smooth muscles (due to Na^+ depletion) → ↓ PVR → ↓ BP.

Restriction of dietary salt intake will reduce the dose of the diuretic needed. Thiazides are the first-line antihypertensives.

They may be combined with a K^+ sparing diuretic to avoid hypokalaemia. Thiazides may be used in combination with other antihypertensives. Loop diuretics are used only in hypertension with chronic renal failure or congestive heart failure.

SYMPATHOLYTICS

I. Drugs Acting Centrally

Clonidine Clonidine is a selective α_2 agonist. Stimulation of α_2 receptors in the CNS (in the vasomotor centre and hypothalamus), decreases central sympathetic outflow, blocks the release of noradrenaline from the nerve terminals leading to a fall in BP and bradycardia.

Adverse effects include drowsiness, dryness of mouth, nose and eyes; parotid gland swelling and pain, fluid retention, constipation and impotence. Sudden withdrawal of clonidine will lead to rebound hypertension, headache, tremors, sweating and tachycardia. Hence the dose should be tapered.

Uses Mild to moderate hypertension.

Other uses

1. In *Opioid withdrawal* Most withdrawal symptoms in opioid addicts are due to sympathetic overactivity and can be benefited by treatment with clonidine.
2. *Diabetic neuropathy* Clonidine controls diarrhoea by improving absorption of NaCl and water in the gut by stimulation of α_2 receptors in the intestines.
3. *With anaesthetics* Clonidine given preoperatively reduces the dose of the general anaesthetic needed due to its analgesic effects.

α-methyl dopa—an analog of dopa, is a prodrug. It is metabolised in the body to α-methyl norepinephrine which is an α_2 agonist and acts like clonidine. Renin levels also fall. Left ventricular hypertrophy is reversed in about 12 weeks of treatment.

Adverse effects are sedation, dryness of mouth and nose, headache, postural hypotension, fluid retention and impotence.

Uses It is used in mild to moderate hypertension along with a diuretic.

Ganglion Blockers-*Trimethaphan*

These drugs block both sympathetic and parasympathetic ganglia resulting in decreased sympathetic tone and a fall in BP. But they produce several side effects as they block both ganglia and are not used now. Trimethaphan is the only ganglion blocker used intravenously to produce controlled hypotension during certain surgeries for its rapid and short action (15 minutes).

Adrenergic Neuron Blockers

Guanethidine depletes the stores of noradrenaline in the adrenergic neurons and also blocks its release. Because of the adverse effects like postural hypotension, diarrhoea and sexual dysfunction, it is not used.

Reserpine is an alkaloid obtained from *Rauwolfia serpentina* (Sarpagandhi) that grows in India. In the neurons, it binds to the vesicles that store monoamines like noradrenaline, dopamine and 5-HT and destroys these vesicles. It thus depletes the stores of these monoamines. Reserpine also causes various side effects like drowsiness, depression, parkinsonism, postural hypotension, oedema and sexual dysfunction. Hence it is generally not preferred.

Adrenergic Receptor Blockers

β-blockers (see Chapter 2) are mild antihypertensives. They reduce the BP due to a fall in the cardiac output. They also lower plasma renin activity and have an additional central antihypertensive action. They are well-tolerated and are of special value in patients who also have arrhythmias or angina. They are also suitable for combination with other antihypertensives. They are thus the first line antihypertensive drugs in mild to moderate hypertension. Atenolol is the preferred β-blocker because of the advantages like once a day dosing, absence of CNS side effects and β_1 selectivity. β-blockers should always be tapered while withdrawing.

α-blockers (see Chapter 2) Prazosin is a selective α_1-blocker; it dilates both arterioles and venules. Peripheral vascular resistance is decreased leading to a fall in BP with only mild tachycardia.

'First dose phenomenon' can be avoided by starting with a low dose (0.5 mg) given at bed time. Dose is gradually increased. Prazosin is used in mild to moderate hypertension; it may be combined with diuretics and β-blockers.

α and β-blockers Labetalol blocks α_1 and β receptors. It is used IV in the treatment of hypertension in pheochromocytoma and in hypertensive emergencies.

Vasodilators

Vasodilators relax the vascular smooth muscles thus reducing BP due to decreased peripheral vascular resistance. Salt and water retention and reflex tachycardia are common with vasodilators.

Hydralazine is a directly acting arteriolar dilator. The fall in BP is associated with tachycardia, renin release and fluid retention. Coronary, cerebral and renal blood flow are increased.

Adverse effects are headache, flushing, palpitation, salt and water retention. It may precipitate angina in some patients. Hypersensitivity reactions like serum sickness and lupus erythematosus may occur.

Uses Hydralazine is used with a β-blocker and/or a diuretic in moderate to severe hypertension not controlled by the first line drugs. It can be given in hypertension in pregnancy.

Minoxidil is a directly acting arteriolar dilator used in severe hypertension not responding to other drugs. It acts by opening K^+ channels in smooth muscles.

Minoxidil stimulates the growth of hair on prolonged use. Hence it is used topically (2% solution) in *alopecia*. Young men with relative alopecia are more likely to respond.

Diazoxide is related to thiazide diuretics and is a potent arteriolar dilator. It's mechanism of action is like minoxidil. It is used in hypertensive emergencies where monitoring of infusion is not possible. Diazoxide has a long duration of action (24 hours) and is suitable in such situations.

Sodium nitroprusside is a rapidly acting vasodilator and it relaxes both arterioles and venules. Both peripheral resistance and cardiac output are reduced resulting in lower myocardial oxygen consumption. Nitroprusside acts through the release of nitric oxide which relaxes the vascular smooth muscles. On IV administration, it is rapid (acts within 30 seconds) and short-acting (duration 3 minutes) allowing titration of the dose. This makes it suitable for use in hypertensive emergencies with close monitoring. It decomposes on exposure to light; the infusion bottle and tubing should be covered with opaque foil.

Adverse reactions are palpitation, sweating, weakness, nausea, vomiting and in high doses thiocyanate toxicity including psychosis.

Uses

1. Nitroprusside is the drug of choice in hypertensive emergencies.
2. It is used in situations where short-term reduction of myocardial work load is required as in myocardial infarction.

Calcium Channel Blockers

Calcium channel blockers (CCBs) (see page 123) are another important group of antihypertensives. They dilate the arterioles resulting in reduced peripheral vascular resistance. Nifedipine produces some reflex tachycardia while this is not seen with verapamil and diltiazem as they are cardiac depressants. Fluid retention is negligible unlike other arteriolar dilators.

- CCBs are well-tolerated, and effective.
- Sublingual nifedipine used in hypertensive emergencies effectively lowers BP in 10 minutes.
- CCBs are of special value in patients who also have angina.
- Sustained release preparations or long acting CCBs may be used for smoother control of BP.
- CCBs may be used in combination with other antihypertensives in moderate to severe hypertension.

Angiotensin Converting Enzyme (ACE) Inhibitors

Angiotensin II is a powerful vasoconstrictor. Aldosterone also raises the BP by increasing the plasma volume (Fig 5.2). ACE inhibitors prevent the formation of angiotensin II and (indirectly) aldosterone. There is vasodilation and decrease in PVR resulting in ↓ BP. As ACE also degrades bradykinin, ACE inhibitors raise the bradykinin levels which is a potent vasodilator. This also contributes to the fall in BP.

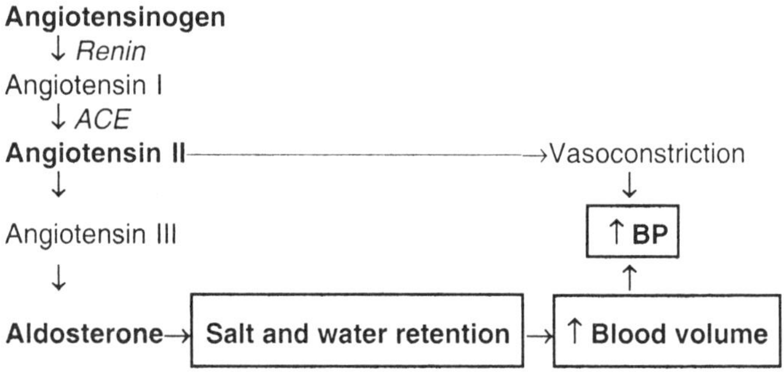

Fig 5.2: Renin-angiotensin system

The blood flow to the kidneys, brain and heart increases due to selective vasodilation and thus maintains adequate blood supply to these vital organs.

Pharmacokinetics ACE inhibitors are generally well-absorbed. Except captopril and lisinopril all others are prodrugs. Duration of action varies (Table 5.6).

TABLE 5.6: Dose and duration of action of some commonly used ACE inhibitors

Drug	*Duration of action (in hrs)*	*Daily dose in hypertension (mg)*
Captopril	6-12	12.5-50 mg BD
Enalapril	24	2.5-20 mg OD
Lisinopril	>24	5-40 mg OD
Ramipril	8-48	1.25-10 mg OD

Adverse effects ACE inhibitors are well-tolerated. Adverse effects include persistent dry cough (due to ↑ bradykinin levels), hyperkalaemia, alteration of taste sensation, skin rashes, hypotension, headache, nausea, abdominal pain and blood disorders. Angiooedema though rare can be severe. At the first sign of angiooedema ACE inhibitors should be stopped.

Uses

1. *Hypertension* ACE inhibitors are useful in the treatment of hypertension of all grades due to all causes. Addition of a diuretic potentiates their efficacy. They are presently the first line antihypertensives. They are specially indicated as antihypertensives in:
   a. patients with diabetes as ACE-I slow the development of nephropathy.
   b. renal diseases—ACE inhibitors slow the progression.
   c. left ventricular hypertrophy—is gradually reversed by ACE inhibitors.
2. *CCF* ACE inhibitors are the first line drugs (see page 115).
3. *Myocardial infarction* ACE inhibitors started within 24 hours and given for several weeks prevent the development of CCF and reduce mortality.

Angiotensin II Receptor Antagonists

Losartan is an angiotensin II receptor antagonist. AT_1 receptors present in vascular and myocardial tissue, brain, kidney and adrenal glomerular cells are blocked by losartan. Losartan relaxes vascular smooth muscles, promotes salt and water excretion and reduces plasma volume. The advantage of AT II antagonists over ACE inhibitors is that there is **no** increase in bradykinin levels and its associated adverse effects like dry cough and angiooedema.

Adverse effects include hypotension and hyperkalaemia. It is contraindicated in pregnancy and lactation.

Uses Losartan (50 mg OD) is used in the treatment of hypertension in similar indications as that of ACE inhibitors. Others like candesertan and valsartan can also be used.

Drug interactions of antihypertensives

1. Sympathomimetics and tricyclic antidepressants can antagonise the effects of sympatholytics.
2. Antihistamines add to sedation produced by clonidine and methyldopa.
3. NSAIDs tend to cause salt and water retention and may blunt the effect of antihypertensives.

TABLE 5.7: Dose and route of administration of some commonly used antihypertensives

Antihypertensives	*Daily doses*	*Routes*
Hydrochlorothiazide + Amiloride	12.5-25 mg + 1.25-2.5 mg daily	Oral
Clonidine	100-300 μg	Oral
Methyldopa	250-500 mg q 6-12 hr	Oral
Atenolol	25-100 mg OD	Oral
Prazosin	2-20 mg daily	Oral
Hydralazine	25-50 mg q 8-24 hr	Oral
Diazoxide	50-100 mg every 5-10 min	IV
Sodium nitroprusside	0.2-0.3 mg/min	IV
Nifedipine	10 mg	SL
	5-20 mg q 8-12 hr	Oral
Losartan	50 mg OD	Oral

For ACE inhibitors see Table 5.6

Treatment of Hypertension

Mild hypertension Treatment is started with low dose of a single drug—a thiazide diuretic or a β-blocker. If the patient does not adequately respond in 3-4 weeks, an ACE inhibitor or a calcium channel blocker should be tried. If BP is not controlled by one drug, another should be added.

Moderate hypertension A combination of a diuretic with a sympatholytic may be given. If response is inadequate add a third drug.

Severe hypertension may be associated with cardiac or renal disorder. A vasodilator with a diuretic and a β-blocker is useful.

Hypertensive emergencies Conditions like hypertensive encephalopathy and acute cardiac failure due to hypertension require immediate reduction of BP. Parenteral drugs are preferred. IV sodium nitroprusside under close monitoring is the drug of choice (in some conditions BP should be lowered gradually to avoid ischaemia to vital organs). IV esmolol, diazoxide and sublingual nifedipine are alternatives. As soon as possible switch over to oral drugs.

Hypertension in pregnancy The drugs found safe are—methyldopa orally for maintenance and hydralazine (parenteral) for reduction of BP in emergency. However they should be used only after the first trimester. Cardio-selective β-blockers (atenolol) can also be used.

Combination of antihypertensives When it is not possible to achieve adequate control of BP with a single drug, a combination may be used. Antihypertensives may also be combined to overcome the side effects of one another. This also allows use of lower doses of each drug.

Sympatholytics and vasodilators cause fluid retention which can be overcome by adding a diuretic.

Vasodilators like nifedipine and hydralazine evoke reflex tachycardia. This can be countered by β-blockers, while propranolol may cause initial rise in PVR which is countered by vasodilators.

Combination of ACE inhibitors and diuretics is synergistic.

Non-pharmacological measures Low salt diet, weight reduction, transidental meditation, all go a long way in controlling the blood pressure. Smoking and alcohol should be given up. These measures also help in reducing the dose of the antihypertensive needed.

❑ PHARMACOTHERAPY OF SHOCK

Shock is acute circulatory failure with underperfusion of tissues. Symptoms of sympathetic overactivity of tissues are generally seen—like pallor, sweating, cold extremities and tachycardia. Shock may be:

1. *Hypovolaemic shock* Decreased fluid volume due to sudden loss of plasma or blood as in haemorrhage, burns or dehydration—results in hypovolaemic shock.
2. *Septic shock* is precipitated by severe bacterial infection. It may be due to release of bacterial toxins.
3. *Cardiogenic shock* is due to failure of heart as a pump as in myocardial infarction.
4. *Anaphylactic shock* Type I hypersensitivity reaction causing release of massive amounts of histamine which is triggered by antigen-antibody reaction (page 48).
5. *Neurogenic shock* is due to venous pooling as following spinal anaesthesia, abdominal or testicular trauma.

Shock of any type needs immediate treatment:

a. The cause should be identified and treated
b. Maintain BP and plasma volume
c. Correct the acid base and electrolyte disturbances
d. Ensure adequate urine output.

In shock due to myocardial infarction, IV morphine is the drug of choice to relieve pain and anxiety. Thrombolytic therapy (see Chapter 8) and oxygen inhalation should be started immediately. Absolute bed rest, prevention of arrhythmias and maintenance of cardiac output are all important.

Septic shock should be treated with appropriate antibiotics.

❑ PLASMA EXPANDERS

To restore the intravascular volume, the component lost should ideally be replaced like—plasma in burns and blood after haemorrhage. But in emergency, immediate volume replacement is important. In such situations plasma expanders are used. These are high molecular weight substances which when infused IV exert oncotic pressure and remain in the body for a long time to increase the volume of circulating fluid.

An ideal plasma expander should exert oncotic pressure comparable to plasma, be long-acting, non-antigenic and pharmacologically inert.

The plasma expanders used are dextran, gelatin polymer, hydroxyethyl starches and polyvinyl pyrrolidone.

Dextrans (Dextran 70 mol. wt. 70,000 and dextran 40 mol. wt. 40,000) are commonly used. Allergic reactions are common.

Gelatin products have a mol. wt. of 30,000 and a duration of action of 12 hours. Allergic reactions are rare.

Hydroxyethyl starch (Hetastarch) maintains blood volume for a long period and allergic reactions are rare.

Polyvinyl pyrrolidone (PVP) is a synthetic polymer. It is not preferred due to various disadvantages like—it provokes histamine release and interferes with blood grouping.

Uses of plasma expanders These are used as plasma substitutes in hypovolaemic shock, burns and extensive fluid loss—as an emergency measure to restore plasma volume.

VASOACTIVE DRUGS

Drugs that affect the vascular smooth muscles are vasoactive drugs. They are vasoconstrictors and vasodilators. Some prostaglandins, angiotensin and antidiuretic hormone are natural vasoconstrictors released in the body (endogenous). They are released in hypotension and hypovolemia. Drugs that cause vasoconstriction are listed below. Vasodilators include natural vasodilators released in the body like some prostaglandins, acetylcholine, nitric oxide and drugs like nitrates and others (see below).

Vasoconstrictors

Endogenous Noradrenaline, PGs (TXA_2)
Antiotensin, ADH, 5-HT

Drugs

α-agonists—adrenaline, ephedrine, phenylephrine, mephenteramine, metaraminol methoxamine

5HT agonist—sumatriptan, ergot alkaloids

Vasodilators

Endogenous—PGs, acetylcholine, nitric oxide

Drugs

ACE inhibitors—captopril, enalapril, ramipril

Angiotensin II receptor antagonists—losartan, candesartan

Ca^{++} channel blockers—nifedipine, nimodipine

α blockers—prozosin, phentolamine, phenoxybenzamine

Nitrates—nitroglycerine, sodium nitroprusside

K^{+} channel openers—minoxidil, cromakalim, nicorandil

Others—hydralazine, theophylline

Vasoconstrictors: In general vasoconstrictors bring about a rise in blood pressure with bradycardia. α_1 agonists are used in hypotension and topically as nasal decongestants.

Vasodilators: In general the effects of vasodilators include hypotension and reduced cardiac workload. However, they may cause reflex tachycardia. Adverse effects to vasodilators generally include palpitation, flushing, dizziness, headache, hypotension, and edema.

Vasodilators are used in the treatment of hypertension, angina pectoris, cardiac failure, myocardial infarction and peripheral vascular diseases.

6

Central Nervous System

- General anaesthetics
- Local anaesthetics
- Sedative hypnotics
- Alcohols
- Antiepileptics
- Drugs used in Parkinsonism
- Opioid analgesics and antagonists
- Nonsteroidal anti-inflammatory drugs (NSAIDs)
- Drugs used in rheumatoid arthritis and gout
- Drugs used in psychiatric disorders—Antipsychotics, Antidepressants and Antianxiety agents
- Antidepressants
- CNS stimulants

GENERAL ANAESTHETICS

General anaesthetics are agents that bring about reversible loss of sensation and consciousness. Before 1846, alcohol, opium, packing a limb with ice and concussion, i.e. making the patient unconscious by a blow on the head were used to relieve surgical pain. Dr Horace Wells a dentist, tried to demonstrate the effect of nitrous oxide as an anesthetic in 1844 but was unsuccessful as he removed the gas bag too early. Dr William Morton who was present at the demonstration, worked on it and in 1846 demonstrated ether anaesthesia successfully. Since then several anaesthetics have been synthesized over the decades.

Ideal anaesthetic should be pleasant, non-irritating, provide adequate analgesia, immobility and muscle relaxation; should be non-inflammable and administration should be easy and controllable and have a wide margin of safety. Induction and recovery should be smooth and should not affect cardiovascular functions. It should be inexpensive.

CLASSIFICATION

I. Inhalational

A. *Gases* – Nitrous oxide, Cyclopropane

B. *Liquids* – Ether, Halothane, Enflurane, Isoflurane, Methoxyflurane

II. Intravenous

A. *Inducing agents* – Thiopentone sodium, Methohexitone, Propofol, Etomidate

B. *Dissociative anaesthesia* – Ketamine

C. *Neuroleptanalgesia* – Fentanyl + Droperidol

D. *Benzodiazepines* – Diazepam, Lorazepam, Midazolam

INHALATIONAL ANAESTHETICS

Nitrous oxide is a gas with a slightly sweetish odour. It produces light anaesthesia without significant depression of respiration or vasomotor centre.

Advantages

1. Strong analgesic
2. Induction is rapid and smooth
3. It is non-irritating and non-inflammable
4. Recovery is rapid
5. Postoperative nausea is not significant
6. Has little effect on respiration and cardiovascular functions, hence ideal for combination
7. It is non-toxic to liver, kidney and brain and is quickly removed from lungs.

Disadvantages

1. It is less potent and should be used with other agents.
2. Poor muscle relaxant.

Status in anaesthesia Nitrous oxide is used as an adjuvant to other anaesthetics. It is used along with oxygen (30%).

Ether is a colourless volatile liquid. It is highly inflammable; vapours are irritating.

Advantages

1. Potent and reliable anaesthetic.
2. Good analgesic.
3. Effect on cardiovascular and respiratory functions are not significant; reflexes are well-maintained.
4. It is a bronchodilator.
5. Provides full muscle relaxation in deep anaesthesia.
6. Does not sensitize the heart to adrenaline.
7. Easy to administer as complicated equipment is not necessary.
8. Inexpensive.

Disadvantages

1. It is inflammable—hence diathermy is contraindicated.
2. Induction is slow and unpleasant.
3. It is irritating and therefore enhances respiratory secretions.
4. Postoperative nausea and vomiting are frequent.
5. Recovery is slow.

Status in anaesthesia Ether is now not preferred because of flammability and irritant property. But it is still used in developing countries like India because it is cheap, easy to administer (by open drop method) and relatively safe.

Halothane is a colourless volatile liquid with a sweet odour. It is non-irritant and non-inflammable.

Advantages

1. Potent, non-inflammable anaesthetic.
2. Induction is smooth and rapid—in 2-5 minutes anaesthesia can be produced
3. Non-irritant—therefore does not increase salivary or bronchial secretions.
4. Recovery is rapid.
5. Postoperative nausea and vomiting is of low incidence.

Disadvantages

1. Not a good analgesic; not a muscle relaxant.
2. Halothane is a direct cardiac depressant. Cardiac output and BP start falling and heart rate may decrease. It sensitizes the heart to the action of adrenaline.
3. It also causes some respiratory depression.
4. Severe hepatitis which may be fatal occurs rarely.
5. Malignant hyperthermia—a genetically determined reaction occurs rarely. Succinylcholine accentuates this effect of halothane. It is due to intracellular release of calcium which causes muscle contraction and increased heat production. It is treated with dantrolene.
6. Expensive.

Status in anaesthesia Halothane is one of the most popular anaesthetics. Analgesics and muscle relaxants are used along with it. Non-flammability, non-irritant property, rapid induction and recovery has made halothane an important and preferred anaesthetic—most widely used.

Enflurane and **isoflurane** are similar to halothane except that:

1. they are safer regarding the liver toxicity.
2. they do not sensitize the heart to adrenaline.

Isoflurane is extensively used in European countries. It is expensive.

Desflurane and sevoflurane are newer agents which allow very rapid induction and recovery. But they too have some disadvantages. Desflurane is pungent—may induce coughing and sometimes laryngospasm. A special vapourizer is required for its administration. Sevoflurane is chemically unstable. A metabolite of sevoflurane may cause renal damage. If these disadvantages of sevoflurane could be overcome, we may have found an ideal anaesthetic.

Oxygen in anaesthesia Oxygen should be added routinely to inhalational agents to protect against hypoxia (especially when halothane is used). When O_2 is not available, ether is the safest agent for maintenance of anaesthesia.

INTRAVENOUS ANAESTHETICS

Intravenous anaesthetics allow an extremely rapid induction because the blood concentration can be raised rapidly—in one arm-brain circulation (~ 11 sec) there is loss of consciousness. These are used for induction because of the rapid onset of action and anaesthesia is maintained by an inhalational agent.

INDUCING AGENTS

Thiopentone sodium is an ultrashort-acting barbiturate which when administered IV, rapidly induces anaesthesia without analgesia.

On IV injection it produces unconsciousness in 20-30 sec. It is highly lipid soluble; duration of action is 4-7 minutes. It gets rapidly redistributed in the body tissues.

Advantages Quick onset of action; induction is smooth, rapid and pleasant.

Disadvantages Not a good analgesic nor muscle relaxant. Thiopentone sodium cannot be used alone as the dose required results in, respiratory and circulatory depression.

Uses For induction of anaesthesia prior to administration of inhalational anaesthetics.

Precautions Equipment for resuscitation should be kept ready.

Adverse effects include respiratory depression, hypotension and hiccoughs.

Methohexitone is similar to thiopentone but is more potent.

Propofol is an oily liquid; quick induction (30 sec) and recovery (4 min) is possible from a single dose. It is used for induction and maintenance for short procedures of up to 1 hour duration.

DISSOCIATIVE ANAESTHESIA

Ketamine is a phencyclidine derivative. In anaesthetic doses it produces a trans-like state known as *dissociative anaesthesia* characterised by intense analgesia, immobility, amnesia (loss of memory) and a feeling of dissociation from ones own body and surroundings. Ketamine hydrochloride given 1-2 mg/kg slow IV or 10 mg/kg IM produces dissociative anaesthesia within 3-5 min which lasts for 10-15 min after a single injection. Amnesia lasts for 1-2 hr. Premedication with atropine is needed. Return to consciousness is gradual. Delirium may be accompanied. If diazepam is administered pre and postoperatively, delirium can be avoided. Heart rate, CO and BP are increased due to sympathetic stimulation.

Advantages

- Provides profound analgesia and can be used as a single agent for minor procedures
- Respiration is not depressed, does not induce hypotension
- Less likely to induce vomiting
- Pharyngeal and laryngeal reflexes are only slightly affected
- It is particularly useful in children and poor-risk patients and also in asthmatic patients since it does not induce bronchospasm.

Disadvantages

- Hallucinations and involuntary movements may occur during recovery
- May be dangerous in hypertensives as it raises the BP.

Contraindications Hypertension, CCF, cerebral haemorrhage, increased intracranial tension, psychiatric disorders and pregnancy before term.

NEUROLEPTANALGESIA

A combination of fentanyl and droperidol is used.

Fentanyl is a short-acting (30-50 min) and potent opioid analgesic (page 184).

Droperidol is a rapidly acting, potent neuroleptic related to haloperidol.

When the combination is given IV, a state of 'neuroleptanalgesia' is produced. This is characterised by calmness, psychic indifference and intense analgesia without loss of consciousness. It lasts for 30-40 min. Fentanyl 0.05 mg + droperidol 2.5 mg/ml—4 to 6 ml is infused IV over 10 min. Patient is drowsy but cooperative. Respiratory depression is present. There is a slight fall in BP and HR. During recovery extrapyramidal symptoms may be seen—due to droperidol. It is employed for endoscopies, burn dressing, angiographies and other diagnostic and minor surgical procedures.

Neuroleptanaesthesia Addition of 65% N_2O + 35% O_2 to the above combination produces neuroleptanaesthesia.

BENZODIAZEPINES

Benzodiazepines like diazepam, lorazepam and midazolam are used to induce or supplement anaesthesia. They cause sedation, amnesia and reduce anxiety which are beneficial in such patients. BZD may be employed alone in procedures like endoscopies, reduction of fractures, cardiac catheterisation and cardioversion. IV midazolam is particularly preferred as it is faster and shorter-acting, more potent and does not cause pain or irritation at the injection sites. BZDs are also used as preanaesthetic medication.

PREANAESTHETIC MEDICATION

Prior to anaesthesia, certain drugs are administered in order to make anaesthesia safer and more pleasant and is known as preanaesthetic medication. It is given in order to:

1. decrease anxiety
2. provide amnesia for the preoperative period
3. relieve preoperative pain if present
4. make anaesthesia safer
5. reduce side effects of anaesthetics
6. reduce gastric acidity.

To achieve the above purpose, more than one drug is required. An informative, supportive, preoperative visit by the anaesthesiologist is very much essential.

Sedative hypnotics Antianxiety agents like benzodiazepines are used extensively as preanaesthetic medication. They reduce anxiety and produce sedation. Diazepam 5-10 mg is given orally. It also produces amnesia. Barbiturates are not preferred due to the disadvantages like respiratory depression.

Antihistamines have sedative, antiemetic and anti-cholinergic properties and are useful, e.g. promethazine.

Antiemetics Metoclopromide, domperidone or ondansetron may be used. Antihistamines with antiemetic properties may also be used for this purpose.

Anticholinergic drugs Some irritant anaesthetics like ether increase the salivary and respiratory secretions. The secretions from the oral cavity may enter into the larynx causing various problems including laryngospasm and aspiration pneumonia. Hence we need drugs that reduce these secretions. But we now have less irritant anaesthetics and secretions are less of a problem. Atropine, scopolamine or glycopyrrolate can be used. They

- reduce the secretions
- prevent bradycardia due to vagal stimulation
- prevent laryngospasm which is due to excessive secretions.

Scopolamine produces more sedation. Glycopyrrolate is a derivative of atropine. As compared to atropine glycopyrrolate is longer acting, and is less likely to cause significant tachycardia. It also produces less sedation than scopolamine.

Drugs that reduce acidity H_2 blockers like ranitidine decrease gastric acid secretion and are given on the night before surgery. Decrease in gastric secretions reduces the damage to lungs if aspiration occurs when the patient is on anaesthesia.

Gastrokinetic agents—metoclopramide is a dopamine antagonist that promotes gastrointestinal motility and increases the tone of oesophageal end of the stomach. This speeds gastric emptying. The combination of H_2 blocker + metoclopramide provides best protection against aspiration.

Opioids—like morphine and pethidine reduce anxiety and apprehension, provide analgesia and reduce the dose of the anaesthetic required. But they depress respiration and may cause hypotension, postoperative constipation, and urinary retention; precipitate asthma and delay recovery.

Balanced anaesthesia Since it is not possible to achieve ideal anaesthesia with a single drug, multiple drugs are employed to attain this—preanaesthetic medication, IV anaesthetics for induction, inhalational agents for maintenance, oxygen, skeletal muscle relaxants and analgesics. This is termed *balanced anaesthesia*.

❑ LOCAL ANAESTHETICS

Local anaesthetics are drugs that block nerve conduction when applied locally to nerve tissue in appropriate concentrations. Their action is completely reversible. They act on every type of nerve fibre and can cause both sensory and motor paralysis in the innervated area. They act on axons, cell body, dendrites, synapses and other excitable membranes that utilize sodium channels as the primary means of action potential generation.

Cocaine was the first agent to be isolated by Niemann in 1860. Inspite of its addiction potential, cocaine was used for 30 years as a surface anaesthetic. In an effort made to improve the properties of cocaine, procaine was synthesized in 1905. It ruled the field for the next 50 years. In 1943, Lignocaine was synthesized and it continues to dominate the field till today.

Classification of local anaesthetics (LAs) based on the route of administration and duration of action.

I. **Injectable**

1. *Short-acting* — Procaine, Chloroprocaine
2. *Intermediate-acting* — Lignocaine, Prilocaine
3. *Long-acting* — Tetracaine (amethocaine), Bupivacaine,
   — Dibucaine (cinchocaine), Ropivacaine, Etidocaine.

II. **Surface anaesthetics** — Lignocaine, Cocaine, Tetracaine, Benzocaine, Oxethazaine, Dibucaine, Dyclonine

Depending on the linking chain in their structure, LAs can be classified as:

Ester linked – Cocaine, Procaine, Tetracaine, Benzocaine, Chloroprocaine

Amide linked – Lignocaine (Lidocaine), Mepivacaine, Bupivacaine, Etidocaine, Prilocaine and Ropivacaine

MECHANISM OF ACTION

Local anaesthetics prevent the generation and the conduction of nerve impulses. The primary mechanism of action is blockade of voltage-gated sodium channels.

Local anaesthetics directly interact with specific site on voltage-sensitive Na^+ channels and gradually raise the threshold for excitation. With increasing concentration, impulse conduction slows, rate of rise of action potential (AP) declines, AP amplitude decreases and finally the ability to generate an AP is abolished. These result from binding of LA to more and more sodium channels. Thus, it prevents the generation of an AP and its conduction.

Small nerve fibres are more susceptible as it presents a greater surface area per unit volume. Thus, smaller fibres are blocked first—autonomic fibres are blocked first followed by sensory fibres conducting pain, temperature sense, then touch, pressure and vibration sensations in the same order. Sensory and motor fibres are equally sensitive. Non-myelinated fibres are blocked more readily than the myelinated.

Addition of a vasoconstrictor like adrenaline (1:1,00,000 to 1: 2,00,000) or phenylephrine (1:20,000):

1. prolongs the duration of action of LAs by slowing the rate of absorption from the site of administration.
2. reduces systemic toxicity of LAs since the absorption rate is reduced and as it gets absorbed, it gets metabolised.

SYSTEMIC ACTIONS

Depending on the concentration attained in the plasma, any LA can produce systemic effects. LAs interfere with the function of all organs in which conduction or transmission of impulses occur. Thus CNS, autonomic ganglia, NMJ and all muscles are affected.

CNS Local anaesthetics depress the inhibition from the cerebral cortex. This loss of inhibition results in unopposed excitatory activity which is manifested as restlessness, tremors and may proceed to convulsions. This central stimulation is followed by generalised CNS depression and death may result from respiratory failure.

CVS The primary site of action is the myocardium—lignocaine decreases excitability, conduction rate and force of contraction (quinidine like effects). It also causes arteriolar dilatation. Since procaine is short-acting, procainamide is used as an antiarrhythmic. Bupivacaine is more cardiotoxic than other LAs.

Smooth muscle LAs depress contractions in the intact bowel. They also relax vascular and bronchial smooth muscles.

PHARMACOKINETICS

Local anaesthetics are rapidly absorbed from the mucous membranes and abraded skin. Rate of absorption is dependent on the vascularity of the area. Thus, vasoconstriction decreases the absorption. Toxicity depends on the balance between absorption and metabolism, i.e. if it gets metabolised as it gets absorbed, then toxicity is less. Ester-linked LAs are rapidly hydrolysed by plasma pseudocholinesterase and in the liver. Amide linked LAs are metabolised by the liver. They undergo extensive first pass metabolism.

ADVERSE EFFECTS (Table 6.1)

1. *Hypersensitivity reactions*—Skin rashes, dermatitis, asthma or rarely anaphylaxis. These reactions are more common with ester type of drugs. Intradermal sensitivity test should be done before using these drugs. Moreover, allergy is most often due to the preservative methylparaben. Preparations that do not contain this preservative are now available.
2. *CNS*—Dizziness, auditory and visual disturbances, mental confusion, disorientation, anxiety, muscle tremors, convulsions and respiratory failure can result from large doses. Intravenous diazepam controls convulsions. Infact, these can be prevented by preanaesthetic administration of diazepam, especially if large doses are to be used.
3. *CVS*—Hypotension, bradycardia, arrhythmias may be encountered. Rarely cardiac arrest can occur.
4. *Local irritation*—can be seen with bupivacaine. Wound healing may be delayed.

TABLE 6.1: Adverse effects of local anaesthetics

CNS	:	Dizziness, confusion, anxiety, tremors, occasionally convulsions and respiratory depression
CVS	:	Hypotension, bradycardia, arrhythmias
Hypersensitivity reactions	:	Rashes, dermatitis, asthma, rarely anaphylaxis

INDIVIDUAL COMPOUNDS

A. *INJECTABLE* (Table 6.2)

1. ***Lignocaine***—most widely used LA. It is faster and longer-acting. Action is seen in 3 minutes for nerve block. It is useful for all types of blocks. In contrast to other LAs, lignocaine causes drowsiness and mental clouding.

XYLOCAINE 4% topical solution, 2% Jelly, 5% ointment, 1% and 2% injection, 5% for spinal anaesthesia.

2. ***Bupivacaine HCl***—widely used. But it can cause more cardiotoxicity than others. Injection 0.25-0.5% with or without adrenaline.

3. ***Ropivacaine***—is similar to bupivacaine except that it is less cardiotoxic.

4. ***Chloroprocaine HCl***—potency is twice that of procaine and its toxicity is lower because of its more rapid metabolism.

5. ***Etidocaine HCl***—its analgesic action lasts 2-3 times longer. It is used for epidural and all types of infiltration and regional anaesthesia.

6. ***Mepivacaine***—action is more rapid in onset and more prolonged than that of lignocaine.

7. ***Prilocaine HCl***—onset of action and duration are longer. Because of it's toxicity, its use is restricted to dental procedures.

8. ***Cocaine***—produces euphoria and is a drug of dependence and abuse. It is a surface anaesthetic. It is a protoplasmic poison and hence cannot be injected. Cocaine is not preferred now due to toxicity.

9. ***Procaine***—was widely used once. But is now replaced by other agents. It is hydrolysed to PABA which interferes with sulfonamides. It is rapidly absorbed following parenteral administration. It is ineffective when applied topically—thus not useful as a surface anaesthetic.

10. ***Tetracaine***—is a PABA derivative and is 10 times more toxic and more active than procaine. It is used on the eye as 0.5% drops, ointments 0.5% and cream 1% for topical use. 0.25 to 0.5% injection is used for spinal anaesthesia.

TABLE 6.2: Preparations and uses of some local anaesthetics

	Drug	*Preparation*	*Uses*
1.	Tetracaine	1-2% ointment, eye drops, cream, powder	Topical, spinal anaesthesia
2.	Lignocaine	2-4% drops, spray, jelly, ointment, cream, 1-10% Inj	Topical, infiltration, nerve block, spinal, epidural and IV regional anaesthesia
3.	Benzocaine	1-2% dusting powder, 5% suppository, cream, gels, ointments, 20% spray	Topical anaesthesia
4.	Oxethazaine	0.2% suspension	Topical anaesthesia (used in peptic ulcer)
5.	Prilocaine	5% Cream, 4% Inj	Topical, nerve block anaesthesia
6.	Dibucaine	0.5-1% Cream	Topical anaesthesia
7.	Mepivacaine	1-3% Inj	Nerve block, epidural anaesthesia
8.	Bupivacaine	0.25-0.75% Inj	Infiltration, nerve block, spinal, epidural anaesthesia
9.	Ropivacaine	2-10% Inj	Infiltration, nerve block, spinal, epidural anaesthesia
10.	Etidocaine	1% Inj	Epidural anaesthesia

B. *LOCAL ANAESTHETICS USED ONLY ON THE EYE*

Benoxinate HCl—within 60 seconds of administration it produces corneal anaesthesia enough to perform tonometry.

Proparacaine HCl—produces little or no initial irritation—0.5% ophthalmic solution is used.

C. *LOCAL ANAESTHETICS USED ON THE SKIN AND MUCOUS MEMBRANES*

LAs used on the skin and mucous membranes are dibucaine, dyclonine hydrochloride and pramoxine hydrochloride. These drugs are effective when used topically in the symptomatic relief of anal and genital pruritus, poison ivy rashes, acute and chronic dermatoses. Dibucaine is the most potent, most toxic and longest-acting LA. It is available as cream and ointment.

D. *POORLY SOLUBLE ANAESTHETIC*

These are too slowly absorbed to be toxic. They can be applied to wounds directly and ulcerated surfaces as they produce sustained anaesthetic effect, e.g. benzocaine.

USES OF LOCAL ANAESTHETICS

Local anaesthesia is the loss of sensation without the loss of consciousness or impairment of central control of vital functions. Depending on the site and technique of administration, LA can be:

Surface anaesthesia Anaesthesia of mucous membrane of the eye, nose, mouth, tracheobronchial tree, oesophagus and genitourinary tract can be produced by direct application of the anaesthetic solution. Tetracaine 2%, lignocaine 2-10% are most often used. Phenylephrine (but not adrenaline) produces vasoconstriction on topical application and prolongs the duration of action. Anaesthesia is entirely superficial and does not extend to submucosal structures. But LAs are absorbed from mucous membranes and may result in systemic toxicity. Local anaesthetics can also be used on abraded skin. Surface anaesthesia is useful in the eye for tonometry, surgery, nasal lesions, stomatitis, sore throat, tonsillectomy, endoscopies, intubation, gastric ulcer, burns and proctoscopy.

Infiltration anaesthesia Injection of a local anaesthetic solution directly into the tissue can be (i) superficial—only into the skin, or (ii) into deeper structures including intra-abdominal organs. Duration of anaesthesia can be increased by adrenaline (1:2,00,000). Adrenaline should not be used (i) around end arteries to avoid necrosis, and (ii) intradermally to avoid sloughing. Drugs used are lignocaine, procaine, bupivacaine.

Advantage By using infiltration anaesthesia, it is possible to provide anaesthesia without disturbing normal body activities.

Disadvantage Large amounts of the anaesthetic is required in major surgeries which may result in systemic toxicity.

Uses For minor procedures like incisions, drainage of an abscess, excision, etc.

Field block Subcutaneous injection of a LA solution proximal to the site to be anaesthetised, interrupts nerve transmission in the region distal to the injection. Sites such as forearm, scalp, anterior abdominal wall and lower limbs are used for field block. Knowledge of the neuroanatomy of the area is essential.

Advantages lesser dose can be used to provide a greater area of anaesthesia.

Nerve block Injection of a solution of a LA around individual peripheral nerves or nerve plexuses produces larger areas of anaesthesia with a smaller amount of the drug than the above techniques. Anaesthesia starts a few centimeters distal to the injection.

Nerve block anaesthesia is useful for:

1. blocks of brachial plexus for procedures on the arm (distal to deltoid).
2. intercostal nerve blocks to anaesthetise anterior abdominal wall.
3. cervical plexus block for surgery of the neck.
4. sciatic and femoral nerve blocks for surgeries distal to the knee.
5. blocks of nerves at wrist and ankle.
6. radial and ulnar nerve block at the elbow.
7. sensory cranial nerve blocks.
8. facial and lingual nerve blocks.
9. inferior alveolar nerve block for extraction of lower jaw teeth.

Onset of action is within 3 minutes with lignocaine. Duration depends on lipid solubility and protein binding. Anaesthesia by nerve block lasts longer than by field block or infiltration techniques. Nerve blocks are done for tooth extraction, operations on the eye, limbs and in neuralgias.

Spinal anaesthesia (SA) Local anaesthetic solution is injected into the subarachnoid space between L2-3 or L3-4 below the lower end of the spinal cord. The drug acts on nerve roots.

Lower abdomen and lower limbs are anaesthetised and paralysed. The level of anaesthesia can be altered by changing the volume of injection, specific gravity of the solution and posture of the patient. Level of sympathetic block produced is 2 segments higher and motor paralysis 2 segments lower than sensory or cutaneous anaesthesia. Duration depends on the concentration, dose and the drug itself.

Advantages Safer, provides good analgesia and muscle relaxation and there is no loss of consciousness. In cardiac, pulmonary and renal diseases, SA may be preferred over general anaesthesia whenever possible.

Uses Surgical procedures on the lower limb, pelvis, lower abdomen, obstetric procedures, caesarean section and other operations are done on spinal anaesthesia.

Complications of SA

1. *Hypotension and bradycardia* due to sympathetic blockade.
2. *Respiratory paralysis*—hypotension and ischaemia of the respiratory centre results in respiratory failure. Due to paralysis of the abdominal muscles, cough reflex is less effective resulting in stasis of respiratory secretions → respiratory infections.
3. *Headache* due to seepage of CSF, can be treated with analgesics.
4. *Cauda equina syndrome* is uncommon—control over bladder and bowel sphincters is lost because of damage to nerve roots.
5. Infection—resulting in meningitis
6. Nausea and vomiting—premedication can be given to prevent this.

Epidural Anaesthesia

LA is injected into the spinal extradural space and it acts on the nerve roots. It is technically more difficult and comparatively larger volumes of the anaesthetic are needed.

Advantages

1. Sensory blockade is 4-5 segments higher than motor blockade. This is useful in childbirth, as the mother has no labour pain and can still cooperate in the process of labour and is conscious throughout.

2. As there is no risk of injecting into SA space, there are no chances of infection.

Intravenous Regional Anaesthesia

This type of anaesthesia is useful for rapid anaesthetization of an extremity. A rubber bandage is used to force the blood out of the limb (veins) and a tourniquet is applied to prevent the re-entry of the blood. A dilute solution of the local anaesthetic is then injected intravenously. It diffuses into extravascular tissues. Onset of anaesthesia is in 2 minutes. Because of the pain produced by the tourniquet, this type of anaesthesia is used for procedures lasting less than one hour. About 25% of the drug enters into the systemic circulation. This type of anaesthesia is commonly used on the upper limbs though it can also be used on the legs and the thighs.

❑ SEDATIVE HYPNOTICS

Sedative is a drug that produces a calming or quietening effect and reduces excitement. It may cause drowsiness. Hypnotic is a drug that induces sleep resembling natural sleep. Both sedation and hypnosis may be considered as different grades of CNS depression. All human beings need sleep. Insomnia is sleeplessness. Since centuries man has sought the help of drugs and other remedies for insomnia.

Sleep can be classified into two types depending on the physiological characteristics.

1. NREM (Non-rapid eye movement) sleep
2. REM (Rapid eye movement) sleep.

Throughout the night, NREM and REM sleep cycles repeat alternately for brief periods. Approximately one-third of our life is spent in sleep.

CLASSIFICATION

1. **Benzodiazepines**

Long-acting	Diazepam, Chlordiazepoxide, Flurazepam, Chlorazepate.

Short-acting	Temazepam, Lorazepam, Triazolam, Midazolam, Nitrazepam, Clonazepam, Alprazolam
2. **Barbiturates**	Phenobarbitone, Mephobarbitone, Secobarbitone, Pentobarbitone, Thiopentone, Hexobarbitone
3. **Newer agents**	Zolpidem, Zopiclone
4. **Miscellaneous**	Paraldehyde, Chloral hydrate, Glutethimide.

BENZODIAZEPINES (BZD) Based on primary use

Chlordiazepoxide was the first BZD to be introduced into clinical medicine in 1961 and since then thousands of BZDs have been synthesized of which 35 are now in clinical use.

Pharmacological actions The most important actions of BZDs are on the CNS and include.

1. Sedation and hypnosis
2. Reduction in anxiety
3. Muscle relaxation
4. Anticonvulsant effects.

Sedation and hypnosis BZDs hasten the onset of sleep and increase the duration of sleep. The quality of sleep resembles natural sleep more closely when compared to other hypnotics. Tolerance develops to this effect gradually.

Anxiolytic or antianxiety effects BZDs reduce anxiety and aggression and thus produce a calming effect.

Muscle relaxant action BZDs reduce muscle tone by a central action. Generally anxiety is associated with an increased muscle tone and may be responsible for aches and pains in these patients. The muscle relaxation by BZDs adds to its beneficial effects in such patients.

Anticonvulsant effects BZDs have anticonvulsant properties (see page 168).

Mechanism of action BZDs bind to the BZD receptors and enhance the effect of GABA—the inhibitory neurotransmitter.

BZDs as hypnotics—when compared to barbiturates:

1. BZDs induce sleep which more closely resembles natural sleep and has less hangover.
2. In hypnotic doses they do not affect respiration or cardiovascular functions.
3. BZDs have a higher safety margin and are safer than barbiturates even in overdoses. The respiratory depression in overdoses is milder.
4. In case of BZD overdosage, a specific BZD antagonist—flumazenil can be used to reverse the symptoms.
5. BZDs do not cause microsomal enzyme induction and therefore do not alter the blood levels of other drugs.
6. BZDs have lower abuse liability.

Because of the above reasons, BZDs are the most preferred sedative hypnotics.

Pharmacokinetics There are significant pharmacokinetic differences among BZDs due to their difference in lipid solubility.

Adverse effects BZDs are generally well tolerated. The common side effects include drowsiness, confusion, amnesia, lethargy, ataxia, day time sedation and impaired motor coordination such as driving skills—therefore, while on BZDs driving should be avoided.

In some patients it may cause irritability and anxiety.

Tolerance and dependence Both tolerance and risk of dependance are less with BZDs as compared to barbiturates. Patients develop tolerance to the sedative effects. If BZDs are suddenly stopped after long-term administration, withdrawal symptoms like anxiety, sleeplessness, irritability and sweating can occur.

Uses of BZDs

1. **Insomnia** When drugs are to be used to treat sleeplessness, BZDs are the agents of choice.
2. **In anxiety states** BZDs are the most commonly used anxiolytics for the treatment of anxiety states and anxiety neuroses.
3. **As anticonvulsants** IV diazepam is the drug of choice in the treatment of status epilepticus. Clonazepam is used with other antiepileptic drugs.

4. **Muscle relaxant** BZDs are centrally acting muscle relaxants used in chronic muscle spasm and spasticity.
5. **As preanaeshetic medication** BZDs are useful for their sedation and anxiolytic effects (page 145).
6. **During alcohol withdrawal**—BZDs are useful in patients during withdrawal of alcohol or other sedative-hypnotics.

Flumazenil is a BZD receptor antagonist which competes with BZDs for the receptor.

Uses

1. To reverse BZD sedation/anaesthesia
2. In BZD overdosage.

BARBITURATES

Barbiturates are derivatives of barbituric acid and were the largest group of hypnotics in clinical use until the 1960s.

Classification

Barbiturates can be classified based on their duration of action as:

Long-acting	Phenobarbitone, Mephobarbitone
Short-acting	Pentobarbitone, Butobarbitone
Ultrashort-acting	Thiopentone, Hexobarbitone, Methohexitone

Mechanism of Action

Barbiturates bind to GABA receptors and enhance the inhibitory activity of GABA.

PHARMACOLOGICAL ACTIONS

1. CNS

Sedation Barbiturates cause sedation and induce sleep. They reduce anxiety and impair memory.

They can produce euphoria and are drugs of addiction while some people may experience dysphoria. Barbiturates produce hyperalgesia (increased sensitivity to pain). Therefore barbiturates, when given as hypnotics for a patient in pain may be more troublesome than being of any benefit.

Anaesthesia In higher doses barbiturates produce general anaesthesia. The ultra short-acting barbiturates like thiopentone sodium are used intravenously for this effect.

Anticonvulsant effects All barbiturates have anticonvulsant action. Phenobarbitone is used in the treatment of epilepsy.

2. Respiratory system Barbiturates depress the respiration.

3. Cardiovascular system Barbiturates cause mild hypotension.

4. Skeletal muscles Higher doses of barbiturates depress the excitability of the neuromuscular junction.

PHARMACOKINETICS

Barbiturates are well-absorbed and widely distributed in the body. Barbiturates are metabolised in the liver. They are hepatic microsomal enzyme inducers. The metabolites are excreted in urine.

ADVERSE REACTIONS

Hangover may be accompanied by nausea, vomiting, vertigo and diarrhoea. Changes of mood, impaired judgement and fine motor skills may be seen. Respiratory depression and hypersensitivity reactions are common.

Tolerance and dependance On repeated administration, tolerance develops to the effects of barbiturates.

Development of dependence to barbiturates make them one of the drugs of abuse. Withdrawal symptoms include anxiety, restlessness, abdominal cramps, hallucinations, delirium and convulsions.

Acute barbiturate poisoning In acute barbiturate poisoning, there is respiratory depression, hypotension and shock. It can be fatal. There is no specific antidote for treatment. Stomach wash, forced alkaline diuresis and haemodialysis should be done.

Uses Because of respiratory depression and risk of abuse, barbiturates are generally not preferred.

1. *Sedation and hypnosis* Benzodiazepines are preferred to barbiturates as sedative hypnotics.

2. *Anaesthesia* Thiopentone sodium is used IV for the induction of general anaesthesia.
3. *Preanesthetic medication* Barbiturates were used earlier for the sedative-hypnotic property, but are not preferred now.
4. *Antiepileptic* Phenobarbitone is used as an antiepileptic (page 124).
5. *Neonatal jaundice* Phenobarbitone is a microsomal enzyme inducer. It enhances the production of the enzyme required for metabolism and excretion of bilirubin. It therefore helps in the clearance of jaundice in the neonates.

NEWER AGENTS

Zolpidem is a newly developed hypnotic—non-benzodiazepine drug. It is claimed to be a better hypnotic. Adverse effects are similar to BZD.

Zopiclone is another new hypnotic. Its actions resemble those of BZDs.

MISCELLANEOUS

Chloral hydrate is used as an alternative to BZD. It has a bad taste and is an irritant—causes nausea and vomiting. It produces hypnosis without affecting respiratory and cardiovascular functions. Not preferred now.

Paraldehyde is a colourless, transparent, pungent, inflammable liquid. It is an irritant and can dissolve plastic—cannot be given by a plastic syringe. It is a good hypnotic causing little hangover. It can be given rectally, intramuscularly or orally.

It also has anticonvulsant properties.

Uses

1. As an anticonvulsant
2. Hypnotic—rarely used.

❑ ALCOHOLS

ETHYL ALCOHOL (Ethanol)

Ethyl alcohol is manufactured by fermentation of sugars. It is a colourless, volatile, inflammable liquid. The ethanol content of various alcoholic beverages ranges from 4-55%.

Actions

1. *Local* On topical application, ethanol evaporates quickly and has a cooling effect. It is an astringent—precipitates surface proteins and hardens the skin. 40-50% alcohol is rubefacient and counter irritant. Alcohol is also an antiseptic. At 70%, it has maximum antiseptic properties which decrease above that. It is not effective against spores.

2. *CNS* Alcohol is a CNS depressant. Small doses cause euphoria, relief of anxiety and loss of social inhibitions. Moderate doses impair muscular coordination and visual acuity making driving dangerous. With higher doses mental clouding, impaired judgement, drowsiness and loss of self control result. High doses cause coma. Death is due to respiratory depression.

Alcohol may precipitate convulsions in epileptics. Tolerance develops on long-term use.

Chronic consumption of moderate amounts of alcohol results in accumulation of fat in the liver, liver enlargement, followed by fatty degeneration and cirrhosis.

Alcohol induces microsomal enzymes.

Other effects Alcohol causes vasodilation in the skin causing warmth. But this increases heat loss and should not be used in cold weather. Alcohol also increases gastric secretion. It is an appetizer. Low doses taken over a long-time increases HDL and lowers LDL cholesterol. Alcohol is a diuretic (↓ADH secretion). Food value is 7 calories/gram.

Uses

1. *Antiseptic* 70% alcohol is applied topically.
2. *Bed sores* When rubbed onto the skin, alcohol hardens the skin and prevents bed sores.
3. Alcoholic sponges are used for reduction of body temperature *in fevers*.
4. *Appetite stimulant* About 50 ml of 6-10% alcohol given before meals is an appetite stimulant.
5. *Neuralgias* In severe neuralgias like trigeminal neuralgia, injection of alcohol around the nerve causes permanent loss of transmission and relieves pain.
6. *In methanol poisoning*

Disulfiram

Disulfiram inhibits the enzyme aldehyde dehydrogenase. If alcohol is consumed after taking disulfiram, acetaldehyde accumulates and within few minutes it can produce flushing, throbbing headache, nausea, vomiting, sweating, hypotension and confusion called **the antabuse reaction,** due to accumulation of acetaldehyde. The effect lasts for 7-14 days after stopping disulfiram. The reactions can sometimes be very severe and therefore treatment should be given in a hospital.

Other drugs that cause antabuse reaction are metronidazole, chlorpropamide, tolbutamide, griseofulvin, cephalosporins and phenylbutazone.

Contraindications Patients with liver disease, patients physically dependant on alcohol.

METHYL ALCOHOL (Methanol, Wood Alcohol)

Methanol is used to denature ethyl alcohol. Ingestion results in methanol poisoning.

$$\text{Methanol} \xrightarrow[\textit{dehydrogenase}]{\textit{Alcohol}} \text{Formaldehyde} \xrightarrow[\textit{dehydrogenase}]{\textit{Aldehyde}} \text{Formic Acid}$$

Toxic effects are due to formic acid. Manifestations are vomiting, headache, vertigo, severe abdominal pain, hypotension, delirium, acidosis and coma. Formic acid has affinity for optic nerve and causes retinal damage resulting in blindness. Death is due to respiratory failure.

Treatment

1. *Correction of acidosis* As acidosis hastens retinal damage, immediate correction of acidosis with IV sodium bicarbonate infusion helps in preventing blindness.
2. Patient should be kept in a dark room to protect the eyes.
3. Gastric lavage should be given.
4. BP and ventilation should be maintained.
5. Ethyl alcohol is given as infusion. It competes with methanol for alcohol dehydrogenase, slows the metabolism of methanol and thus prevents the formation of toxic metabolites.

❑ ANTIEPILEPTICS

Epilepsy is a common neurological abnormality that affects about 0.5-1% of the population. Epilepsy is a chronic disorder characterised by recurrent seizures often accompanied by episodes of unconsciousness and/or amnesia. It is a disorder of brain function.

Seizure is an alteration in behaviour because of abnormal firing of some brain neurons. In most of the cases, the cause is not known. It may be due to various reasons including trauma during birth process, head injury, childhood fevers, brain tumors, meningitis or drug induced.

Seizures have been classified into partial and generalised seizures.

Partial seizures are classified as simple partial in which there is no impairment of consciousness and complex partial seizures with impairment of consciousness.

Simple partial seizures There is no impairment of consciousness. The symptoms depend on the site that is affected in the cortex, e.g. if the motor cortex representing the right thumb is involved, there is recurrent contractions of the right thumb. If the sensory area representing the left palm is involved, there is numbness or paraesthesia of the left palm. This type of seizures last for 20-60 seconds.

Complex partial seizures This is characterised by purposeless movements like lipsmaking, hand wringing or swallowing that lasts for 30 sec to 2 minutes. Consciousness is impaired.

Generalised seizures They may be:

Absence seizures (petitmal) In this, there is sudden onset of impaired consciousness and the person is staring. He stops all activities and the episode lasts for a short period usually less than 30 seconds.

Myoclonic seizures involve a sudden, brief, shock-like contraction of muscles. It may be limited to a part of the body or may affect the whole body.

Atonic seizures (Drop attacks) are characterised by sudden loss of postural tone and the head may drop for a few seconds or the person may drop to the ground for no reason.

Tonic-clonic seizures (Grandmal epilepsy) is characterised by sudden loss of consciousness followed by sustained contraction of muscles throughout the body (known as tonic phase), lasting for 1 minute and then, a series of jerks, i.e. periods of muscle contraction alternating with periods of relaxation (clonic phase) lasting for 2-4 minutes follow. CNS depression then occurs and the person goes into sleep. Injury may occur during the convulsive episode.

Status epilepticus is continuous or repeated seizures of any variety without recovery of consciousness between the attacks.

Classification of Antiepileptic Drugs

Hydantoins	Phenytoin, Mephenytoin
Barbiturates	Phenobarbitone, Mephobarbitone
Deoxybarbiturate	Primidone
Iminostilbene	Carbamazepine
Succinimide	Ethosuximide
GABA transaminase inhibitors	Valproic acid, Vigabatrin
Benzodiazepines	Diazepam, Clonazepam, Lorazepam, Clorazepate
Miscellaneous	Gabapentin, Lamotrigine, Acetazolamide, Amphetamine.

PHENYTOIN (Diphenylhydantoin)

Phenytoin was synthesized in 1908, but its anticonvulsant property was discovered only in 1938.

Pharmacological actions

CNS Phenytoin has good antiseizure activity. It is one of the most effective drugs against generalised tonic-clonic seizures and partial seizures.

Mechanism of action Phenytoin causes blockade of the sodium channels and stabilizes the neuronal membrane. It inhibits the generation of repetitive action potentials.

Pharmacokinetics Phenytoin is poorly water-soluble—hence absorption is slow. Phenytoin is 90% bound to plasma proteins. It is metabolised in the liver initially by first order and later by zero order kinetics (see page 27) as the dose increases. Therefore, monitoring of plasma concentration is useful. Phenytoin is an enzyme inducer.

Adverse effects depend on the dose, duration and route.

1. Nausea, vomiting, epigastric pain, anorexia.
2. Nystagmus, diplopia, ataxia are common.
3. Gingival hyperplasia is more common in children on prolonged use.
4. Peripheral neuropathy.
5. Endocrine
   i. Hirsutism, acne, coarsening of facial features.
   ii. Hyperglycaemia—as phenytoin inhibits insulin release.
   iii. ↓ release of ADH.
   iv. Osteomalacia, hypocalcaemia due to altered metabolism of vitamin D and inhibition of intestinal absorption of Ca^{++} Phenytoin also reduces target tissue sensitivity to vitamin D.
6. Hypersensitivity—rashes, SLE, hepatic necrosis, lymphadenopathy and neutropenia.
7. Megaloblastic anaemia—as phenytoin decreases absorption and increases excretion of folates.
8. Teratogenicity—when taken by the pregnant lady, phenytoin produces foetal hydantoin syndrome characterised by hypoplastic phalanges, cleft palate, harelip and microcephaly in the offspring.

Toxic doses—cerebellar and vestibular effects are prominent; drowsiness, delirium, confusion, hallucinations, altered behaviour and coma follow.

Uses

1. Generalised tonic-clonic seizures and partial seizures (not useful in absence seizures).
2. Status epilepticus—phenytoin is used by slow IV injection.
3. Trigeminal neuralgia—as an alternative to carbamazepine.
4. Cardiac arrhythmias—Phenytoin is useful in digitalis induced arrhythmias.

Drug interactions

- Phenytoin is an enzyme inducer. Given with phenobarbitone, both increase each other's metabolism. Also phenobarbitone competitively inhibits phenytoin metabolism.
- Carbamazepine and phenytoin enhance each other's metabolism.
- Valproate displaces protein bound phenytoin.
- Cimetidine and chloramphenicol inhibit the metabolism of phenytoin resulting in toxicity.
- Antacids ↓ absorption of phenytoin.

PHENOBARBITONE (page 158-160)

Phenobarbitone was the first effective antiepileptic drug to be introduced in 1912. It still remains one of the widely used drugs.

Antiepileptic actions Phenobarbitone has specific antiepileptic activity and raises the seizure threshold. Primidone which is rarely used now is metabolised to phenobarbitone.

Mechanism of action Barbiturates enhance the inhibitory activity of GABA in the CNS.

Pharmacokinetics Oral absorption of phenobarbitone is slow but complete. It is a microsomal enzyme inducer.

Uses Phenobarbitone is one of the widely used antiepileptic because of its efficacy and low cost. It is used in:

1. Generalised tonic-clonic seizures.
2. Partial seizures.
3. In neonatal jaundice (see page 160)

CARBAMAZEPINE

Carbamazepine is closely related to imipramine.

Antiseizure activity Carbamazepine has good anti-seizure activity. It's mechanism of action is similar to phenytoin, i.e. it blocks sodium channels.

Carbamazepine is also useful in the treatment of trigeminal neuralgia (severe pain along the distribution of the trigeminal nerve) and glossopharyngeal neuralgia.

Carbamazepine is also found to be beneficial in mood disorders.

Pharmacokinetics Absorption is slow and erratic; has a t½ of 10-20 hours. It is a microsomal enzyme inducer.

Adverse effects Drowsiness, vertigo, ataxia, diplopia, blurring of vision, nausea, vomiting and dizziness are common. Driving is dangerous for patients on carbamazepine. Hypersensitivity reactions—like skin rashes may occur. Haematological toxicity includes leukopenia, thrombocytopenia and rarely agranulocytosis and aplastic anaemia. It is a teratogen.

Uses

1. Generalised tonic clonic seizures (grand mal epilepsy).
2. Simple and complex partial seizures—especially temporal lobe epilepsy.
3. Trigeminal neuralgia and glossopharyngeal neuralgia—carbamazepine is the drug of choice for these neuralgias and has to be given for several months.
4. Bipolar mood disorder—carbamazepine is used as an alternative to other antidepressants.

ETHOSUXIMIDE

Ethosuximide is the primary agent for absence seizures. It raises the seizure threshold.

Mechanism of action Ethosuximide reduces the calcium currents (T-currents) in the thalamic neurons.

Pharmacokinetics Absorption is complete on administration of oral dosage forms. It is metabolised in the liver.

Adverse effects The most common adverse effects are nausea, vomiting, epigastric pain, gastric irritation and anorexia. These can be avoided by starting with a low dose and gradually increasing it. CNS effects like drowsiness, fatigue, lethargy, euphoria, dizziness, headache and hiccough are dose-related effects. Hypersensitivity reactions like rashes, urticaria, leukopenia, thrombocytopenia or pancytopenia have been reported.

Uses Ethosuximide is the drug of choice for absence seizures.

VALPROIC ACID

Valproic acid (salt→sodium valproate) is a very effective antiepileptic drug useful in many types of epilepsies including absence seizures, partial and generalised tonic-clonic seizures.

Mechanism of action Valproic acid acts by multiple mechanisms.

1. It enhances the level of GABA by:
   i. increasing the synthesis of GABA—by increased activity of GABA synthetase enzyme.
   ii. decreasing the metabolism of GABA—by inhibiting GABA transaminase enzyme.
2. Like phenytoin, it blocks the sodium channels.

Adverse effects Gastrointestinal symptoms like nausea, vomiting, epigastric distress occur initially. Tremors, sedation, ataxia, rashes and alopecia are rare. Valproic acid can cause fulminant hepatitis—though rare can be fatal. Hence careful monitoring of liver functions is mandatory. Valproic acid is teratogenic, it can cause neural tube defects.

Uses Useful in partial and generalised seizures. Valproic acid is particularly useful in absence seizures. In patients with both absence seizures and generalised tonic-clonic attacks, valproate is the drug of choice.

BENZODIAZEPINES

Benzodiazepines have useful anticonvulsant properties. **Diazepam** is the drug of choice in status epilepticus. **Clonazepam** is a potent antiepileptic useful in absence and myoclonic seizures. But tolerance develops to its antiepileptic effects. **Clobazam** causes less sedation and is effective in most types of epilepsies.

Treatment of Epilepsies (Table 6.3)

TABLE 6.3: Choice of antiseizure drugs

Types of epilepsy	*Preferred drugs*
1. Generalised tonic-clonic and simple partial seizures	Carbamazepine, Phenytoin
2. Absence seizures	Ethosuximide, Valproic acid
3. Tonic-clonic + absence seizures	Valproic acid
4. Complex partial seizures	Carbamazepine, Phenytoin, Valproic acid
5. Febrile convulsions	Diazepam
6. Status epilepticus	Diazepam, Phenytoin, General anaesthesia

Febrile convulsions Two to four per cent of children experience convulsions during fever; of them 2-3 per cent become epileptics. Treatment is controversial. Children < 18 months developing febrile convulsions, those with neurological abnormalities and those with seizures lasting for > 15 minutes, complex seizures—all these have greater risk of recurrence. Diazepam (0.5 mg/kg) given orally or rectally at the onset of fever prevents convulsions. Timely use of paracetamol and tepid sponging prevents high fever. If convulsions occur, diazepam rectally or intravenously can be used.

Status epilepticus is a neurological emergency which may be fatal. Diazepam IV (5-10 mg every 10-15 minutes up to 30 mg) is the drug of choice. Phenytoin given intravenously takes 15-20 minutes to act. Some prefer to combine diazepam and phenytoin. If seizures continue—general anaesthesia is the last resort. Airway maintenance is important. After the control of seizures, long-term antiepileptic therapy is needed.

In pregnancy—antiepileptics should be continued because abrupt discontinuation increases the risk of status epilepticus which is hazardous to the foetus.

❑ DRUGS USED IN PARKINSONISM

Parkinsonism is a chronic, progressive, motor disorder characterised by rigidity, tremors and bradykinesia. Other symptoms include excessive salivation, abnormalities of posture and gait, seborrhoea and mood changes. It was described by James Parkinson in 1817 and is therefore named after him.

The incidence is about 1 per cent of population above 65 years of age. It is usually idiopathic in origin but can also be drug induced. In idiopathic parkinsonism, there is degeneration of nigrostriatal neurons in the basal ganglia resulting in dopamine deficiency. The balance between inhibitory dopaminergic neurons and excitatory cholinergic neurons is disturbed.

Antiparkinsonian drugs can only help to reduce the symptoms and improve the quality of life. The two strategies in the treatment are (i) to enhance dopamine activity (ii) to depress cholinergic overactivity.

CLASSIFICATION

1. **Drugs that increase dopamine levels**
   - i. *DA precursor* Levodopa.
   - ii. *Drugs that release dopamine* Amantadine
   - iii. *Dopaminergic agonists* Bromocryptine, Lisuride, Ropinirole, pramipexole
   - iv. *Inhibit dopamine metabolism*
     - a. MAO inhibitors—Selegiline
     - b. COMT inhibitors—Tolcapone, entacapone
2. **Drugs influencing cholinergic system**
   - i. *Central anticholinergics* Benztropine, Benzhexol, Biperidine, Trihexyphenidyl
   - ii. *Antihistamines* Diphenhydramine, Orphenadrine, Promethazine.

LEVODOPA

Though parkinsonism is due to dopamine deficiency, dopamine is of no therapeutic value because it does not cross the blood-brain barrier. Levodopa is a prodrug which is converted to dopamine in the body. It crosses the BBB and is taken up by the surviving nigrostriatal neurons.

$$\text{Levodopa} \xrightarrow{\text{decarboxylase}} \text{Dopamine}$$

Antiparkinsonian effect On administration of levodopa, there is an overall improvement in the patient as all the symptoms subside.

Other actions

- *CTZ*—Dopamine stimulates the CTZ to induce vomiting.
- *CVS*—Large amounts of levodopa converted to dopamine in the periphery causes postural hypotension and tachycardia—dopamine is a catecholamine.

Endocrine—Dopamine suppresses the prolactin secretion.

Pharmacokinetics Levodopa is rapidly absorbed. Presence of food delays absorption. It undergoes first pass metabolism in the gut and the liver. Its t½ is 1-2 hours.

Adverse reactions As large amounts (95%) of levodopa is converted to dopamine in the periphery, several adverse effects are expected. Nausea, vomiting, postural hypotension, palpitation and occasionally arrhythmias can occur. Tolerance develops to these effects after sometime. Behavioural effects like anxiety, depression, hallucinations and sometimes psychosis can occur.

Abnormal involuntary movements like facial tics, grimacing, choreoathetoid movements of the limbs may develop after a few months of use and require reduction in the dose of levodopa.

Fluctuation in response to levodopa can occur after 2-5 years of use—known as 'on-off' phenomenon—where the patient has alternately good response and severe disease.

Uses Levodopa is the most effective drug in idiopathic parkinsonism but is not useful in drug induced parkinsonism.

Drug interactions

1. Pyridoxine enhances the peripheral decarboxylation of levodopa and thus reduces its availability to the CNS.

2. Phenothiazines, metoclopramide and reserpine are DA antagonists. They reverse the effects of levodopa.

Carbidopa and benserazide are peripheral dopa decarboxylase inhibitors. When carbidopa or benserazide are given with levodopa, they prevent the formation of dopamine in the periphery. They do not cross the BBB and hence allow levodopa to reach the CNS. The combination is synergistic and therefore levodopa is always given with carbidopa/benserazide.

Advantages of combining carbidapa/benzerazide—with levodopa.

1. Dose of L-dopa can be reduced by 75%.
2. Response to L-dopa appears earlier.
3. Side effects like vomiting and tachycardia are largely reduced.
4. Pyridoxine does not interfere with treatment.

Amantadine is an antiviral drug. It enhances the release of DA in the brain and diminishes the re-uptake of DA. The response starts early and its adverse effects are minor. Large doses produce insomnia, dizziness, vomiting, postural hypotension, hallucinations and ankle oedema.

Amantadine is used in mild cases of parkinsonism. It can also be used along with levodopa.

Dopamine receptor agonists Bromocriptine and pergolide are ergot derivatives having dopamine agonistic activity. The newer agents ropinirole and pramipexole are selective D_2 agonists, are better tolerated, quickly attain therapeutic levels and adverse effects are milder except that they may cause some sleep disorders.

Dopamine agonists are all longer acting because of which they are useful in the treatment of 'on-off' phenomenon.

Adverse effects include nausea, vomiting, hallucinations and skin eruptions. Ergot derivatives can cause postural hypotension and 'first dose phenomenon'—that is sudden cardiovascular collapse.

DA agonists are used in:

1. In the treatment of 'on-off' phenomenon
2. As alternatives in the initial treatment of parkinsonism.

Lisuride and pergolide are similar to bromocriptine.

Drugs that Inhibit DA Metabolism

Selegiline (Deprenyl) is a selective MAO-B inhibitor. MAO-B is present in DA containing regions of the CNS. Selegiline prolongs the action of levodopa by preventing its destruction. Selegiline may delay the progression of parkinsonism.

Adverse effects include nausea, postural hypotension, confusion and hallucinations.

Uses Mild cases of parkinsonism are started on selegiline. It is also used along with levodopa.

COMT inhibitors—tolcapone and entacapone inhibit the peripheral metabolism of levodopa thereby increasing its bioavailability. Tolcapone crosses the BBB and enhances the availability of levodopa in the brain.

Adverse effects are nausea, orthostatic hypotension, confusion and hallucinations. Tolcapone can also cause hepatotoxicity.

Anticholinergics The cholinergic overactivity is overcome by anticholinergics. Tremors, seborrhoea and sialorrhoea are reduced more than rigidity. Atropine derivatives like benzhexol, benztropine, trihexyphenidyl are used. Antihistamines are useful in parkinsonism because to their anticholinergic properties. Atropine-like side effects such as dry mouth, constipation, blurred vision may be encountered.

Uses Anticholinergics are used as (i) adjunct to levodopa, (ii) drugs of choice in drug-induced parkinsonism.

Drug induced parkinsonism Drugs like reserpine, metoclopramide and phenothiazines can induce parkinsonism. Reserpine depletes catecholamine stores, metoclopramide and phenothiazines are dopamine antagonists.

Treatment Withdrawal of the drug usually reverses the symptoms. When drugs are needed, one of the anticholinergics are effective.

❑ OPIOID ANALGESICS AND ANTAGONISTS

Pain or algesia is an unpleasant sensation. It cannot be easily defined. Pain is a warning signal and indicates that there is some impairment in the body. It is the most important symptom that brings the patient to the doctor or physiotherapist and demands immediate relief. Prompt relief of pain instills enormous confidence in the patient regarding the doctors treating ability.

Pain arising from the skin and integumental structures, muscles, bones and joints is known as **somatic pain.** It is usually caused by inflammation and is well-defined or sharp pain.

Pain arising from the viscera is vague, dull-aching type, difficult to pinpoint to one site and is known as **visceral pain.** It may be accompanied by autonomic responses like sweating, nausea and hypotension. It may be due to spasm, ischaemia or inflammation.

When pain is referred to a cutaneous area which receives nerve supply from the same spinal segment as that of the affected viscera, it is known as **referred pain**, e.g. cardiac pain referred to the left arm.

Pain consists of 2 components—the original 'sensation' and the 'reaction' to it. The original sensation is carried by the afferent nerve fibres and is the same in all. The reaction component differs widely from one person to another.

Analgesic is a drug which relieves pain without loss of consciousness. Analgesics only afford symptomatic relief from pain without affecting the cause.

Analgesics are of 2 classes.

- Opioid or morphine type of analgesics
- Non-opioid or aspirin type of analgesics.

OPIOID ANALGESICS

Opium is the dark brown gummy substance obtained from the poppy capsule *(Papaver somniferum)*. On incising the unripe seed capsule, a milky juice comes out which turns brown on drying and this is crude opium. Opium is the Greek name for juice. Opium has been in use since 4000 BC. It was used both for medicinal and recreational purposes as it causes euphoria. By 18th century, opium smoking had become quite popular in Europe. It was Serturner who isolated a pure opium alkaloid in 1806. He named it *Morphine* after Morpheus, the Greek God of dreams. As the research progressed, opium was found to contain 20 alkaloids. By around 19th century, the pure opium alkaloids were available for therapeutic use. But because they were equally abused, efforts were made to isolate the analgesic property, i.e. to obtain an opioid that is only analgesic and has no euphoric effects. In the process, various agonists, antagonists and partial agonists were synthesized. 'Opioid' is the term used for drugs with morphine-like actions. They were earlier called narcotic analgesics.

CLASSIFICATION

1. *Agonists*
   Natural opium alkaloids, e.g. Morphine, Codeine,
   Synthetic opioids, e.g. Pethidine, Methadone
2. *Antagonists* Naloxone, Naltrexone
3. *Mixed agonist-antagonists* Pentazocine, Nalbuphine, Butorphanol, Buprenorphine, Nalorpine

Chemically the opium alkaloids can be grouped into

1. *The Phenanthrene group* Morphine, Codeine, Thebaine
2. *The Benzylisoquinoline group* Papaverine, Noscapine, Narcine.

Opioids can also be classified depending on their source as

1. *Natural opium alkaloids* Morphine, Codeine, Noscapine
2. *Semisynthetic derivatives* Heroin, Oxymorphone, Pholcodeine
3. *Synthetic opioids* Pethidine, Fentanyl, Diphenoxylate, Loperamide, Methadone, Dextropropoxyphene and Tramadol

Morphine is the most important alkaloid of opium. Many new opioids with actions similar to morphine have been synthesized. But none of them are superior to morphine as an analgesic. Morphine is discussed as the prototype of the group.

Mechanism of Action

Morphine and other opioids produce their effects by acting on specific opioid receptors. These receptors are abundant in the CNS and other tissues. The opioid receptors are *mu* (μ) *kappa* (κ) and *delta* (δ). It is found that there are 3 families of endogenous opioid peptides released in the body viz the *enkephalins,* the *endorphins* and the *dynorphins.* This indicates that we have a natural system in the body that releases various opioid peptides in response to pain.

Pharmacological Actions

Central nervous system

1. **Analgesia** Morphine is a potent analgesic and relieves pain without loss of consciousness. Dull aching visceral pain is relieved better than sharp pricking pain. But, in higher doses it relieves even the severe pain as that of biliary colic. Morphine alters both the perception and reaction to pain. It raises the pain threshold and thus increases the capacity to tolerate pain. Further it alters the emotional reaction to pain.

   Euphoria and sedation contribute to its analgesic effects.
2. **Euphoria, sedation and hypnosis** Morphine produces a feeling of well-being termed *euphoria.* It is this effect which makes it an important drug of abuse. Rapid intravenous injection of morphine produces a warm flushing of the skin and an immensely pleasurable sensation in the lower abdomen lasting for about 45 seconds and is known as 'high', 'rush' or 'kick'. The person loses rational thinking and is lost in colourful day dreams. It also produces drowsiness, a calming effect, inability to concentrate, feeling of detachment and indifference to surroundings.

   But the effects of morphine may not be pleasurable in all. A person has to learn to experience its pleasurable effects. It may produce dysphoria in some.
3. **Respiration** Morphine produces significant respiratory depression. It directly depresses the respiratory centre in the brain stem. This action is dose dependent. Death from morphine poisoning is almost always due to respiratory arrest.

   Sedation and indifference to surroundings add to the respiratory depression.
4. **Cough centre** It directly depresses the cough centre and thereby suppresses cough.

5. **Nausea and emesis** Morphine directly stimulates the CTZ in the medulla causing nausea and vomiting. In higher doses it depresses the vomiting centre and hence there is no vomiting in poisoning. Therefore, emetics should not even be tried in poisoning.
6. **Pupils** Morphine produces constriction of pupil resulting in a characteristic pinpoint pupil in high doses by a central effect.
7. **Vagus** Morphine stimulates vagal centre causing bradycardia.
8. **Heat regulation** Opioids act on heat-regulating centre and body temperature falls slightly.
9. **Excitatory effect** In high doses opioids produce convulsions. They may increase the excitability of the spinal cord.

Cardiovascular system In therapeutic doses, morphine produces hypotension by direct peripheral vasodilatation.

In higher doses it causes depression of the vasomotor centre and also brings about histamine release, both causing a fall in BP. Postural hypotension and fainting may occur.

GIT Opioids decrease the motility of the gut.

Stomach Gastric motility is decreased and gastric acid secretion is reduced. Opioids increase the tone of the antrum and first part of the duodenum which also result in delayed emptying by as much as 12 hours.

Intestines Morphine reduces all intestinal secretions, delays digestion of food in the small intestine; resting tone is increased. There can be spasms of the intestine. The tone of the sphincters is increased leading to spasm. The intestinal motility is markedly diminished. Thus, reduced secretions and motility result in marked constipation.

Other smooth muscles

Biliary tract Morphine causes spasm of the sphincter of Oddi and may cause biliary colic.

Urinary bladder and ureter Tone and contractions of the ureter is increased; tone of external sphincter and volume of the bladder are increased. Opioids inhibit urinary voiding reflex.

All these result in urinary retention especially in elderly male with prostatic hypertrophy.

Bronchi Morphine causes release of histamine from the mast cells leading to bronchoconstriction. This can be dangerous in asthmatics.

Neuroendocrine effects Morphine inhibits the release of gonadotrophin-releasing hormone and CRF.

Pharmacokinetics

Given orally, absorption of morphine is slow and incomplete and undergoes extensive first pass metabolism. Bioavailability is 20 to 40 per cent.

Given subcutaneously, onset of action is in 15-20 min, duration of action is 3-5 hr. Morphine is metabolised in the liver by glucuronide conjugation.

Adverse Effects

Morphine can produce a wide range of adverse effects like- nausea, vomiting, dizziness, mental clouding, respiratory depression, constipation, dysphoria, urinary retention and hypotension.

Allergic reactions including skin rashes, pruritus and wheal at the site of injection and rarely anaphylaxis may be seen. This is because morphine liberates histamine. It is a drug of dependance.

Tolerance and dependance Repeated administration of morphine results in the development of tolerance to some of its effects including respiratory depression, analgesia, sedation and euphoriant effects and other CNS depressant effects. Constipation and miosis show no tolerance. Though lethal dose of morphine is about 250 mg, addicts can tolerate morphine in grams. An addict needs progressively higher doses to get his 'kick' or 'rush'. Patients in pain can also tolerate a higher dose of morphine. Cross-tolerance is seen among different opioids.

Dependance Opium has been a drug of addiction for many centuries. Its ability to produce euphoria makes it a drug of addiction. Opioids produce both psychological and physical dependance. Sudden withdrawal of opioids or administration of opioid antagonists produce significant withdrawal symptoms in such dependent individuals. Manifestations are lacrimation, sweating, yawning, anxiety, apprehension, restlessness, running nose and tremors—seen 8-12 hr after the last dose. The person craves for the drug. As the syndrome progresses, fever, insomnia, abdominal colic, severe sneezing, violent yawning, diarrhoea, blurring of vision due to mydriasis, hypertension, severe dehydration, gooseflesh, palpitation and cardiovascular collapse can occur. There is severe weakness, depression and irritability. Goose flesh is due to pilomotor activity; skin resembles that of a plucked turkey. Hence the word 'cold turkey' is used for sudden withdrawal. Abdominal cramps, pain in the bones and muscles of the back and limbs are also characteristic.

Withdrawal symptoms are generally not fatal. Administration of a suitable opioid, dramatically and completely reverses the symptoms of withdrawal. Without treatment, symptoms disappear in 7-10 days.

Withdrawal in the newborn Babies born to mothers who were addicts prior to delivery—will also be dependent. Withdrawal symptoms seen are irritability, excessive crying, tremors, frantic suckling of fists, diarrhoea, sneezing, yawning, vomiting and fever. Tincture of opium is started and gradually withdrawn.

Management of Addiction

Morphine is slowly withdrawn over several days and oral methadone is given.

Advantages of methadone administration are:

1. Methadone is effective orally and by this route no 'kick' is experienced.
2. It is more potent, long-acting and prevents withdrawal symptoms.

The dose is adjusted based on the degree of dependance. Methadone is then slowly withdrawn.

Most addicts can be completely withdrawn from opioids in about 10 days though mild withdrawal symptoms still remain. Symptoms like insomnia, malaise, restlessness, irritability, fatigue and GI hyperactivity may last up to several months.

Clonidine a central α_2 agonist can suppress some of the autonomic withdrawal symptoms like anxiety, nausea, vomiting and diarrhoea. It is given for 7-10 days and withdrawn over 3-4 days. Night time sedation with a hypnotic is helpful.

Uses of Morphine

Dose Morphine 10 to 20 mg IM/SC; 20 mg tab (ethyl morphine) is now available for oral use.

1. *Analgesic* Morphine is one of the most potent analgesics available. It provides **symptomatic relief of pain** without affecting the underlying disease. It is an excellent analgesic for severely painful conditions such as acute myocardial infarction, fractures, burns, pulmonary embolism, terminal stages of cancer, acute pericarditis, spontaneous pneumothorax and post-operative pain. In excruciating pain, morphine can be given IV.

In **MI,** morphine relieves pain and thereby anxiety. As a result reflex sympathetic stimulation is reduced.

- Morphine is given with atropine to relieve **renal and biliary colic.** Atropine relieves spasm
- Since opiate receptors are present in the spinal cord, epidural morphine can be used to produce **epidural analgesia.** There is no interference with motor function or autonomic changes and no systemic adverse effects
- **Obstetric analgesia** Pethidine is preferred to morphine for this condition
- Opioids can be given to control pain of cancers
- But opioids should *not be* freely used in case of other chronic pain because of the risk of addiction

2. *As preanaesthetic medication* Morphine and pethidine are commonly used as preanaesthetic medication. They reduce anxiety, provide analgesia, allow smoother induction and reduce the dose of the anaesthetic required. But they have certain disadvantages:

- Opioids depress respiration
- Morphine may cause bronchospasm and is dangerous in patients with poor respiratory reserve
- They cause vasomotor depression

- They may induce vomiting
- Postoperative urinary retention and constipation may be troublesome.

3. *Acute left ventricular failure* Morphine relieves the dyspnoea of LVF and pulmonary oedema. The mechanism is not clear. The relief may be due to:

i. reduction in the work of the heart due to decreased anxiety. Reduced anxiety decreases sympathetic stimulation which inturn decreases cardiac work.

iii. cardiovascular effects like decreased PVR reduces the cardiac work load.

4. *Diarrhoea* Opioids are effective for the symptomatic treatment of diarrhoea. Synthetic opioids—diphenoxylate and loperamide are preferred as antidiarrheals.

5. *Cough* Codeine and noscapine are the preferred opioids for this purpose. But now many nonaddictive antitussives are available for the treatment of cough.

6. *Special anaesthesia*
   - High doses of morphine can be used IV to produce general anaesthesia
   - Neuroleptanalgesia—fentanyl an opioid, can be used to produce neuroleptanalgesia with droperidol (page 181)
   - Morphine can be used epidurally for the relief of post operative and chronic pain.

7. *Sedative* Morphine relieves anxiety in threatened abortion without affecting uterine motility. It is an useful sedative in the presence of pain.

Acute morphine poisoning may be accidental, suicidal or homicidal. Lethal dose in non-addicts is about 250 mg but addicts can tolerate grams of morphine. Signs and symptoms include respiratory depression with shallow breathing, pin point pupils, hypotension, shock, cyanosis, flaccidity, stupor, hypothermia, coma and death due to respiratory failure and pulmonary oedema.

Treatment

1. Positive pressure respiration.
2. Maintenance of BP.
3. Gastric lavage with potassium permanganate to remove unabsorbed drug.
4. Specific antidote is naloxone—0.4-0.8 mg IV repeated every 10-15 min.

Precautions and Contraindications

1. Avoid opioids in patients with respiratory insufficiency—COPD.
2. An attack of bronchial asthma can be precipitated by morphine.
3. Head injury—morphine is contraindicated because:
   i. morphine increases CSF pressure.
   ii. causes respiratory depression.
   iii. vomiting, miosis and mental clouding produced by morphine makes it difficult to treat head injuries.
5. In hypovolaemic shock, morphine further decreases the BP.
6. Opioids potentiate CNS depressants.
7. Undiagnosed acute abdomen—morphine relieves pain, may cause vomiting and constipation. All these may interfere with the diagnosis. Hence it can be administered only after the diagnosis is made.

OTHER OPIOIDS

Codeine is a naturally occurring opium alkaloid. Codeine depresses the cough centre even in low doses. It is effective orally and is well-absorbed.

It is less potent (one-sixth) than morphine as an analgesic (60 mg codeine = 10 mg morphine).

It produces less respiratory depression and is less constipating. Codeine has less addiction liability and less chances of tolerance. It is well absorbed on oral administration.

Hence codeine is used as an antitussive. Duration of action is 4-6 hr. Constipation is the most common side effect.

Uses Codeine is a commonly used antitussive. It is also available in combination with paracetamol for analgesia. It is to be given at bedtime (CODOPLUS → Codeine 30 mg + Paracetamol 500 mg).

Papaverine is devoid of opioid and analgesic activity.

Noscapine is a naturally occurring opium alkaloid. In therapeutic doses, it has no other actions on the CNS except for antitussive effects. Hence it has no disadvantages of opioids. *Dose:* 15-30 mg—3-4 times a day. Noscapine is highly effective and safe. The only adverse effect is nausea. It is used as a cough suppressant.

Several other centrally acting antitussives have been synthesized including, pholcodeine and dextromethorphan.

Pholcodeine is structurally related to opioids and is an effective antitussive. It has a long half-life and therefore can be given once a day.

Dextromethorphan has no analgesic or addictive properties. It acts centrally as an antitussive. Toxicity is very low; extremely high doses cause CNS depression. Antitussive dose: 10-30 mg, 3-4 times a day.

PETHIDINE (Meperidine) Pethidine is a derivative of morphine. Many of its actions resemble that of morphine. When compared to morphine:

- pethidine is $^{1}/_{10}$th as potent as morphine (100 mg pethidine = 10 mg morphine). However, as an analgesic pethidine is equal to morphine
- the onset of action is more rapid and duration of action is shorter
- it produces corneal anaesthesia
- it is not a good antitussive
- it is less constipating
- in some patients, it may cause dysphoria
- in toxic doses, pethidine sometimes produces CNS stimulation and convulsions instead of sedation.

Adverse effects are similar to morphine except that constipation and urinary retention are less common.

Uses

Dose 25-100 mg IM/SC is the analgesic dose.

In pain Pethidine is used as an analgesic in visceral pain and also for other indications of morphine. Because of efficacy and less spasmogenic effect, it is preferred to morphine.

During labour Given during labour, pethidine produces less respiratory depression in the newborn when compared to morphine and is therefore preferred to morphine for obstetric analgesia.

Preanaesthetic medication—pethidine can also be used as preanaesthetic medication.

DERIVATIVES OF PETHIDINE

Fentanyl is a pethidine congener. It is about 80 times more potent than morphine as an analgesic and is faster acting. It is used in combination with droperidol, a neuroleptic agent to produce 'neuroleptanalgesia.' The combination is given IV to produce sedation and intense analgesia without loss of consciousness. This state is maintained for 30-40 minutes as both have rapid and short action.

A fixed dose combination is available with 0.05 mg fentanyl + 2.5 mg droperidol per ml. 5 ml is the dose used IV over 10 minutes. Patient is drowsy but responds to commands.

i. neuroleptoanalgesia is useful for short surgical procedures especially in 'poor risk' patients.
ii. epidural fentanyl is used for postoperative and obstetric analgesia.
iii. Fentanyl is also used for chronic pain. Transdermal patches of fentanyl are available.

Other derivatives of pethidine *alfentanil, sufentanil* and *ramifentanil* are similar to fentanyl.

Methadone a synthetic opioid, has actions similar to morphine. It's main features are:

- It is an effective analgesic
- It is effective by oral route
- It has a long duration of action and therefore effectively suppresses withdrawal symptoms in addicts.

Methadone is about 90% bound to plasma proteins; it is firmly bound to proteins in various tissues, including brain. After repeated administration, it accumulates in tissues. When administration is stopped, it is slowly released from these binding sites. Hence, its withdrawal symptoms are mild. As euphoric effects are less intense, abuse potential is less. Tolerance develops more slowly. Even in addicts, withdrawal symptoms are gradual in onset, less intense, but prolonged.

Uses

1. *In opioid dependance.* In morphine addicts oral methadone is given and morphine is stopped. Methadone prevents withdrawal symptoms in them (see page 179).
2. *Opioid maintenance:* Gradually increasing doses of methadone is given orally to produce a high degree of tolerance. Such subjects do not experience the pleasurable effects of IV morphine, because of tolerance, i.e. opioids are not pleasurable in them and they give up the habit.
3. Methadone can also be used as an *analgesic.*

Dextropropoxyphene is a congener of methadone. It binds to the opioid receptors and produces effects similar to morphine. It is less constipating and is orally effective. But dextropropoxyphene is an irritant when given parenterally. Large doses cause CNS stimulation. It also has abuse potential.

Uses Used in mild to moderate pain. It is marketed in combination with aspirin.

Dextropropoxyphene 32 mg + aspirin 600 mg.

Tramadol is a recently developed synthetic analgesic. It is a weak opioid agonist. In addition it inhibits the re-uptake of noradrenaline and serotonin in the CNS. The mechanism of action is not clear.

Adverse effects include drowsiness, dryness of mouth and nausea. It is a drug of dependence. It may precipitate seizures.

Tramadol is used in acute and chronic pain, like post-operative pain and neuralgias.

MIXED AGONISTS AND ANTAGONISTS

They include—pentazocine, nalbuphine, buprenorphine, butarphanol and nalorphine.

Pentazocine In an attempt to develop an analgesic with less risk of addiction and low adverse effects, pentazocine was developed. Pentazocine it is a κ receptor agonist.

- CNS effects of pentazocine are similar to morphine. Euphoria is seen only in low doses. With higher doses—dysphoria can occur due to κ receptor stimulation.
- Sedation and respiratory depression are less.
- It has weak antagonistic properties at μ receptors.
- Tolerance and dependance develop on repeated use.
- CVS—in contrast to morphine, pentazocine causes ↑BP and ↑heart rate and thereby increases cardiac work. It is therefore **not** suitable in MI.
- Biliary spasm and constipation are less severe.
- Pentazocine can be given both orally and parenterally. It undergoes first pass metabolism.
- Dose 50-100 mg oral; 30-60 mg IM (FORTWIN).

Adverse effects Sedation, sweating, dizziness, nausea, dysphoria with anxiety, nightmares and hallucinations, which are unpleasant are seen above 60 mg. As it is an irritant, IM injection can be painful and cause sterile abscesses.

Uses Pentazocine is a commonly used opioid analgesic especially in postoperative and chronic pain—abuse liability is less than morphine.

Nalbuphine is an agonist-antagonist—like pentazocine. It is a good analgesic. Though it produces respiratory depression like morphine, it has a ceiling effect at 30 mg, i.e. an increase in dose beyond 30 mg does not increase respiratory depression further. Higher doses produce dysphoria.

Uses As analgesic—10-20 mg IM.

Buprenorphine is a highly lipid soluble synthetic opioid. It is a partial μ agonist, 25 times as potent as morphine. Though onset of action is slow, duration of analgesia is long. Other CNS effects are similar to morphine while respiratory depression is less. Patients exhibit lower degree of tolerance and dependance liability. Withdrawal syndrome appears late and is mild.

Dose 0.3-0.6 mg SC, IM or sublingual (oral not available).

Uses Chronic pain like terminal cancer.

Butorphanol is similar to pentazocine.

Nalorphine is also an agonist-antagonist. At low doses, it is a good analgesic. But it causes dysphoria (κ agonist) and respiratory depression even in low doses. Hence it cannot be used as an analgesic. At high doses it acts as an antagonist and counters all the actions of opioids.

Uses Nalorphine may be used in acute opioid poisoning. It can also be used for the diagnosis of opioid addiction.

OPIOID ANTAGONISTS

Naloxone is a pure antagonist—acts as a competitive antagonist to all types of opioid receptors. In normal individuals, it does not produce any significant actions. But in opium addicts, given IV, it promptly antagonises all the actions of morphine including respiratory depression and sedation and precipitates withdrawal syndrome. It also blocks the action of endogenous opioid peptides—endorphins, enkephalins and dynorphins. It blocks the analgesia produced by placebo and acupuncture. This suggests that endogenous opioid peptides are responsible for analgesia by these methods.

Given orally it undergoes first pass metabolism and is metabolised by the liver. Duration of action is 3-4 hours.

Uses

1. Naloxone is the drug of choice for morphine overdosage.
2. It is also used to reverse neonatal asphyxia due to opioids used in the mother during labour.
3. Naloxone can also be used for the diagnosis of opioid dependance—it precipitates withdrawal in addicts.
4. Hypotension seen during shock could be due to endogenous opioids released during such stress. Naloxone has been found to be beneficial in reversing such hypotension.

Naltrexone is another pure opioid antagonist. It is

- orally effective
- has a longer duration of action of 1-2 days.

Naltrexone is used for 'opioid blockade' therapy in post addicts so that even if such persons take an opioid, they do not experience the pleasurable effects and therefore lose the liking for opioids.

Alcohol craving is also reduced by naltrexone and is used to prevent relapse of heavy drinking.

❑ NONSTEROIDAL ANTI-INFLAMMATORY DRUGS (NSAIDs)

NSAIDs are aspirin-type or non-opioid analgesics. In addition they have anti-inflammatory, antipyretic and uricosuric properties—without addiction liability.

The medicinal effects of the bark of the willow tree has been known since centuries. The active principle 'salicin' was isolated from the willow bark. This salicin is converted to glucose and salicylic acid in the body. In 1875, sodium salicylate was first used in the treatment of rheumatic fever. After its anti-inflammatory and uricosuric properties were established, efforts were made to synthesize derivatives which were less expensive. Now they have replaced the natural ones in the market.

Mechanism of Action

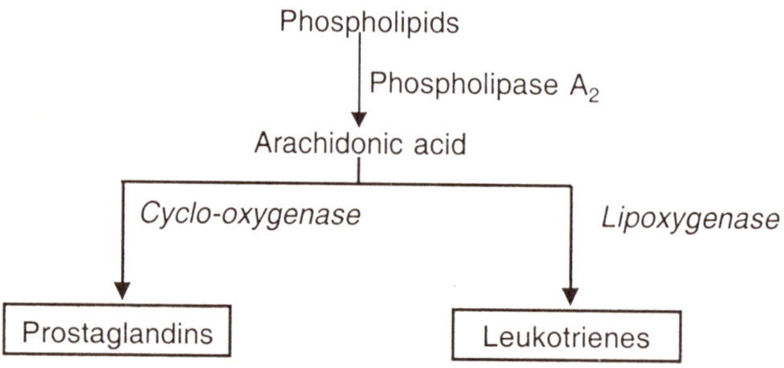

CLASSIFICATION

1. ***Salicylic acid derivatives***—Aspirin, Sodium salicylate, Diflunisal
2. ***Para-aminophenol derivatives***—Paracetamol
3. ***Pyrazolone derivatives***—Phenylbutazone, Azapropazone

4. *Indole acetic acid derivatives*—Indomethacin, Sulindac
5. *Arylacetic acid derivatives*—Diclofenac, Ketorolac, Tolmetin
6. *Propionic acid derivatives*—Ibuprofen, Fenoprofen, Carprofen, Naproxen, Ketoprofen, Oxaprozin
7. *Anthranilic acids (Fenamates)*—Flufenamic acid, Mefenamic acid, Enfenamic acid
8. *Oxicams*—Piroxicam, Tenoxicam
9. *Alkanones*—Nabumetone
10. *Sulfonanilide derivative*—Nimesulide, Celecoxib.

During inflammation, arachidonic acid liberated from membrane phospholipids is converted to prostaglandins (PGs), catalysed by the enzyme cyclo-oxygenase. These prostaglandins produce hyperalgesia—they sensitize the nerve endings to pain and other mediators of inflammation like bradykinin and histamine.

NSAIDs inhibit the PG synthesis by inhibiting the enzyme cyclo-oxygenase.

SALICYLATES

Salicylates are salts of salicylic acid, e.g. methyl salicylate, sodium salicylate, acetyl salicylic acid (aspirin). Aspirin is taken as the prototype.

PHARMACOLOGICAL ACTIONS

1. **Analgesia** Aspirin is a good analgesic and relieves pain of inflammatory origin without euphoria. Pain originating from the integumental structures like muscles, bones, joints, and pain in connective tissues is relieved. But in vague visceral pain, aspirin is relatively ineffective.

The pain is relieved without euphoria and hypnosis. Hence there is no development of tolerance and dependance. But aspirin is a weak analgesic when compared to morphine.

2. **Antipyretic action** In fever, salicylates bring down the temperature to normal level. But, in normal individuals, there is no change in temperature.

In fever, pyrogen—a protein, circulates in the body and this increases the synthesis of PGs in the hypothalamus, thereby raising its temperature set point. The thermostatic mechanism in the hypothalamus is thus disturbed. Aspirin inhibits PG synthesis in the hypothalamus and resets the thermostat at the normal level bringing down the temperature.

Enhanced sweating and cutaneous vasodilatation promote heat loss and assist in the antipyretic action.

3. **Anti-inflammatory action** At higher doses of 4-6 gm/day, aspirin acts as an anti-inflammatory agent. Signs of inflammation like tenderness, swelling, erythema and pain are all reduced or suppressed. But, the progression of the disease in rheumatoid arthritis, rheumatic fever or osteoarthritis is not affected.

Once again the mechanism of action is PG synthesis inhibition—PGs present in inflammatory tissue are responsible for oedema, erythema and pain. In addition, aspirin also interferes with the formation of chemical mediators of the kallikrein system. As a result, it decreases the adherence of granulocytes to the damaged vasculature, stabilizes lysomes and decreases the migration of the polymorphonuclear leukocytes and macrophages into the site of inflammation.

4. **Respiration** In therapeutic doses of 4-6 gm/day—salicylates increase consumption of oxygen by skeletal muscles. As a result there is $\uparrow CO_2$ production. The $\uparrow CO_2$ stimulates respiratory centre. Salicylates also directly stimulate the medullary respiratory centre. Both these actions increase the rate and depth of respiration. These effects are dose dependent.

As a result of this stimulation of respiration, plasma CO_2 is washed out leading to respiratory alkalosis. With toxic doses, the respiratory centre is depressed leading to respiratory failure.

5. **Acid-base and electrolyte balance** In anti-inflammatory doses, salicylates produce significant respiratory stimulation so that CO_2 is washed out resulting in respiratory alkalosis; pH becomes alkaline. This is compensated by increased excretion of HCO_3^- in urine.

With toxic doses, salicylates depress the respiratory centre directly. As a result, CO_2 accumulates, plasma CO_2 level rises and pH decreases, i.e. there is acidosis.

Toxic doses also depress vasomotor centre. This vasomotor depression impairs renal function resulting in accumulation of strong acids of metabolic origin like lactic, pyruvic and acetoacetic acids.

The above effects are accompanied by dehydration due to:

- water lost in urine with HCO_3^-, Na^+ and K^+
- increased sweating
- water lost during hyperventilation.

Thus high doses cause severe dehydration with acidosis.

6. **Metabolic effects** Salicylates enhance the cellular metabolism. More of O_2 is used and more CO_2 is produced, especially in skeletal muscles—leading to increased heat production. Glucose utilization is increased leading to mild hypoglycaemia.

In toxic doses, hyperpyrexia, increased protein catabolism, negative nitrogen balance and hyperglycaemia (due to central sympathetic stimulation which increases adrenaline levels) can occur.

7. **Gastrointestinal tract** Aspirin is a gastric irritant. Irritation of the gastric mucosa leads to epigastric distress, nausea and vomiting. Aspirin also stimulates the CTZ to produce vomiting.

Gastric erosion, ulceration and GI bleeding can occur particularly in higher doses.

Mechanism: Salicylates increase gastric acid secretion and suppress the protective effect of prostaglandins by inhibiting their synthesis (we know that PGs increase mucous production in the stomach and protect from ulceration).

In addition it decreases platelet aggregation which also increases the tendency to bleed.

8. **CVS** In therapeutic doses no significant cardiovascular effects are seen. In toxic doses it depresses the VMC and thus depresses the circulation.

9. **Immunological effects** In higher doses, salicylates suppress several antigen-antibody reactions. It inhibits antibody production, Ag-Ab aggregation and antigen induced release of histamine. These effects might also help in rheumatic fever.

10. **Uric acid excretion** Uric acid is excreted by secretion from the distal tubules. In a dose of 1-2 gm/day, aspirin increases

plasma urate levels because it inhibits urate secretion by the distal tubules.

Large doses of > 5 gm/day increase urate excretion because it inhibits reabsorption of urate by the proximal tubule causing uricosuria. But, its uricosuric effect cannot be used for treatment of Gout because high doses are required and such doses result in many adverse effects.

11. **Blood** Even in small doses aspirin inhibits TXA_2 synthesis by platelets. It therefore interferes with platelet aggregation and prolongs the bleeding time. Even a single dose can irreversibly inhibit TXA_2 synthesis in platelets.

12. **Local effects** Salicylic acid when applied locally is a keratolytic. It also has mild antiseptic and fungistatic properties. Salicylic acid is also an irritant for the broken skin.

PHARMACOKINETICS

Salicylates are absorbed from the stomach and the upper small intestine. But aspirin as such is poorly soluble, hence not well-absorbed. When administered as microfine particles, absorption increases. Thus particle size, pH of the GIT, solubility of the preparation and presence of food in the stomach influence the absorption.

Salicylic acid and methylsalicylate are absorbed from the intact skin. They are extensively bound to plasma proteins. Aspirin is broken down in the liver, plasma and other tissues to release salicylic acid which is the active form. Plasma t½ of aspirin is 3-5 hours. Salicylates are excreted in the urine.

ADVERSE EFFECTS

1. Nausea, epigastric distress, vomiting, erosive gastritis, peptic ulcer, increased occult blood loss in stools are common.
2. Allergic reactions are manifested as rashes, urticaria, angio-oedema, and asthma especially in those with a history of allergies.
3. Salicylates can cause haemolysis in patients with G_6PD deficiency.
4. Nephrotoxicity: Almost all NSAIDs can cause nephrotoxicity after long-term use.

5. Hepatotoxicity can also occur.
6. *Reye's Syndrome* seen in children is a form of hepatic dysfunction which may be fatal. It develops a few days after a viral infection especially influenza and varicella. An increased incidence of this syndrome has been noted when aspirin is used to treat fever. Hence aspirin is contraindicated in children with viral fever.
7. *Pregnancy and infancy* Aspirin when taken in full term pregnancy delays the onset of labour due to inhibition of PG synthesis (PGs play an important role in the initiation of labour).

   Premature closure of ductus arteriosus may occur in the foetus resulting in portal hypertension. It can also increase postpartum bleeding due to inhibition of platelet aggregation.
8. *Salicylism* Prolonged administration of salicylates as in the treatment of rheumatoid arthritis may lead to chronic salicylate intoxication termed 'Salicylism'. The syndrome is characterised by headache, vertigo, dizziness, tinnitus, vomiting, mental confusion, diarrhoea, sweating, difficulty in hearing, thirst and dehydration. These symptoms are reversible on withdrawal of salicylates.

Acute salicylate intoxication Poisoning may be accidental or suicidal. It is more common in children, 15-30 g is the fatal dose of aspirin.

Symptoms and signs Dehydration, hyperpyrexia, GI irritation, vomiting, sometimes haematemesis, acid-base imbalance, restlessness, delirium, hallucinations, metabolic acidosis, tremors, convulsions, coma and death due to respiratory failure and cardiovascular collapse.

Treatment is symptomatic and includes:

1. Stomach wash lavage to eliminate unabsorbed drugs.
2. IV fluids to correct acid-base imbalance and dehydration.
3. Temperature is brought down by external cooling with alcohol or cold water sponges.
4. If there is bleeding, blood transfusion and vitamin K are needed.
5. The IV fluids should contain Na^+, K^+, HCO_3^- and glucose (to treat hypokalaemia and acidosis).

6. In severe cases, forced alkaline diuresis with sodium bicarbonate and a diuretic like frusemide is given along with IV fluids. Sodium bicarbonate make salicylates water soluble and increases their excretion through kidneys.

Precautions and Contraindications

Peptic ulcer, liver diseases, bleeding tendencies, children suffering from viral fever and pregnancy are contraindications for the use of salicylates. Treatment with NSAIDs should be stopped one week before any surgery.

PREPARATIONS

Preparations and dosage of salicylates (Table 6.4).

TABLE 6.4: Preparations and dosage of salicylates

Drug	*Preparation*	*Dose*
Aspirin	300, 350 tab (ASABUF);	Analgesic—300-600 mg every 6-8 hr
	DISPRIN (Apirin 350 mg and Calcium carbonate 105 mg)	Anti-inflammatory—4-6 gm/day Antiplatelet effects—75-300 mg/day
Sodium salicylate	325, 650 mg tablets	325-650 mg every 4-8 hr
Salicylic acid	2% ointment; Whitfield's ointment- – Salicylic acid 3% – Benzoic acid 6%	For topical use
Methylsalicylate (Oil of wintergreen)	Ointment/liniment for topical use	As counter irritant
Diflunisal	250, 500 mg tab (DOLOBID)	250 mg every 8-12 hr

USES

1. *As analgesic* for headache, backache, myalgias, arthralgias, neuralgias, toothache and dysmenorrhoea. The NSAIDs are beneficial in a variety of painful conditions of integumental origin.

2. *Fever* NSAIDs are useful for the symptomatic relief of fever.

3. *For inflammatory conditions* Aspirin is effective in a number of inflammatory conditions such as arthritis and fibromyositis.

4. *Acute rheumatic fever* In a dose of 4-6 g/day, aspirin brings about a dramatic relief of signs and symptoms in 24 to 48 hr. The dose is reduced after 4-7 days and maintenance doses of 2-3 gm/day are given for 2-3 weeks.

5. *Rheumatoid arthritis* Aspirin relieves pain, reduces swelling and redness of joints in rheumatoid arthritis. Joint mobility improves, fever subsides, and there is a reduction in morning stiffness. But NSAIDs do not alter the progress of the disease. The relief is only symptomatic.

   Dose 4-6 g/day in 4-6 divided doses.

6. *Osteoarthritis* It provides symptomatic relief in osteoarthritis.

7. *Postmyocardial infarction and post-stroke* Aspirin in a low dose inhibits platelet aggregation and by this it may prevent reinfarction. It also decreases the incidence of transient ischaemic attacks (TIA) and stroke in such patients.

8. *Miscellaneous uses*
   i. To delay labour—since PGs are involved in the initiation of labour, aspirin delays labour due to PG synthesis inhibition.
   ii. Patent Ductus Arteriosus. Aspirin may bring about closure of PDA in the newborn.

9. *Local* Salicylic acid is used as a keratolytic, fungistatic and mild antiseptic. Methylsalicylate is a counter-irritant used in myalgias.

DRUG INTERACTIONS

- Salicylates compete for protein binding sites and displace other drugs resulting in toxicity with warfarin, heparin, naproxen, phenytoin and sulfonylureas.
- Inhibition of platelet aggregation may increase the risk of bleeding with oral anticoagulants.

Diflunisal is a derivative of salicylic acid. Diflunisal is 3-4 times more potent than aspirin as an anti-inflammatory agent but is a poor antipyretic due to poor penetration into CNS. Gastrointestinal and antiplatelet effects are less intense than aspirin. Side effects are fewer.

Uses Osteoarthritis, strain and sprains. Initial dose 500-1000 mg followed by 250 mg twice or thrice daily.

PARA-AMINOPHENOL DERIVATIVES

Paracetamol (acetaminophen) Phenacetin was the first drug used in this group. But, due to severe adverse effects it is now banned.

Paracetamol, a metabolite of phenacetin is found to be safer and effective.

Actions Paracetamol has analgesic, good antipyretic and weak anti-inflammatory properties. Due to weak PG inhibitory activity in the periphery, it has poor anti-inflammatory actions.

Paracetamol is active on cyclo-oxygenase in the brain because of which it acts as an antipyretic. In the presence of peroxides which are present at the site of inflammation, paracetamol has poor ability to inhibit cyclo-oxygenase. It is therefore a poor anti-inflammatory agent. It does not stimulate respiration, has no actions on acid-base balance, cellular metabolism, cardiovascular system and platelet function; it is not an uricosuric agent and gastric irritation is mild.

Pharmacokinetics Paracetamol is well-absorbed orally, 30% protein bound; metabolised by the hepatic microsomal enzymes: by glucuronide and glutathione conjugation.

Adverse effects In antipyretic doses, paracetamol is safe and well-tolerated. Nausea and rashes may occur. But when large doses are taken, *acute paracetamol poisoning* results. Children are more susceptible because their ability to conjugate by glucuronidation is poor. 10-15 gm in adults cause serious toxicity. Symptoms are—nausea, vomiting, anorexia and abdominal pain during first 24 hrs. Paracetamol is hepatotoxic and causes severe hepatic damage. Manifestations are seen within

2-4 days and include increased serum transaminases, jaundice, liver tenderness and prolonged prothrombin time which may progress to liver failure in some patients. Hepatic lesions are reversible when promptly treated.

Nephrotoxicity may result in acute renal failure in some.

Mechanism A small portion of paracetamol is metabolised to a toxic compound—N-acetyl-benzoquinone-imine which is destroyed generally by conjugation with glutathione. But when large doses of paracetamol are taken, hepatic glutathione gets used up and the levels of toxic compound increase. It causes hepatic necrosis.

Chronic alcoholics and infants are more prone to hepatotoxicity.

Treatment Stomach wash is given. Activated charcoal prevents further absorption. Antidote is N-acetylcysteine which is more effective when given early.

Uses

- Paracetamol is used as an analgesic in painful conditions like toothache, headache and myalgia
- As an antipyretic in fevers.

PYRAZOLON DERIVATIVES

Phenylbutazone has good anti-inflammatory activity, but has poorer analgesic and antipyretic effects. It is an uricosuric agent.

Phenylbutazone causes retention of Na^+ and water. Thus, after 1-2 weeks of use oedema results. It can also precipitate congestive cardiac failure.

Pharmacokinetics Completely absorbed orally; IM injection is not recommended because its absorption is slow as it binds to local tissue proteins and also causes local tissue damage. It is 98% bound to plasma proteins; t½ is 60 hours.

Dose 100-200 mg, BD. Small doses may be given 3-4 times a day to avoid gastric irritation.

Adverse effects

- Phenylbutazone is more toxic than aspirin and is poorly tolerated—dyspepsia, epigastric distress, nausea and vomiting, peptic ulceration and diarrhoea may occur. Oedema and CCF can occur.

- Hypersensitivity reactions like rashes, serum sickness, stomatitis, hepatitis, nephritis, dermatitis and jaundice can occur. Phenylbutazone may cause serious haematological complications such as bone marrow depression, aplastic anaemia, agranulocytosis and thrombocytopenia.
- It may inhibit iodine uptake by thyroid resulting in hypothyroidism and goitre on long-term use.
- CNS effects like insomnia, vertigo, optic neuritis, blurring of vision and convulsions may be encountered.

Because of its toxicity, phenylbutazone is withdrawn from the market in many western countries.

Uses

1. Rheumatoid arthritis
2. Ankylosing spondylitis
3. Osteoarthritis
4. Gout—phenylbutazone produces satisfactory relief from pain and inflammation in acute attacks
5. Other musculoskeletal disorders.

Azapropazone is structurally related to phenylbutazone but is less likely to cause agranulocytosis; t½ is 12-16 hr.

Metamizol is a potent analgesic and antipyretic, but poor anti-inflammatory agent and has no uricosuric properties (ANALGIN, NOVALGIN) 500 mg 3-4 times a day. It offers no advantages over aspirin. Not recommended in children upto 6 years.

Propiphenazone is similar to metamizol.
Dose 300-600 mg 3-4 times a day (SARIDON).

INDOLE ACETIC ACID DERIVATIVES

Indomethacin is a potent anti-inflammatory agent, antipyretic and good analgesic. It is well-absorbed, 90% bound to plasma proteins; t½—4-6 hr.
Dose 25-50 mg BD-TDS.

Adverse effects are high Gastrointestinal irritation with nausea, gastrointestinal bleeding, vomiting, diarrhoea and peptic ulcers can occur.

CNS effects include headache, dizziness, ataxia, confusion, hallucinations, depression and psychosis.

Hypersensitivity reactions like skin rashes, leukopenia, and asthma are common. It can also cause bleeding due to decreased platelet aggregation and oedema due to salt and water retention.

Drug interactions Indomethacin blunts the diuretic action of furosemide and the antihypertensive action of thiazides, furosemide, β-blockers and ACE inhibitors by causing salt and water retention.

Uses

- Rheumatoid arthritis
- Gout
- Ankylosing spondylitis
- Psoriatic arthritis
- For closure of patent ductus arteriosus (PDA).

Sulindac has weaker analgesic, antipyretic and anti-inflammatory actions but is less toxic. Does not antagonize the diuretic and antihypertensive actions of thiazides. It may be used as an alternative drug for inflammatory conditions.

Diclofenac is an analgesic, antipyretic and anti-inflammatory agent. It's tissue penetrability is good and attains good concentration in synovial fluid which is maintained for a long time. Adverse effects are mild.

Dose 50 mg BD–TDS. Gel is available for topical application (INAC GEL). Ophthalmic preparation is available for use in postoperative pain.

Uses

1. Treatment of chronic inflammatory conditions like rheumatoid arthritis and osteoarthritis.
2. Acute musculoskeletal pain.
3. Postoperatively for relief of pain and inflammation.

Ketorolac Another PG synthesis inhibitor having good analgesic and anti-inflammatory properties. It is used to relieve postoperative pain. It is mostly used parenterally though is can also be given orally.

PROPIONIC ACID DERIVATIVES

Ibuprofen is better tolerated than aspirin. Analgesic, antipyretic and anti-inflammatory efficacy is slightly lower than aspirin. It is 99% bound to plasma proteins.

Adverse effects are milder and the incidence is lower. Nausea, vomiting, gastric discomfort, CNS effects, hypersensitivity reactions, fluid retention are all similar but **less severe**.

Dose Ibuprofen—400-800 mg TDS (BRUFEN); Ibuprofen + paracetamol (COMBIFLAM).

Uses

1. As an analgesic in painful conditions.
2. In fever.
3. Soft tissue injuries, fractures, following tooth extraction, to relieve postoperative pain, dysmenorrhoea and osteoarthritis.
4. Gout.

Other propionic acid derivatives like fenoprofen, ketoprofen, corprofen and naproxen are similar to ibuprofen in actions. Oxaprozin is long acting and given once daily.

ANTHRANILLIC ACID DERIVATIVES

Fenamates are analgesic, antipyretic, anti-inflammatory drugs with less efficacy, and are more toxic; contraindicated in children. They should not be used for more than one week. Though they can be used as analgesics they are not preferred.

OXICAMS

Piroxicam is an oxicam derivative. It is long-acting, has good anti-inflammatory, analgesic and antipyretic activity. No clinically significant drug interactions are seen; better tolerated as it is less ulcerogenic. Dose 20 mg OD. It is **long-acting.** Piroxicam is used for rheumatoid arthritis, osteoarthritis, ankylosing spondylitis, acute musculoskeletal pain and postoperative pain.

Meloxicam, pivoxicam and ***tenoxicam*** are other oxicams with action and adverse effects similar to piroxicam.

ALKANONES

Nabumetone is an anti-inflammatory agent with significant efficacy in rheumatoid arthritis and osteoarthritis. It has a relatively low incidence of side effects, it is comparatively less ulcerogenic. Nabumetone is a prodrug and also selectively inhibits COX-2 due to these, nabumetone causes less gastric irritation.

It is used in rheumatoid and osteoarthritis.

SULFONANILIDE DERIVATIVES

Nimesulide a sulfonamide, compound is a weak inhibitor of PG synthesis with a higher affinity for COX-2 than COX-1. It inhibits leukocyte function, prevents the release of mediators and in addition has antihistaminic and antiallergic properties. Nimesulide has analgesic, antipyretic and anti-inflammatory actions like other NSAIDs.

Nimesulide is well-absorbed orally, extensively bound to plasma proteins and has a t½ of 3 hours. It is excreted by the kidney.

Dose 50-100 mg BD

Adverse effects are generally mild; they are nausea, epigastric pain, rashes, drowsiness and dizziness. But it can cause serious hepatotoxicity because of which it is now banned.

Uses Nimesulide was used in headache, toothache, myalgia, dysmenorrhoea, sinusitis, postoperative pain and arthritis. It is beneficial in patients who develop bronchospasm with other NSAIDs.

Celecoxib a sulfonamide, is a highly selective COX-2 inhibitor. It is an effective anti-inflammatory agent useful in rheumatoid arthritis and osteoarthritis. Early studies have shown it to be less ulcerogenic while other adverse effects are similar to other NSAIDs. It does not affect platelet aggregation. **Rofecoxib** has properties similar to celecoxib.

ANTAGONISTS OF LEUKOTRIENE SYNTHESIS AND LEUKOTRIENE RECEPTORS

Zileuton, docebenone, piriprost—Some of them inhibit 5-lipoxygenase and thereby prevent the synthesis of leukotrienes, while others act as competitive antagonists of LT receptor. They are useful in asthma and other inflammatory conditions.

Adverse effects Dyspepsia, diarrhea and headache.

Drugs that block both cyclo-oxygenase and lipoxygenase are tenidap, diclofenac and indomethacin. Tenidap also blocks IL-1 formation.

❑ DRUGS USED IN RHEUMATOID ARTHRITIS AND GOUT

Rheumatoid arthritis (RA) is a chronic, progressive, autoimmune, inflammatory disease, mainly affecting the joints and the periarticular tissues. The antigen-antibody complexes trigger the pathological process. Mediators of inflammation released in the joints initiate the inflammatory process. The earliest lesion is vasculitis, followed by synovial oedema and infiltration with inflammatory cells. There is local synthesis of prostaglandins and leukotrienes. Prostaglandins cause vasodilation and pain. The inflammatory cells release lysosomal enzymes which cause damage to bones and cartilage.

Drugs Used in the Treatment of Rheumatoid Arthritis

1. NSAIDs
2. DMDs — Gold, d-penicillamine, Chloroquine and Hydroxychloroquine, Sulphasalazine, TNF blocking drugs
3. Immunosuppressants — Methotrexate, Cyclophosphamide, Azathioprine, Leflunomide
4. Adjuvants — Glucocorticoids

Nonsteroidal Anti-inflammatory Drugs (NSAIDs)

Nonsteroidal anti-inflammatory drugs are the first line drugs in rheumatoid arthritis. NSAIDs afford symptomatic relief but do not modify the course of the disease.

Disease Modifying Drugs (DMDs)

Disease modifying drugs are also called *disease modifying anti-rheumatic drugs (DMARDs).* These are the second line drugs

TABLE 6.5: Properties of some commonly used NSAIDs

Drugs	*Properties*	*Advantages*	*Uses*
Aspirin	Good analgesic, antipyretic, anti-inflammatory and uricosuric agent	Antiplatelet activity even in low doses; Powerful anti-inflammatory activity	As analgesic—headache backache, neuralgias, dysmenorrhea; pyrexia, rheumatic fever, rheumatic, psoriatic and osteoarthritis, for anti-platelet activity in post-stroke and post-MI; closure of PDA; to delay labour
Paracetamol	Good analgesic, antipyretic but poor anti-inflammatory	Less gastric irritation	As analgesic; in fever
Diclofenac	Analgesic, antipyretic, anti-inflammatory	Good concentration in synovial fluid; adverse effects mild	Chronic inflammatory conditions; rheumatoid arthritis, osteoarthritis, acute musculoskeletal pain and postoperative pain
Piroxicam	Analgesic, antipyretic, anti-inflammatory	Long-acting (given once a day), less ulcerogenic, better tolerated	Arthritis, musculoskeletal pain, postoperative pain
Phenylbutazone	Good anti-inflammatory; poor analgesic, antipyretic; salt and water retention causes oedema; more toxic than aspirin	Powerful anti-inflammatory agent	Rheumatoid and osteoarthritis; gout, ankylosing spondylitis
Indomethacin	Good analgesic, anti-inflammatory and antipyretic but toxicity is high	Potent anti-inflammatory and analgesic	Rheumatoid, psoriatic and osteoarthritis, gout, ankylosing spondylitis, closure of PDA
Ibuprofen	Analgesic, anti-inflammatory, antipyretic all actions milder than aspirin	Adverse effects milder therefore better tolerated	As analgesic in painful conditions, antipyretic, soft tissue injuries, fractures, post-operative pain, arthritis and gout

and are reserved for patients with progressive disease who do not obtain satisfactory relief from NSAIDs. They are capable of arresting the progress of the disease and inducing remission in these patients. Recent studies have shown that RA causes significant systemic effects that shorten life expectancy. This has renewed interest in the use of DMDs in RA. The effects of these drugs may take 6 weeks to 6 months to become evident and are therefore called *slow-acting anti-rheumatic drugs* (SAARDs).

Gold salts were introduced for the treatment of RA in 1920s, but only in 1960s their beneficial effects were clearly shown. They are considered to be the most effective agents for arresting the disease process.

On treatment, a gradual reduction of the signs and symptoms are seen. It brings about a decrease in the rheumatoid factor and immunoglobulins.

Mechanism of action is not exactly known. But gold depresses cell-mediated immunity (CMI). Gold salts concentrate in tissues rich in mononuclear phagocytes, selectively accumulate in the lysosomes of synovial cells and other macrophages in the inflamed synovium. They alter the structure and functions of the macrophages, depress their migration and phagocytic activity. They also inhibit lysosomal enzyme activity. Thus gold salts depress CMI.

Preparations Aurothiomalate sodium and auronofin are given orally, aurothioglucose is given parenterally.

Adverse effects Treatment with gold is associated with several adverse effects and only 60% of patients remain on treatment at the end of 2 years.

Adverse effects include:

1. *On skin and mucous membrane* dermatitis, pruritus, stomatitis, pharyngitis, glossitis, gastritis, colitis and vaginitis. A grey blue pigmentation on exposed parts of the skin may be seen.
2. *Renal toxicity* Haematuria, glomerulonephritis.
3. *Nervous system* Encephalitis, peripheral neuritis.
4. *Liver* Hepatitis, cholestatic jaundice.
5. *Blood* Thrombocytopenia, leukopenia, agranulocytosis, aplastic anaemia.

6. *CVS* Postural hypotension.
7. *Lungs* Pulmonary fibrosis.

Contraindications Kidney, liver and skin diseases; pregnancy and blood dyscrasias.

Uses

1. *Rheumatoid arthritis*—gold is used in active arthritis that progresses even after treatment with an adequate course of NSAIDs, rest and physiotherapy. In most patients gold salts arrest the progression of the disease, improve grip strength, reduce morning stiffness and prevent involvement of unaffected joints.
   Gold is also beneficial in:
2. Juvenile rheumatoid arthritis
3. Psoriatic arthritis
4. Pemphigus
5. Lupus erythematosus.

d-penicillamine is an analog of the amino acid cysteine and a metabolite of penicillin. It is a chelating agent that chelates copper. Its actions and toxicities are similar to gold but is less effective than gold. Hence it is not preferred. It is used as an alternative to gold in early, mild and non-erosive disease.

Adverse effects include drug fever, skin rashes, proteinuria, leucopenia, thrombocytopenia, aplastic anaemia, a variety of autoimmune diseases including lupus erythematosus, thyroiditis and haemolytic anaemia. Anorexia, nausea, vomiting, loss of taste perception and alopecia may also be seen.

Chloroquine and hydroxychloroquine These antimalarial drugs are found to be useful in mild non-erosive rheumatoid arthritis. They induce remission in 50% of patients. They are less effective but are better tolerated than gold.

Mechanism of action is not exactly understood but they are known to depress cell-mediated immunity.

Toxicity Chloroquine and hydroxychloroquine accumulate in tissues leading to toxicity. The most significant side effect is the retinal damage on long-term use. This toxicity is less common and reversible with hydroxychloroquine which is therefore preferred over chloroquine in rheumatoid arthritis.

Every 3 months eyes should be tested. Other adverse effects include myopathy, neuropathy and irritable bowel syndrome.

Dose Hydroxychloroquine 400 mg/day for 4-6 weeks; maintenance dose is 200 mg/day.

Sulphasalazine is a compound of sulphapyridine and 5-amino salicylic acid. In the colon, sulphasalazine is split by the bacterial action and sulphapyridine gets absorbed. This has anti-inflammatory actions though the mechanism is not known. *Adverse effects* include gastrointestinal upset and skin rashes.

TNF blocking agents Cytokines, particularly tumor necrosis factor (TNF) plays an important role in the process of inflammation. TNF produced by macrophages and activated T cells, acts through TNF receptors to stimulate the release of other cytokines. TNF blocking drugs are found to be useful in rheumatoid arthritis. **Infliximab** is a monoclonal antibody which specifically binds to human TNF. When given in combination with methotrexate, it slows the progression of rheumatoid arthritis. It is given intravenously. Adverse effects of the combination include increased susceptibility to upper respiratory infections, nausea, headache, cough, sinusitis and skin rashes. Antinuclear and anti-DNA antibodies may develop.

Etanercept is a recombinant fusion protein that binds to TNF molecules. It is given subcutaneously and is found to slow the progression of the disease in rheumatoid arthritis patients. It is also found to be useful in psoriatic and juvenile arthritis. Etanercept can be given with methotrexate and the combination has a better effect.

Pain, itching and allergic reactions at the site of injection, anti-etanercept antibodies and anti-DNA antibodies have been detected.

Immunosuppressants

Immunosuppressants are cytotoxic drugs and are reserved for patients having seriously crippling disease with reversible lesions after conventional therapy has failed. Among the immunosuppressants, methotrexate is the best tolerated. Toxicity includes nausea, mucosal ulcers, bone marrow suppression and hepatotoxicity. Weekly regimens of low oral doses are better tolerated.

Leflunomide is a prodrug. The active metabolite inhibits autoimmune T cell proliferation and production of auto-antibodies by B cells. Leflunomide is orally effective, and has a long t½ of 5-40 days. *Adverse effects* include diarrhoea and raised hepatic enzymes.

Leflunomide is used with methotrexate in rheumatoid arthritis patients who are not responding to methotrexate alone.

Corticosteroids

Detailed pharmacology is discussed in chapter. Glucocorticoids have anti-inflammatory and immunosuppressant activity. They produce prompt and dramatic relief of symptoms but do not stop the progress of the disease. However, long-term use of these drugs leads to several adverse effects. Moreover, on withdrawal of glucocorticoids, there may be an exacerbation of the disease. Therefore glucocorticoids are used as adjuvants. They may be used to treat exacerbations. Low dose long-term treatment with prednisolone is used in some patients (5-10 mg/day).

Intra-articular corticosteroids are helpful to relieve pain in severely inflamed joints.

Immunoadsorption Apheresis

Extracorporeal immunoadsorption of plasma for the removal of IgG-containing immunocomplexes has been approved for the treatment of moderate to severe rheumatoid arthritis. The duration of benefit varies from few months to several years. Adverse effects are mild and tolerable.

Diet and Inflammation

Clinical studies have shown that when patients of rheumatoid arthritis are given a diet rich in unsaturated fatty acids (such as marine fish), there is a decrease in morning stiffness, pain and swelling of the joints. Unsaturated fatty acids compete with arachidonic acid for uptake and metabolism and their metabolic products are only weak inflammatory mediators when compared to the products of arachidonic acid metabolism. Adequate consumption of marine fish should be recommended.

For people who do not eat fish, eicosapentaenoic acid 1-4 g/day may be given as tablets. It serves as an adjuvant.

Pharmacotherapy of Gout

Gout is a familial metabolic disorder characterised by recurrent episodes of acute arthritis due to deposits of monosodium urate in the joints and cartilage. There is an inherent abnormality of purine metabolism resulting in over production of uric acid—a major end product of purine metabolism. As uric acid is poorly water soluble, it gets precipitated—especially at low pH and deposited in the cartilages of joints and ears, subcutaneous tissues, bursae and sometimes in kidneys. An acute attack of gout occurs as an inflammatory reaction to crystals of sodium urate deposited in the joint tissue. There is infiltration of granulocytes which phagocytize the urate crystals and release a glycoprotein that causes joint destruction. The joint becomes red, swollen, tender and extremely painful.

Secondary hyperuricaemia may be drug induced or may occur in lymphomas and leukaemias. Gout may also be due to decreased excretion of uric acid.

Strategies in the treatment of gout is either to decrease the biosynthesis of uric acid or enhance the excretion of uric acid.

Drugs Used in Gout

In acute gout:	Colchicine, NSAIDs.	
In chronic gout:	*Uric acid synthesis inhibitor*	Allopurinol
	Uricosuric drugs	Probenecid, Sulphinpyrazone.

Colchicine is an alkaloid of *colchicum autumnale*. It is an unique anti-inflammatory agent effective only against gouty arthritis. It is not an analgesic.

Actions In gout, colchicine is highly effective in acute attacks and it dramatically relieves pain within a few hours.

Mechanism of action Colchicine inhibits the migration of granulocytes into the inflamed area and the release of glycoprotein by them.

Other actions Colchicine binds to microtubules and arrests cell division in metaphase. It increases gut motility by neurogenic stimulation.

Pharmacokinetics Colchicine is rapidly absorbed orally, metabolised in the liver and undergoes enterohepatic circulation.

Adverse effects are dose related. Nausea, vomiting, diarrhoea and abdominal pain are the earliest side effects and may be avoided by giving colchicine intravenously. Anaemia, leukopenia and alopecia may be seen. In high doses haemorrhagic gastroenteritis, nephrotoxicity, CNS depression, muscular paralysis and respiratory failure can occur.

Uses

1. Acute gout—colchicine 1 mg orally initially followed by 0.5 mg every 2-3 hours relieves pain and swelling within 12 hours. But diarrhoea limits its use.
2. Prophylaxis—Colchicine may also be used for the prophylaxis of recurrent episodes of gouty arthritis.

NSAIDs afford symptomatic relief in the treatment of gout. Indomethacin is the most commonly used agent in acute gout. Piroxicam, naproxen and other newer NSAIDs are also used. They relieve an acute attack in 12-24 hours and are better tolerated than colchicine. But NSAIDs are not recommended for long-term use due to their toxicity.

Allopurinol is an analog of hypoxanthine and inhibits the biosynthesis of uric acid.

Mechanism of action Purine nucleotides are degraded to hypoxanthine. Uric acid is produced as shown in Figure 6.1. Allopurinol and its metabolite alloxanthine both inhibit the enzyme xanthine oxidase and thereby prevent the synthesis of uric acid. The plasma concentration of uric acid is reduced.

Pharmacokinetics Allopurinol is 80% absorbed orally; t½ of allopurinol is 2-3 hr; t½ of alloxanthine is 24 hours.

Adverse effects are mild. Hypersensitivity reactions include fever and rashes. Gastrointestinal irritation, headache, nausea and dizziness may occur.

Attacks of acute gouty arthritis may be seen frequently during the initial months of treatment with allopurinol.

Drug interactions The anticancer drugs—6-mercaptopurine and azathioprine are metabolised by xanthine oxidase. Hence when allopurinol is used concurrently the dose of these anticancer drugs should be reduced.

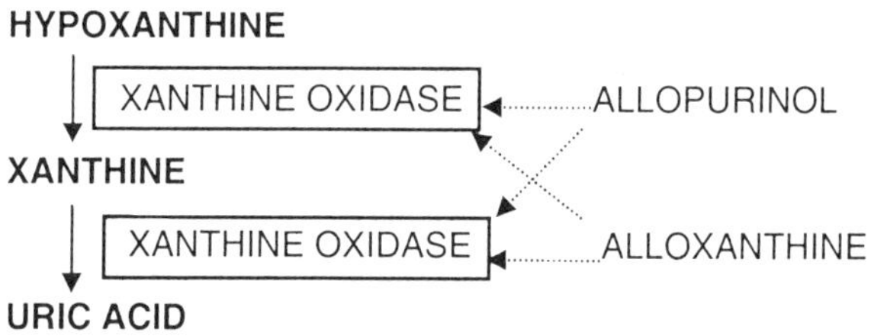

Fig. 6.1: Biosynthesis of uric acid

Uses Allopurinol is used in chronic gout and secondary hyperuricaemia. Initial dose is 100 mg/day and may be gradually increased to 300 mg/day depending on the response. Colchicine or an NSAID should be given during the first few weeks of allopurinol therapy to prevent the acute attacks of gouty arthritis. On treatment with allopurinol, tophi are gradually resorbed and the formation of renal stones are prevented. In patients with large tophaceous deposits, both allopurinol and uricosuric drugs can be given.

Uricosuric Drugs

Probenecid is an organic acid developed to inhibit the renal tubular secretion of penicillin in order to prolong its action.

Probenecid blocks tubular reabsorption of uric acid and thereby promotes its excretion. It is well-absorbed and well-tolerated. Adverse effects include gastrointestinal irritation and skin rashes. Large amounts of water should be given to prevent the formation of renal stones.

Probenecid is indicated in chronic gout and secondary hyperuricaemia. It is started with 500 mg once a day and gradually increased to 1 g/day. Probenecid may also precipitate acute attacks of gout due to fluctuating urate levels.

Sulphinpyrazone A pyrazolone derivative is another uricosuric drug which has actions and adverse effects similar to probenecid. It is used in chronic gout in an initial dose of 200 mg/day and gradually increased to 400-800 mg/day.

❑ DRUGS USED IN PSYCHIATRIC DISORDERS—ANTIPSYCHOTICS, ANTIDEPRESSANTS AND ANTIANXIETY AGENTS

Since ages, man has sought the help of drugs to modify behaviour, mood and emotion. Psychoactive drugs were used both for recreational purposes and for the treatment of mental illnesses (Psyche = mind).

In 1931 Sen and Bose showed that *Rawolfia serpentina* is useful in the treatment of insanity. ECT was introduced in 1937 for the treatment of depression. In 1950 chlorpromazine was synthesized in France and its usefulness in psychiatric patients was demonstrated in 1952. During the second half of the twentieth century, extensive research has been carried out in psychopharmacology and we now have several useful drugs in this branch of pharmacology.

Psychiatric conditions are broadly divided into psychoses, neuroses and personality disorders.

Psychoses are the more severe psychiatric disorders of the three and involve a marked impairment of behaviour, inability to think coherently, and to comprehend reality. Patients have no 'insight' into these abnormalities.

Psychoses could be due to:

i. An organic cause, i.e. there is a definable toxic, metabolic or pathological change—as following head injury.
ii. Functional or idiopathic disorders—where there is no definable cause like in schizophrenia, paranoia and affective disorders.

Schizophrenia (split mind) affects about 1% of population, starts in an early age and is highly incapacitating. It is characterised by delusions, hallucinations, irrational conclusions, interpretations and withdrawal from social contacts. Patients with chronic schizophrenia have shrinkage of the brain.

Neuroses are the milder forms of psychiatric disorders and include anxiety, mood changes, panic disorders, obsessions, irrational fears and reactive depression as seen following tragedies.

Personality disorders include paranoid, schizoid,histrionic, avoidant,antisocial and obsessive compulsive personality types.

Drugs used in psychiatric illnesses may be grouped as:

1. *Antipsychotics or neuroleptics*—used in psychoses.
2. *Antidepressants or psychotropic drugs*—used in affective disorders.
3. *Antianxiety drugs.*

Neuroleptic is a drug that reduces initiative, brings about emotional quietening and induces drowsiness. **Tranquilliser** is a drug that brings about tranquillity by calming, soothing and quietening effects. This is the older terminology. Neuroleptics or antipsychotics were called 'major traquillisers' and antianxiety drugs were called 'minor tranquillisers'. These terminologies are no longer used.

ANTIPSYCHOTICS (NEUROLEPTICS)

CLASSIFICATION

1. **Classical/typical neuroleptics**
   a. *Phenothiazines*—Chlorpromazine, Triflupromazine, Thioridazine, Mesoridazine, Trifluoperazine, Fluphenazine.
   b. *Butyrophenones*—Haloperidol, Droperidol, Trifluperidol.
   c. *Thioxanthenes*—Thiothixene, Chlorprothixene.
2. **Atypical neuroleptics**—Clozapine, Olanzapine, Risperidone, Quetiapine
3. **Miscellaneous**—Reserpine.

Chlorpromazine (CPZ)

Pharmacological Actions

CNS Behavioural effects—in normal subjects CPZ reduces motor activity, produces drowsiness and indifference to surroundings. In psychotic agitated patients, it reduces aggression, initiative and motor activity, relieves anxiety and brings about emotional quietening and drowsiness. It normalises the sleep disturbances characteristic of psychoses.

Other CNS Actions

1. *Cortex* CPZ lowers seizure threshold and can precipitate convulsions in untreated epileptics.
2. *Hypothalamus* CPZ decreases gonadotrophin secretion and may result in amenorrhoea in women. It increases the secretion of prolactin resulting in galactorrhoea and gynaecomastia.
3. *Basal ganglia* CPZ acts as a dopamine antagonist and therefore results in extrapyramidal motor symptoms (drug induced parkinsonism).
4. *Brainstem* Vasomotor reflexes are depressed leading to a fall in BP.
5. *CTZ* Neuroleptics block the dopamine (DA) receptors in the CTZ and thereby act as antiemetics.

Autonomic nervous system The actions on the ANS are complex. CPZ is an alpha blocker. The alpha blocking potency varies with each neuroleptic. CPZ also has anticholinergic properties which leads to side effects like dryness of mouth, blurred vision, reduced sweating, decreased gastric motility, constipation and urinary retention. The degree of anticholinergic activity also varies with each drug.

CVS Neuroleptics produce orthostatic hypotension due to alpha blockade action and reflex tachycardia. CPZ also has a direct myocardiac depressant effect like quinidine.

Local anaesthetic CPZ has local anaesthetic properties—but is not used for the purpose since it is an irritant.

Kidney CPZ depresses ADH secretion and has weak diuretic effects.

Tolerance develops to the sedative and hypotensive actions while no tolerance is seen to the antipsychotic actions.

Pharmacokinetics CPZ is incompletely absorbed following oral administration and also undergoes significant first pass metabolism (bioavailability is 30%). It is highly protein bound; has a t½ of 20 to 24 hr and is therefore given once a day.

Adverse reactions Antipsychotics have a high therapeutic index and are fairly safe drugs.

1. Cardiovascular and autonomic effects—postural hypotension, palpitation, blurred vision, dry mouth, constipation, nasal stuffiness and urinary retention.
2. CNS effects—drowsiness and mental confusion, a variety of neurological syndromes involving the extrapyramidal system including parkinsonism, dyskinesias, dystonias, akathesia and malignant neuroleptic syndrome are troublesome side effects.
3. Endocrine disturbances—gynaecomastia, amenorrhoea and galactorrhoea.
4. Hypersensitivity reactions—jaundice, agranulocytosis and skin rashes.

Drug interactions Neuroleptics enhance the sedative effects of CNS depressants, and the effects of anticholinergic drugs and alpha blockers. When combined with these groups of drugs, the effects may be additive.

Neuroleptics inhibit the actions of dopamine agonists and L-dopa.

Uses

Neuroleptics are given orally (chlorpromazine 100-800 mg). In acute psychosis they may be given intramuscularly and the response is seen in 24 hours. In chronic psychosis it takes 2-3 weeks of treatment to obtain the response.

1. *Psychiatric conditions* Psychoses including schizophrenia and organic brain syndromes like delirium and dementia all respond to antipsychotics.
2. *Nausea, vomiting* CPZ is a good antiemetic and is used in vomiting due to radiation sickness and drug induced vomiting.
3. *Hiccough* CPZ can control intractable hiccough though the mechanism of action is not known.
4. *Other neuropsychiatric syndromes* Neuroleptics are useful in the treatment of several syndromes with psychiatric features

like psychoses associated with chronic alcoholism and Huntington's disease.

Atypical Antipsychotics

Clozapine In addition to blocking DA receptors, clozapine also blocks 5-HT_2, α adrenergic and muscarinic receptors. Clozapine is an effective antipsychotic.

It has the following advantages over conventional antipsychotics:

1. Very low incidence of extrapyramidal side effects.
2. Sedation is low.
3. No endocrine side effects, i.e. no galactorrhoea and gynaecomastia.
4. It is effective in patients not responding to conventional antipsychotics.

Disadvantage May cause agranulocytosis in some patients which can be fatal.Hence use should be restricted to patients who are not responding to other drugs.Clozapine can also cause sedation, weight gain and hypotension.

Olanzepine Has the advantage that it causes no EPS dysfunction and no agranulocytosis has been reported.

Risperidone It blocks serotonin and dopamine receptors.

Advantages

1. At low doses no EPS dysfunction
2. Low sedation.

❑ ANTIDEPRESSANTS

Affective disorders are a group of psychoses associated with changes of mood, i.e. depression and mania.

Depression is a common psychiatric disorder and could be:

1. *Reactive* Due to distressing circumstances in life.
2. *Endogenous* Major depression due to a biochemical abnormality in the brain.
3. *Bipolar mood disorder* Mania and depression occur alternately causing cyclic mood swings.

Endogenous depression is thought to be due to deficiency of monoamine activity (NA, 5-HT) in the CNS.

Drugs Used in Affective Disorders

CLASSIFICATION

1. *Tricyclic antidepressants (TCA)*—Imipramine, Desipramine, Amitriptyline, Nortriptyline Doxepin
2. *Selective serotonin (5-HT) reuptake inhibitors (SSRI)*—Fluoxetine, Fluoxamine, Paroxetine, Citalopram, Sertraline, Venlafaxine
3. *Monoamine oxidase (MAO) inhibitors*—Phenelzine, Tranylcypromine.
4. *Atypical antidepressants*—Trazodone, Nefazodone, Bupropion, Mianserine.

Tricyclic Antidepressants

PHARMACOLOGICAL ACTIONS

1. ***CNS*** In normal subjects, TCA cause dizziness, drowsiness, confusion and difficulty in thinking. In depressed patients, after 2-3 weeks of treatment, elevation of mood occurs; the patient shows more interest in the surroundings and the sleep pattern becomes normal.

   Mechanism of action TCAs block the reuptake of amines (noradrenaline or 5-HT) into the presynaptic terminal, and thereby prolong their action on the receptors. Thus they potentiate amine neurotransmission in the CNS.

2. ***CVS*** Postural hypotension and tachycardia (due to blockade of α_1 adrenergic and muscarinic receptors) can be severe in overdosage.

3. ***ANS*** TCAs have anticholinergic properties and cause dry mouth, blurred vision, constipation and urinary retention.

PHARMACOKINETICS

TCAs are rapidly absorbed, highly protein bound and metabolised in the liver. They have a long t½ and can be given once daily.

ADVERSE EFFECTS

Sedation, postural hypotension, tachycardia, sweating and anticholinergic side effects like dry mouth, constipation, blurred vision and urinary retention are relatively common. TCA may precipitate convulsions in epileptics; may cause hallucinations and mania in some patients. Many TCAs may also cause weight gain due to increased appetite.

Acute toxicity is manifested by (mimic symptoms of atropine poisoning) delirium, excitement, hypotension, convulsions, fever, arrhythmias, respiratory depression and coma.

Treatment Physostigmine is given to overcome atropine-like effects; sodium bicarbonate for acidosis, phenytoin for seizures and arrhythmias - with other supportive measures.

Tolerance and dependence—tolerance develops gradually to the sedative and anticholinergic effects over 2-3 weeks.

Following long-term treatment, TCAs should be gradually withdrawn as withdrawal symptoms like headache, anxiety and chills can occur due to physical dependance.

Drug interactions

1. Tricyclics potentiate sympathomimetics—even small amounts of adrenaline used with local anaesthetics can cause serious hypertension.
2. Highly protein bound drugs like phenytoin, aspirin and phenylbutazone displace TCAs from binding sites resulting in toxicity.
3. TCAs potentiate the effects of alcohol and other CNS depressants.

Selective serotonin reuptake inhibitors (SSRI) Fluoxetine, fluoxamine, paroxetine, citalopram, sertraline, venlafaxine.

Antidepressant actions are similar to TCA but differ as follows:

- Low cardiovascular side effects
- Anticholinergic side effects are less
- Less sedation
- Preferred in elderly
- Safer in overdose
- Fluoxetine is the most commonly used SSRI.

MAO inhibitors Tranylcypromine, phenelzine:

- Irreversibly inhibit the enzyme MAO inhibitors and enhance neuronal levels of noradrenaline, dopamine and 5-HT.
- Antidepressant actions develop slowly over weeks of treatment.
- Side effects are hypotension, weight gain, CNS stimulation and atropine-like effects.
- They interact with many drugs and food.
- Patients on MAOI taking tyramine containing foods like cheese, beer, wines, yeast, buttermilk and fish—develop severe hypertension and is known as *'cheese reaction.'* Tyramine is normally metabolised by MAO in the gut wall. On inhibition of MAO by drugs, tyramine escapes metabolism and displaces NA from nerve endings leading to hypertension. Similar interaction with SSRI can result in severe hypertension (serotonin syndrome).
- Because of the side effects and drug interactions, MAO inhibitors are not the preferred antidepressants.

Atypical antidepressants Trazodone, bupropion, mianserin.

Advantages

- Fewer side effects—particularly sedation and anticholinergic effects
- Safer in overdose
- Effective in patients not responding to TCA.

Uses of Antidepressants

1. *Endogenous depression* Antidepressants are used over a long period. The response appears after 2-3 weeks of treatment. The choice of the antidepressant depends on the side effects and patient factors like age. In severe depression with suicidal tendencies, electroconvulsive therapy (ECT) is given.
2. *Panic attacks* Post-traumatic stress disorders and other anxiety disorders—all respond to antidepressants (acute episodes of anxiety are known as panic attacks).

3. *Obsessive compulsive disorders* SSRIs and clomipramine are effective.
4. *Nocturnal enuresis* in children may be treated with antidepressants only when other measures fail and drugs are to be given.
5. *Psychosomatic disorders* Newer antidipressants are tried in fibromyalgia, irritable bowel syndrome, chronic fatigue, tics, migraine and sleep apnoea.
6. *Other indications* Attention deficit hyperactivity disorder, chronic pain and chronic alcoholism—may result in depression—antidepressants are tried.

MOOD STABILIZERS

Lithium is a monovalent cation. On prophylactic use in bipolar mood disorder (manic-depressive illness), lithium acts as a mood stabilizer. It prevents swings of mood and thus reduces both the depressive and manic phases of the illness. Given in acute mania, it gradually suppresses the episode over weeks.

The mechanism of action of lithium is complex and not fully understood. It inhibits the synthesis of second messengers IP_3 and DAG and thereby blocks the respective receptor-mediated effects. This is the most accepted mechanism of action.

Pharmacokinetics Lithium is a small ion and mimics the role of sodium in excitable tissues. Given orally it is well-absorbed. It is filtered at the glomerulus but reabsorbed like sodium. Steady state concentration is reached in 5-6 days. Since safety margin is narrow, **plasma lithium concentration needs to be monitored.**

Adverse effects Lithium is a drug of low therapeutic index and side effects are common. Nausea, vomiting, mild diarrhoea, thirst and polyuria occur initially in most patients. As the plasma concentration rises, hypothyroidism, CNS effects like coarse tremors, drowsiness, giddiness, confusion, ataxia, blurred vision and nystagmus are seen. In severe overdosage, delirium, muscle twitchings, convulsions, arrhythmias and renal failure develop.

Precautions

1. Minimum effective dose should be used.
2. Patients should always use the same formulation.
3. Patients should be aware of the first symptom of toxicity.
4. Lithium is contraindicated in pregnancy.

Drug interactions

1. Diuretics enhance Na^+ loss and lithium absorption from the kidney. This increases plasma lithium levels resulting in toxicity.
2. NSAIDs ↓ lithium elimination and enhance toxicity.

Uses

1. Prophylaxis of bipolar mood disorder—episodes of mania and depression are reduced.
2. Acute mania—since the response to lithium is slow, neuroleptics are preferred.
3. Other uses—lithium is tried in recurrent neuropsychiatric disorders, hyperthyroidism and inappropriate ADH secretion syndrome.

Other mood stabilizers Because of difficulty in using lithium, other drugs are being tried. Carbamazepine and sodium valproate are found to be useful, less toxic alternatives.

ANTIANXIETY DRUGS (ANXIOLYTICS)

Anxiety is tension or apprehension which is a normal response to certain situations in life. It is a universal human emotion. But when it becomes excessive and disproportionate to the situation, it becomes disabling and needs treatment.

CLASSIFICATION

Benzodiazepines Diazepam, Chlordiazepoxide, Lorazepam, Alprazolam.

5-HT agonist-antagonists Buspirone, Gepirone, Ipsapirone.

β-blockers Propranolol.

Others Meprobamate, Hydroxyzine.

Benzodiazepines (page 155) have good antianxiety actions and are the most commonly used drugs for anxiety. They are CNS depressants. Alprazolam in addition has antidepressant properties.

Buspirone is an azapirone with good anxiolytic properties. It is a selective 5-HT_{1A} partial agonist and a weak D_2 antagonist. It is useful in mild to moderate anxiety. Antianxiety effect develops slowly over 2 weeks. Unlike diazepam, it is not a muscle relaxant, not an anticonvulsant, does not produce significant sedation, tolerance or dependence and is not useful in panic attacks.

Buspirone is rapidly absorbed and metabolised in the liver. *Dose* 5-15 mg OD or TDS.

Side effects are mild including headache, dizziness, nausea and rarely restlessness.

β-blockers (page 85) In patients with prominent autonomic symptoms of anxiety like tremors, palpitation and hypertension, propranolol may be useful. β-blockers are also useful in anxiety inducing states like public speaking and stage performance. They can be used as adjuvants to benzodiazepines.

Meprobamate has anxiolytic property but is not preferred now as it is less effective and causes high sedation.

Hydroxyzine is an antihistaminic with anxiolytic actions. But due to high sedation it is not preferred.

❑ CNS STIMULANTS

Drugs that have a predominantly stimulant effect on the CNS may be broadly divided into:

1. *Respiratory stimulants* Doxapram, Nikethamide
2. *Psychomotor stimulants* Amphetamine, Cocaine and Methylxanthines
3. *Convulsants* Leptazol, Strychnine.

Respiratory stimulants are also called analeptics. These drugs stimulate respiration and are sometimes used to treat respiratory failure. Though they may bring about temporary improvement in respiration, the mortality is not reduced. They have a low safety margin and may produce convulsions.

Doxapram Appears to act mainly on the brainstem and spinal cord and increase the activity of respiratory and vasomotor centres.

Adverse effects are nausea, cough, restlessness, hypertension, tachycardia, arrhythmias and convulsions.

Uses

1. Doxapram is occasionally used IV as an analeptic in acute respiratory failure
2. Apnoea in premature infants not responding to theophylline.

Nikethamide is not used because of the risk of convulsions.

Psychomotor stimulants Amphetamine and dextroamphetamine are sympathomimetic drugs (Chapter 2).

Cocaine is a CNS stimulant, produces euphoria and is a drug of abuse (page 150).

Methylxanthines Caffeine, theophylline and theobromine are the naturally occurring xanthine alkaloids. The beverages—coffee contains caffeine; tea contains theophylline and caffeine; cocoa has caffeine and theobromine. Caffeine and theophylline are CNS stimulants. They bring about an increase in mental alertness, a reduction of fatigue produce a sense of well being and improve motor activity and performance, with a clearer flow of thought. Caffeine stimulates the respiratory centre. Higher doses produce irritability, nervousness, restlessness, insomnia, excitement, and headache. High doses can result in convulsions.

CVS Methylxanthines increase the force of contraction of the myocardium and increase the heart rate and therefore increase the cardiac output. But, they also produce peripheral vasodilatation which tends to decrease the BP. The changes in BP are therefore not consistent. Caffeine causes vasoconstriction of cerebral blood vessels.

Kidneys The xanthines have a diuretic effect and thereby increase the urine output.

Smooth muscle Xanthines cause relaxation of smooth muscles especially the bronchial smooth muscle (page 235).

Skeletal muscle Xanthines enhance the power of muscle contraction and thereby increase the capacity to do muscular work by both a central stimulant effect and the peripheral actions.

GI tract Xanthines increase the secretion of acid and pepsin in the stomach and are gastric irritants.

Adverse effects include nervousness, insomnia, tremors, tachycardia, hypotension, arrhythmias, headache, gastritis, nausea, vomiting, epigastric pain and diuresis. High doses produce convulsions. Tolerance develops after sometime. Habituation to caffeine is common.

Uses

i. *Headache* Because of the effect of caffeine on cerebral blood vessels, it is combined with ergotamine for the relief of migraine headache. Caffeine is also combined with aspirin/paracetamol for the treatment of headache.
ii. *Bronchial asthma* Theophylline is used in the treatment of bronchial asthma.

NOOTROPICS are drugs that improve memory and cognition (cognition enhancers).

Piracetam – described as a 'nootropic agent' is thought to protect cerebral cortex from hypoxia and improve learning and memory. In higher doses it also inhibits platelet aggregation. Adverse effects include insomnia, weight-gain, nervousness, depression and gastrointestinal disturbances.

It has been tried in dementia, myoclonus, stroke and other cerebrovascular accidents; alcoholism, behavioural disorders and learning problems in children and in vertigo. The beneficial effects in all these is not proved.

7

Autacoids

- HISTAMINE AND ANTIHISTAMINES
- 5-HYDROXYTRYPTAMINE, ERGOT ALKALOIDS, ANGIOTENSIN AND KININS
- EICOSANOIDS

Autacoids are substances formed in various tissues, have complex physiologic and pathologic actions and act locally at the site of synthesis. They have a brief action and are destroyed locally. Hence they are called *'local hormones'* and differ from true hormones which are produced by specific cells and reach their target tissues through circulation. The word autacoid is derived from Greek: *autos*-self *akos*-remedy. Histamine, 5-hydroxytryptamine (serotonin), endogenous peptides like bradykinin and angiotensin; prostaglandins and leukotrienes are autacoids.

HISTAMINE AND ANTIHISTAMINES

HISTAMINE

Histamine (tissue amine) (*Histos* = tissue) is a biogenic amine formed in many tissues. It is also found in the venoms of bees, wasps and other stinging secretions.

Synthesis, storage, distribution and degradation In humans, histamine is formed from the amino acid histidine. Large amounts are found in the lungs, skin and intestines. Histamine

AUTACOIDS AND THEIR ANTAGONISTS

HISTAMINE (H_1 H_2)

H_1 blockers
- Diphenhydramine
- Chlorpheniramine
- Cetirizine, Loratadine

H_2 blockers
- Ranitidine
- Famotidine
- Roxatidine

5-HT OR SEROTONIN ($5\text{-}HT_{1\text{-}7}$)

Agonists
- Sumatriptan
- Buspirone
- Dexfenfluramine

Blockers
- Cyproheptadine
- Ketanserin
- Ondensetran

ANGIOTENSIN (AT1, AT2)

Blockers
- Losartan

ACE inhibitors
- Captopril
- Enalapril
- Ramipril

PROSTAGLANDINS

Analogs
- Misoprostol
- Dinoprostone
- Carboprost

Synthesis inhibitors
- Aspirin
- Indomethacin
- Paracetamol

KININS (B_1 B_2)
- Bradykinin
- Kallidin
- Antagonists are being developed

LEUKOTRIENES

Antagonists
- Moutelukast
- Zafirlukast

Lipoxygenase Inhibitors
- Zileuton

Some autacoids with examples of agonists and antagonists. Receptor types are given in brackets

is stored in the granules of the mast cells and basophils in an inactive form. Histamine found in brain serves as a neuro transmitter. Degranulation of the mast cells release histamine which is quickly degraded at the site.

Mechanism of Action

Histamine produces its effects by acting on the histamine receptors. Three subtypes are known.

- H_1—present in lungs, gut, blood vessels, nerve endings and brain.
- H_2—stomach (gastric glands), heart, blood vessels and brain.
- H_3—CNS.

Actions

1. **CVS** Histamine dilates small blood vessels resulting in hypotension accompanied by reflex tachycardia. Cerebral blood vessels dilate—producing severe throbbing headache.

Triple response Intradermal injection of histamine elicits triple response comprising of:

i. *red spot at the site* (flush)—due to local capillary dilation.

ii. *flare*—redness surrounding the 'flush' due to arteriolar dilatation.

iii. *wheal*—local oedema due to the escape of fluid from the capillaries.

This response is accompanied by pain and itching.

2. **Smooth muscle** Histamine causes contraction of the non-vascular smooth muscles. Thus bronchospasm and increased intestinal motility are produced.

3. **Glands** Histamine is a powerful stimulant of the gastric acid secretion-acts through H_2 receptors (chapter 9). It also stimulates pepsin and intrinsic factor secretion.

4. **CNS** Histamine functions as a neurotransmitter in the CNS.

5. **Nerve endings** Histamine stimulates sensory nerve endings causing pain and itching.

Adverse reactions include hypotension, flushing, tachycardia, headache, wheal, bronchospasm and diarrhoea.

Uses

Histamine is of no therapeutic value. It is occasionally used in some diagnostic tests like to test the acid secreting ability of the stomach, diagnosis of pheochromocytoma, and to test for bronchial hyperreactivity.

Histamine Substitutes

Betazole is a H_2 agonist and can be used in gastric function tests. *Betahistine* is a H_1 agonist used to control vertigo in Meniere's disease.

ANTIHISTAMINES

Histamine antagonists can be H_1 receptor blockers and H_2 receptor blockers.

Drugs that competitively block H_1 histamine receptors are conventionally called the '*antihistamines*'. H_2 blockers are used in the treatment of peptic ulcer (see Chapter 9).

CLASSIFICATION OF H_1 BLOCKERS

Sedative: Diphenhydramine, Dimenhydrinate, Promethazine.

Less sedative: Pheniramine, Chlorpheniramine, Cyclizine, Meclizine, Buclizine, Mepyramine, Tripelennamine.

Newer non-sedative Terfenadine, Astemizole, Loratadine, Cetirizine.

Actions

1. *Blockade of actions of histamine* H_1 receptor antagonists block the actions of histamine on H_1 receptors. They block the histamine induced effects on smooth muscles of the gut, bronchi, blood vessels and triple response.
2. *Sedation* Antihistamines cause CNS depression; sedation, dizziness, inability to concentrate and disturbances of coordination are common. Alcohol and other CNS depressants potentiate this action. Some patients may experience CNS stimulation resulting in tremors, restlessness and insomnia.
3. *Antimotion sickness effects* Several antihistamines prevent motion sickness and vomiting due to other labyrinthine disturbances. Some of them also control vomiting of pregnancy.
4. *Antiparkinsonian effects* Some of them suppress tremors, rigidity and sialorrhoea probably due to their anticholinergic properties.
5. *Anticholinergic actions* Many of the H_1 blockers have anticholinergic property.
6. *Other actions* Antihistamines also have local anaesthetic effects in high doses. Some of them also block α_1 adrenergic and 5-HT receptors.

Pharmacokinetics Antihistamines are well-absorbed, widely distributed in the body, metabolised in the liver and are excreted in the urine. Route of administration and preparation are given in Table 7.1.

Adverse reactions are mild and on continued use tolerance develops.

Sedation, dizziness, motor incoordination, inability to concentrate make driving dangerous while on antihistamines. Anticholinergic effects like dryness of mouth, blurred vision, constipation and urinary retention may be troublesome. Epigastric distress and headache can also occur. Many of them are teratogenic.

TABLE 7.1: Dose and preparations of some antihistamines

Antihistamine	*Route*	*Trade name*
Diphenhydramine HCl	Oral IM	BENADRYL Cap, Syr
Dimenhydrinate	Oral, IM	DRAMAMINE Tab, Syr Inj
Promethazine	Oral, IM	PHENERGAN Tab, Syr, Inj
Promethazine chlortheophyllinate	Oral	AVOMINE Tab
Pheniramine maleate	Oral, IM	AVIL Tab, Syr, Inj
Chlorpheniramine	Oral, IM	ZEET Tab, Syr, Inj
Cyclizine HCl	Oral	MAREZINE Tab
Meclizine HCl	Oral	ANCOLAN Tab
Buclizine	Oral	LONGIFENE Tab, Syr
Cinnarizine	Oral	STUGERON Tab
Nonsedative (II generation) antihistamines		
Terfenadine	Oral	TREXYL Tab, Syr
Astemizole	Oral	ASTELONG, Tab, Syr
Loratadine	Oral	LORFAST, Tab, Syr
Cetirizine	Oral	ALERID, Tab, Syr

Newer non-sedative antihistamines also called II generation antihistamines have the following advantages over classical antihistamines:

- No sedation because they poorly cross the blood-brain barrier.
- No anticholinergic side effects as these are pure H_1 blockers and do not block cholinergic receptors.
- Some of them like astemizole are long-acting.

However, the therapeutic indications of these agents are limited to allergic disorders like allergic rhinitis and chronic urticaria. They are more expensive. Terfenadine can very rarely cause fatal ventricular arrhythmias; erythromycin and ketoconazole potentiate this cardiotoxicity.

Uses

1. *Allergic reactions* Antihistamines are useful for the prevention and treatment of symptoms of allergic reactions. They are effective in allergic rhinitis, conjunctivitis, hayfever, urticaria, pruritus, some allergic skin rashes and pollinosis.
2. *Common cold* Antihistamines reduce rhinorrhoea and afford symptomatic relief in common cold.
3. *Motion sickness* Given 30-60 minutes before journey, antihistamines prevent motion sickness. They are also useful in treating vertigo of Meniere's disease and other vestibular disturbances. Cinnarizine is preferred.
4. *Antiemetic* Promethazine is used to prevent drug induced and postoperative vomiting. It has also been used in 'morning sickness.'
5. *Preanaesthetic medication* For its sedative, anticholinergic and antiemetic properties, promethazine has been used as pre-anaesthetic medication.
6. *Hypnotic* The sedative antihistamines are sometimes used to induce sleep. Hydroxizine has been used as an anxiolytic.
7. *Parkinsonism* Some of them are useful in drug induced parkinsonism due to their anticholinergic action.
8. *Cough* due to postnasal drip can be controlled by antihistamines like diphenhydramine.

❑ 5-HYDROXYTRYPTAMINE, ERGOT ALKALOIDS, ANGIOTENSIN AND KININS

5-HYDROXYTRYPTAMINE

5-Hydroxytryptamine (serotonin) was isolated in 1948. A large volume of information on 5-HT is now available and has been of great pharmacological interest. It is found in various plant and animal tissues. In human body, 5-HT is present in the intestines, platelets and brain. It is synthesized from the amino acid tryptophan and stored in granules. It is degraded mainly by MAO.

5-HT Receptors The actions of serotonin are mediated through its receptors. Seven types of 5-HT receptors (5-HT_{1-7}) with further subtypes of 5-HT_1 and 5-HT_2 receptors are presently known. Many receptor selective agonists and antagonists are being developed.

Actions

1. *CVS* The action on blood vessels is complex. Large vessels are constricted while arterioles dilate. A characteristic triphasic response is seen on blood pressure following IV injection.

   Initial fall in BP in followed by a rise and then fall.
2. *GI tract* 5-HT increases gastrointestinal motility and contraction resulting in diarrhoea.
3. *Other actions* Weak bronchoconstriction, platelet aggregation; stimulation of sensory nerve endings—causes pain if injected into the skin. 5-HT is a neurotransmitter in the CNS.

Physiological and pathophysiological role 5-HT is postulated to be having a role in peristalsis, vomiting, platelet aggregation, homoeostasis and inflammation. It is also thought to initiate the vasoconstriction in migraine.

Drugs acting on 5-HT receptors Serotonin has no therapeutic uses. However its receptor agonists and antagonists have been used in various conditions.

Serotonin Agonists

Sumatriptan—a 5-HT_{1D} agonist is effective in the treatment of acute migraine and cluster headache. Given at the onset of an attack, sumatriptan relieves headache and also suppresses nausea and vomiting of migrane. It is short-acting.

Other Agonists

Buspirone (see page 221) is a 5-HT_{1A} agonist-antagonist used as an antianxiety agent.

Dexfenfluramine (see page 80) is used as an appetite suppressant.

Serotonin Antagonists

Cyproheptadine blocks 5-HT_2, H_1 histamine and cholinergic receptors. It increases appetite and is used to promote weight gain especially in children.

Ketanserin blocks 5-HT_2 receptors and antagonises vasoconstriction and platelet aggregation promoted by 5-HT. It is used in hypertension.

Ondansetron is a 5-HT_3 antagonist (see page 269) used in the prevention and treatment of vomiting.

Many other drugs including some antihistamines also block serotonin receptors.

ERGOT ALKALOIDS

Ergot alkaloids are produced by a fungus *claviceps purpurea*. Consumption of such grains results in 'ergotism' manifested as gangrene of hands and feet, hallucinations and other CNS effects.

Natural ergot alkaloids include ergometrine, ergotamine and ergotoxine. The semisynthetic dehydrogenated derivatives are also available.

Actions Ergot alkaloids have agonist, partial agonist and antagonistic actions at 5-HT and alpha adrenergic receptors and agonistic actions at CNS dopamine receptors. Thus their actions are complex. Some of them are powerful hallucinogens, e.g. lysergic acid diethylamide (LSD). They cause stimulation of smooth muscles—some mainly vascular smooth muscles and others mainly uterine smooth muscles. The vasoconstrictor effect is responsible for gangrene.

Adverse effects like nausea, vomiting and diarrhoea are common. Prolonged use results in gangrene due to persistent vasospasm.

Uses *(Table 7.2).*

1. Migraine
2. Postpartum haemorrhage—ergometrine is used for the prevention and treatment.

TABLE 7.2: Serotonin agonists, antagonists and their therapeutic uses

	Uses
AGONISTS	
Sumatriptan	• Acute migraine • Cluster headache
Buspirone	Anxiolytic
Dexfenfluramine	Appetite suppressant
ANTAGONISTS	
Cyproheptadine	• Appetite stimulant • Carcinoid tumours
Ketanserin	Hypertension
Ondansetron	Antiemetic
ERGOT ALKALOIDS	
Ergotamine	Acute attack of migraine
Ergometrine	Postpartum haemorrhage
Methysergide	Prophylaxis of migraine

Drugs Used in the Treatment of Migraine

Migraine is a common disorder characterised by severe, throbbing, unilateral, headache often associated with nausea, vomiting and fatigue lasting for several hours. In the classical migraine, a brief 'aura' of visual disturbances occurs prior to the headache. An attack is triggered by factors like stress, anxiety, excitement, food (like chocolate and cheese) and hormonal changes. These triggering factors stimulate the release of vasoactive substances from nerve endings which are responsible for the events that follow. However the exact pathophysiology is not understood and several hypotheses have been put forward.

Aspirin, paracetamol or other NSAIDs, ergotamine and sumatriptan are effective in acute attacks. Drug should be taken at the initiation of an attack.

When the attacks are frequent and severe, prophylaxis is needed. Drugs used for the prophylaxis are: propranolol, flunarizine, cyproheptadine and amytriptyline.

ANGIOTENSIN

Angiotensins are peptides synthesized from the precursor angiotensinogen. Angiotensin II, the most potent angiotensin, acts through angiotensin receptors (AT_1 and AT_2) present on the tissues.

Actions

Angiotensin II causes vasoconstriction resulting in increased blood pressure. It stimulates the synthesis of aldosterone by the adrenal cortex which increases sodium reabsorption by the kidneys. By these actions, renin- angiotensin system regulates the fluid and electrolyte balance and blood pressure.

Inhibitors of ACE and blockers of angiotensin II receptors are now used in the treatment of hypertension, congestive heart failure and other conditions that are due to excess of angiotensin II activity (see Chapter 4).

KININS

Kinins are vasodilator peptides formed from the precursor kininogen by the action of the enzymes called kallikreins. The most important of kinins is bradykinin.

Kinins are potent vasodilators and cause a brief fall in BP. They stimulate contraction of other smooth muscles—thus they induce bronchospasm in asthmatics, slow contraction of intestines (*Brady*= slow) and uterus. Kinins mediate inflammation, and stimulate the pain nerve endings. Kinins produce their actions by acting through B_1 and B_2 receptors.

Drugs affecting the kallikrein-kinin system—B_1 and B_2 antagonists are now being developed.

❑ EICOSANOIDS

Eicosanoids are 20-carbon (eicosa referring to the 20-C atoms) unsaturated fatty acids derived mainly from arachidonic acid in the cell walls. The principal eicosanoids are the prostaglandins (PG), the thromboxanes (TX), and the leukotrienes (LT).

Biosynthesis

Eicosanoids are synthesized locally in most tissues from arachidonic acid. The pathway for synthesis is shown in Figure 7.1.

The cyclo-oxygenase (COX) pathway generates PGs and TXs while lipoxygenase (LOX) pathway generates LTs. There are 2 cyclo-oxygenase isozymes *viz.* COX-1 and COX-2. Eicosanoids produced by COX-1 mainly take part in physiological functions while those produced by COX-2 result in inflammatory and pathological changes.

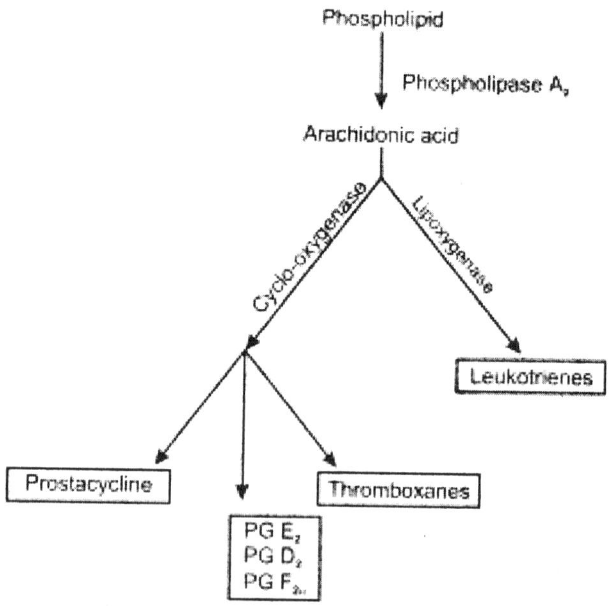

Fig. 7.1: Biosynthesis of eicosanoids

PROSTAGLANDINS AND THROMBOXANES

In 1930s it was found that human semen contains a substance that contracts uterine smooth muscle. As this substance was thought to originate in the prostate, they called it 'Prostaglandin'. But it was later found to be produced in many tissues.

Actions

The eicosanoids act through their specific receptors present on the tissues.

CVS Prostacycline causes vasodilation while TXA_2 causes vasoconstriction. PGE_2 and $PGF_{2\alpha}$ are weak cardiac stimulants.

Other actions PGs (TXA_2, $PGF_2\alpha$) contract gastrointestinal and bronchial smooth muscles. TXA_2 induces platelet aggregation while PGI_2 inhibits it. PGE_2 and $PGF_{2\alpha}$ contract uterus. PGs also stimulate bone turnover and sensitize the nerve endings to pain.

Adverse effects depend on the type of PG, dose and route. Diarrhoea, nausea, vomiting, fever, hypotension and pain due to uterine contractions are common.

Uses

1. *Gynaecological and obstetrical*
   a. *Abortion* For I and II trimester abortion and ripening of cervix during abortion, PGE_2 and $PGF_{2\alpha}$ are used. They are also used with mifepristone to ensure complete expulsion of the products of conception.
   b. *Facilitation of labour* As alternative to oxytocics in patients with renal failure.
   c. *Cervical priming* Intravaginal PGE_2 is used.
   d. *Postpartum haemorrhage* Intramuscular $PGF_{2\alpha}$ is used as an alternative to ergometrine.

2. *Gastrointestinal*

Peptic ulcer PGE_1 (misoprostol) and PGE_2 (enprostil) are used for the prevention of peptic ulcer in patients on high dose NSAIDs.

3. *Cardiovascular*
   a. *Patent ductus arteriosus* Patency of foetal ductus arteriosus depends on local PG synthesis. In neonates with some congenital heart diseases, patency of the ductus arteriosus is maintained with PGs until surgery is done.
   b. To prevent platelet aggregation during haemodialysis.

4. *Other uses* PGs are used in pulmonary hypertension and some peripheral vascular diseases. They can also be used in open angle glaucoma to lower intraocular pressure.

LEUKOTRIENES

Leukotrienes (LT) are products of arachidonic acid metabolism synthesized by the lipoxygenase pathway and are found in the lungs, platelets, mast cells and white blood cells. ('Leuko'—because they are found in white cells; 'trienes'—they contain triene system of double bonds). LTA_4 is the precursor from which LTB_4, LTC_4, LTD_4, LTE_4 and LTF_4 are derived. LTC_4, LTD_4 and LTE_4 are together known as slow reacting substances (SRS-A) of anaphylaxis. The LTs produce their effects through specific receptors.

Actions

Leukotrienes cause vasoconstriction, increase vascular permeability leading to oedema, increase airway mucous secretion and are potent bronchiolar spasmogens. Given subcutaneously they cause wheal and flare. Leukotrienes have a role in inflammation including rheumatoid arthritis, psoriasis and ulcerative colitis. They also contribute to bronchial hyperresponsiveness in bronchial asthma.

Drugs that inhibit lipoxygenase and thus block the synthesis of leukotrienes are under investigation in the treatment of bronchial asthma.

PLATELET ACTIVATING FACTOR (PAF)

PAF is an important mediator in acute and chronic, allergic and inflammatory phenomena. PAF is released from inflammatory cells and acts on specific receptors. It causes local vasodilatation resulting in oedema, hyperalgesia and wheal formation. It is a potent chemotaxin for leukocytes and a spasmogen on bronchial and intestinal smooth muscles. It is a mediator of inflammation.

8

Respiratory System

- Drugs used in the treatment of bronchial asthma
- Drugs used in the treatment of cough

DRUGS USED IN THE TREATMENT OF BRONCHIAL ASTHMA

Bronchial asthma is characterised by dyspnoea and wheeze due to increased resistance to the flow of air through the bronchi. Bronchospasm, mucosal congestion and oedema result in increased airway resistance. The bronchial smooth muscle is hyperresponsive to various stimuli like dust, allergens, cold air, infection and drugs. These trigger factors—trigger an acute attack. Antigen-antibody interaction on the surface of mast cells cause (Fig. 8.1):

i. degranulation of mast cells releasing stored mediators of inflammation

ii. synthesis of other inflammatory mediators which are responsible for bronchospasm, mucosal congestion and oedema. *Inflammation is the primary pathology.*

CLASSIFICATION

1. *Bronchodilators*
   a. *Sympathomimetics* Salbutamol, Terbutaline, Salmeterol, Adrenaline, Ephedrine.
   b. *Methylxanthines* Theophylline, Aminophylline.
   c. *Anticholinergics* Ipratropium bromide, Atropine.

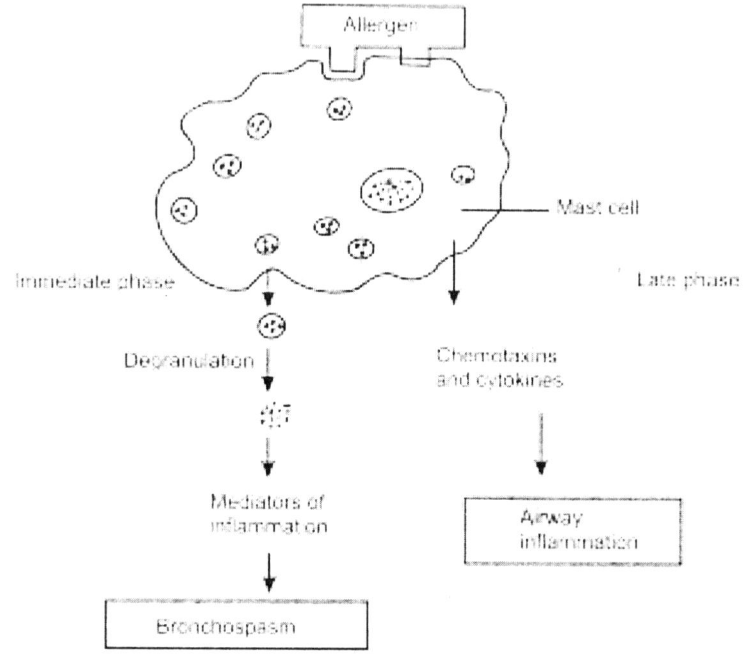

Fig. 8.1: Immediate and late responses of mast cell activation by antigen

2. *Anti-inflammatory agents*
   a. *Systemic* Glucocorticoids, Hydrocortisone, Prednisolone
   b. *Inhalational* Beclomethasone, Budesonide, Flunisolide, Triamcinolone
3. *Mast cell stabilizers*
   Disodium cromoglycate, Nedocromil, Ketotifen.

Sympathomimetic Drugs (see page 73)

These drugs are potent bronchodilators. They stimulate β_2 receptors in bronchial smooth muscles resulting in increased cAMP levels. This increased cAMP leads to bronchodilatation. The increased cAMP in mast cells inhibit the release of inflammatory mediators. They also reduce bronchial secretions and congestion (by acting on α receptors).

Salbutamol and terbutaline are selective β_2 agonists. Given by inhalation, they are fastest-acting bronchodilators with peak effect in 10 minutes. The action lasts for 6 hours. Adverse effects to β_2 agonists include muscle tremors, palpitation and nervousness.

Selective β_2 agonists are the most commonly used bronchodilators as they are the most effective, fast-acting, convenient and relatively safe bronchodilators. They are available as metered dose inhalers, nebulizers and also tablets for oral use. The proper technique in using the inhaler should be taught. 'Spacers' can be used in children and adults who cannot follow the right technique of inhalation.

Oral β_2 agonists have higher adverse effects and are used only in small children who cannot use inhalers and have occasional wheezing (1-4 mg 6 hourly).

Salmeterol is a long-acting selective β_2 agonist. The onset of action is slow (hence not useful in acute attacks) but the effect remains for 12 hours. It is therefore used for long-term maintenance and for prevention of nocturnal asthmatic attacks.

Newer agents like fenoterol, adrenaline, ephedrine and isoprenaline. Though adrenaline and isoprenaline produce prompt bronchodilation, they are not preferred due to the risk of adverse effects.

Ephedrine produces bronchodilation but is slow in onset. Because of low efficacy, side effects and availability of better drugs, ephedrine is not preferred.

Methylxanthines (page 222) are similar to salmeterol.

Theophylline and its derivatives like ***aminophylline*** are good bronchodilators.

Mechanism of action Phosphodiesterase (PDE) is the enzyme that degrades cyclic AMP. Methylxanthines inhibit PDE and thereby enhance cAMP levels which brings about bronchodilation. cAMP also inhibits the release of mediators of inflammation.

cAMP
$\downarrow$ PDE $\leftarrow$ - - - Methylxanthines
5′AMP

Aminophylline is given intravenously, slowly in acute attacks of asthma not responding to β_2 agonists. In an acute attack, drugs given by inhalation may sometimes fail to reach the bronchioles because of severe bronchospasm. Intravenous aminophylline may then be tried. 250 mg aminophylline should be injected slow IV over 15-20 minutes. Rapid IV injection may cause collapse and death due to hypotension and arrhythmias. Convulsions can also occur and should be carefully watched for.

Adverse effects Theophylline is a drug of low therapeutic index. Gastric irritation, vomiting, insomnia, tremors, diuresis, palpitation, and hypotension are quite common. Higher doses cause restlessness, delirium, convulsions and arrhythmias. Children may develop behavioural abnormalities on prolonged use—should be avoided in children.

Status in bronchial asthma Theophylline is a second line drug in bronchial asthma.

1. *Chronic asthma* Oral theophylline can be used to control mild to moderate asthma. Etophylline + 80% theophylline (Deriphylline) injections (IM) are used to relieve acute attacks.
2. *Acute severe asthma (status asthmaticus)* Intravenous aminophylline is tried when, sympathomimetics fail to relieve bronchospasm—but are found to be less effective.

Anticholinergics (see chapter 2)—relax bronchial smooth muscles but response is slower than sympathomimetics. ***Ipratropium bromide*** is given by inhalation and its actions are largely limited to the respiratory tract. It is more effective in chronic bronchitis. It is safe and well-tolerated.

Uses

1. As an adjunct to β_2 agonists.
2. As a bronchodilator in some cases of chronic bronchitis.

ANTI-INFLAMMATORY DRUGS

Glucocorticoids Since inflammation is the primary pathology in bronchial asthma, antiinflammatory agents afford significant benefit.

Mechanism of action Steroids are not bronchodilators. They suppress the inflammatory response to antigen-antibody reaction and thereby reduce mucosal oedema and hyper-irritability. They restore response to β_2 agonists if tolerance has developed. Oral prednisolone is commonly used.

Inhaled steroids The use of inhalational steroids largely minimizes the adverse effects of steroids because of the small dose required. But they are not effective in acute attacks and are only of prophylactic value. They prevent episodes of acute asthma and bronchial hyperreactivity and effectively control symptoms. The effect develops after 1 week of treatment.

Side effects of inhaled steroids include hoarseness of voice, sore throat and oropharyngeal candidiasis. Rinsing the mouth and throat with water after each use can reduce the incidence of candidiasis and sore throat. No HPA axis suppression is seen in the recommended doses.

Beclomethasone dipropionate, budesonide, flunisolide and ***triamcinolone*** are used as inhalers.

Dose Beclomethasone, BECLATE INHALER 50, 100 and 200 μg per metered dose → 1-2 Puffs 3-4 times a day.

Use of glucocorticoids in asthma

1. *Acute exacerbation* A short course (5-7 days) of oral prednisolone is given in addition to β_2 agonists.
2. *Chronic asthma* Beclomethasone/Budesonide inhalation for a long period as prophylaxis.
3. *Status asthmaticus* IV hydrocortisone hemisuccinate followed by oral prednisolone.

MAST CELL STABILIZERS

Cromolyn sodium (disodium cromoglycate) was synthesized in 1965.

Mechanism of action Cromolyn inhibits the degranulation of mast cells and thereby inhibits the release of mediators of inflammation. It thus prevents bronchospasm and inflammation following exposure to allergens. It is therefore used for *prophylaxis*. It is not a bronchodilator - hence not useful in acute episodes.

Cromolyn sodium is used as an inhaler; it takes 2-4 weeks of treatment for the beneficial effects to develop.

Adverse effects are rare. Throat irritation, cough and sometimes bronchospasm can occur on inhalation due to the fine powder.

Uses

1. *Prophylaxis of bronchial asthma*—Cromolyn sodium is used over a long period—2 puffs—3-4 times daily reduces the episodes of acute asthma. Young patients are more likely to be benefitted.
2. *Allergic rhinitis*—Prophylactic nasal spray is used.
3. *Allergic conjunctivitis*—Eye drops are used prophylactically.

Nedocromil is similar to cromolyn sodium in its actions and uses. It is given twice daily.

Ketotifen is an antihistaminic with actions like cromolyn sodium. It inhibits airway inflammation but it is not a bronchodilator. It is given orally. Beneficial effects are seen after 6-12 weeks of use. It is used for the prophylaxis of bronchial asthma and other allergic disorders like allergic rhinitis and conjunctivitis. Drowsiness and dry mouth are common side effects.

Treatment of Asthma

Mild asthma—Inhaled β_2 stimulants.

Moderate asthma—Regular prophylaxis with cromoglycate. If symptoms persist—inhaled steroids for prophylaxis. Acute episodes are managed with inhaled β_2 agonists.

Severe asthma

a. Regular inhaled steroids
b. Inhaled β_2 agonists 3-4 times a day
c. Oral steroids may be considered
d. Additional inhaled ipratropium bromide or oral theophylline may be given.

Status asthmaticus or acute severe asthma is an acute exacerbation. It is a medical emergency; may be triggered by an acute respiratory infection, abrupt withdrawal of steroids, drugs, allergens or emotional stress.

Treatment

1. Nebulization of β_2 agonist and ipratropium alternately—every 30 minutes. Additional salbutamol injection (IM/SC) may be given. Severe tachycardia should be watched for.
2. Hydrocortisone hemisuccinate IV followed by a course of oral prednisolone.
3. Oxygen inhalation.
4. Antibiotics.
5. IV fluids to correct dehydration.
6. Aminophylline 250 mg slow IV over 15-20 minutes may be given carefully—watch for adverse effects.
7. Artificial ventilation may be required in extreme cases.

❑ DRUGS USED IN THE TREATMENT OF COUGH

Cough is a protective reflex that removes the irritant matter and secretions from the respiratory tract. It could be due to infection, allergy, pleural diseases and malignancy. Since it is a protective mechanism, undue suppression of cough can cause more harm than benefit. Only in some conditions as in dry annoying cough, it may serve no useful purpose. In such situations, antitussive or cough suppressants may be used. Antitussives only provide symptomatic relief and do not alter the cause.

ANTITUSSIVES

1. *Central cough suppressants*	Codeine, Noscapine, Dextromethorphan, Antihistamines, Benzonatate.
2. *Pharyngeal demulcents*	Lozenges, Cough drops, Linctuses
3. *Expectorants*	Potassium iodide, Guaiphenesin, Ammonium chloride, Ipecacuanha

Central Cough Suppressants

Central cough suppressants act by inhibiting cough centre in the medulla.

Codeine is a good antitussive with less addiction liability; nausea, constipation and drowsiness are common. *Dose* 10-15 mg every 6 hours (page 182).

Noscapine is a potent antitussive; no other CNS effects are prominent in therapeutic doses. Nausea is the only occasional side effect. *Dose* 15-30 mg every 6 hours.

Dextromethorphan and pholcodeine are synthetic opioid derivatives with antitussive actions like codeine but with less side effects. Pholcodeine is longer-acting—given twice daily.

Benzonatate is chemically related to the local anaesthetic procaine. It acts on the cough receptors in the lungs and also has a central effect. It is given orally.

Antihistamines are useful in cough due to allergy except that due to bronchial asthma.

Pharyngeal Demulcents

These drugs increase the flow of saliva which produces a soothing effect on the pharyngeal mucosa (*demulcere* = to caress soothingly—in LATIN) and reduce afferent impulses arising from the irritated mucosa. Dry cough due to irritation of the pharyngeal mucosa is relieved. Candy sugar or a few drops of lemon also serve this purpose.

Expectorants

Expectorants (Latin—*expectorate* = to drive from the chest) increase the production of respiratory tract secretions which cover the irritated mucosa. As the secretions now become thin and less viscid, they can be easily coughed out. Expectorants may increase the secretions directly or reflexly.

Direct stimulants Volatile oils like eucalyptus oil; creosotes, alcohol, cidar wood oil—when administered by inhalation with steam can increase respiratory secretions.

Reflex expectorants are given orally, they are gastric irritants and reflexly increase respiratory secretions.

Potassium iodide acts both directly and reflexly. Ipecacuanha is an emetic. In sub-emetic doses it is used as an expectorant.

Bronchodilators like salbutamol and terbutaline relieve cough that is resulting from bronchospasm.

The antitussive preparations generally have a combination of a central cough suppressant, an expectorant, an antihistaminic and sometimes a bronchodilator and a mucolytic agent.

MUCOLYTICS

Normally the respiratory mucous is watery. The glycoproteins in the mucous are linked by disulphide bonds to form polymers making it slimy. In respiratory diseases, the glycoproteins form larger polymers with plasma proteins present in the exudate and the secretions become thick and viscid. Mucolytics liquefy the sputum making it less viscid so that it can be easily expectorated.

Bromhexine obtained from the plant *Adhatoda vasica* is a good mucolytic. It depolymerises the mucopolysaccharides in the mucous. It is given orally (8-16 mg thrice daily). Side effects are minor—may cause rhinorrhoea.

Ambroxol is a metabolite of bromhexine with actions similar to it. Ambroxol may be given orally by inhalation. It can be used as an alternative to bromhexine.

Acetylcysteine opens disulfide bonds in the mucoproteins of the sputum reducing its viscosity. It is given by aerosol. Side effects are common and hence not preferred.

Carbocysteine is similar to acetylcysteine and is used orally.

Pancreatic dornase Deoxyribonucleoprotein is a major component of the purulent respiratory tract secretions. Pancreatic dornase is a deoxyribonuclease obtained from the bovine pancreas. It breaks the deoxyribonucleic acid (DNA) into smaller parts thus making the secretions thin and less viscid. It is administered by inhalation.

Pancreatic dornase can cause allergic reactions.

Steam inhalation offers an effective and inexpensive alternative to drugs. In presence of dehydration, just rehydrating the patient is found to be beneficial.

9

Blood

- HAEMATINICS
- DRUGS USED IN THE DISORDERS OF COAGULATION
- HYPOLIPIDAEMIC DRUGS

❑ HAEMATINICS

Haematinics are compounds required in the formation of blood and are employed in the treatment of anaemias. Iron, vitamin B_{12} and folic acid are essential for normal erythropoiesis.

IRON

Iron is essential for haemoglobin production. It is also present in myoglobin, the cytochromes and other enzymes. Total body iron is about 2.5 to 5 grams.

Daily requirement of iron

Adult male	0.5-1 mg
Adult female	1-2 mg
Pregnancy and lactation	3-5 mg

Dietary sources of iron Food that is rich in iron are liver, egg yolk, meat, fish, chicken, spinach, dry fruits, wheat and apple.

Absorption The average Indian diet provides about 10-20 mg of iron. Ten per cent of this iron is absorbed. It is mostly absorbed from the upper gut in the ferrous form. During deficiency, absorption is better.

Factors that influence iron absorption

Ascorbic acid, Amino acids, meat, ↑gastric acidity	*Increase absorption*	Antacids, phosphates, phytates, tetracyclines, presence of food in the stomach	*Decrease absorption*

Transport and distribution Iron is transported with the help of a glycoprotein *transferrin* and stored as *ferritin* and *haemosiderin*, in liver, spleen and bone marrow.

Preparations of Iron

Iron is generally given orally—but can be given parenterally.

Oral iron preparations

1. Ferrous sulphate—200 mg tab
2. Ferrous fumarate—200 mg tab
3. Ferrous gluconate—300 mg tab
4. Ferrous succinate—100 mg
5. Iron calcium complex—5% iron
6. Ferric ammonium citrate—45 mg.
   - Ferrous salts are better absorbed than ferric salts and are cheaper.
   - Expensive preparations of iron with vitamins, liver extract, amino acids, etc. are available but have no clear advantages.
   - *Dose* Ferrous sulphate 3-4 tablets daily.

Adverse effects of oral iron Epigastric pain, nausea, vomiting, gastritis, metallic taste, constipation (due to astringent effect) or diarrhoea (irritant effect) are the usual adverse effects. Liquid preparations of iron cause staining of the teeth.

Parenteral iron Iron is given parenterally only in some situations. Intramuscular injection of iron is given deep IM. Intravenous iron is given slowly over 5-10 minutes or as infusion after a test dose. **Iron dextran** can be given IM and IV. Iron sorbitol citric acid is given IM.

Indications for parenteral iron

1. When oral iron is not tolerated
2. Failure of absorption—as in malabsorption, chronic bowel disease

3. When patients do not take regularly.
4. Severe deficiency with bleeding.

Adverse effects of parenteral iron

Local Pain at the site of injection and pigmentation of the skin.

Systemic Fever, headache, joints pain, palpitation, and rarely anaphylaxis.

Acute iron poisoning is common in infants and children in whom about 10 tablets (1-2 g) can be lethal. Manifestations include vomiting, abdominal pain, haematemesis, bloody diarrhoea, shock, drowsiness, cyanosis, acidosis, dehydration, cardiovascular collapse and coma. Immediate diagnosis and treatment are important as death may occur in 6-12 hr.

Treatment

- Stomach wash with sodium bicarbonate solution.
- Desferrioxamine is the antidote.
- Correction of acidosis and shock.

Uses of Iron

1. Iron deficiency anaemia. The cause for iron deficiency should be identified. Treatment should be continued depending on the response for 3-6 months to replenish the iron stores.
2. Iron is given in conditions with increased iron requirement as in pregnancy, infancy and professional blood donors.

VITAMIN B_{12} AND FOLIC ACID

Vitamin B_{12} and folic acid are water soluble vitamins, belonging to the B-complex group. They are essential for normal DNA synthesis. Their deficiency leads to impaired DNA synthesis and abnormal maturation of RBCs and other rapidly dividing cells. This results in megaloblastic anaemia, characterised by the presence of red cell precursors in the blood and bone marrow. Other manifestations of deficiency include glossitis, stomatitis and malabsorption; neurological manifestations can also result.

Vitamin B_{12}

Vitamin B_{12} (Cyanocobalamin) is synthesized by microorganisms. Liver, fish, egg yolk, meat, cheese and pulses are the dietary sources of B_{12}.

Vitamin B_{12} or extrinsic factor is absorbed with the help of intrinsic factor, a protein secreted by the stomach. It is carried in the plasma by B_{12} binding proteins called *transcobalamin* and is stored in the liver.

Deficiency

B_{12} deficiency may be due to:

1. *Pernicious anaemia* There is deficiency of intrinsic factor resulting in failure of B_{12} absorption.
2. *Other causes* Chronic gastritis, malabsorption and fish tapeworm infestation (consumes B_{12}).

Uses

1. *Vitamin B_{12} deficiency* Prevention and treatment of megaloblastic anaemia due to B_{12} deficiency.
2. *Vitamin B_{12} neuropathies* like subacute combined degeneration respond to vitamin B_{12}.

TABLE 9.1: Daily requirement of vitamin B_{12} and folic acid

	Adults	*Pregnancy and lactation*
Vitamin B_{12}	1-3 μg	3-5 μg
Folic acid	50-100 μg	200-400 μg

Folic Acid

Folic acid was first isolated from spinach and therefore named as folic acid (from leaf).

Dietary source Green vegetables, liver, yeast, egg, milk and some fruits. Prolonged cooking with spices destroys folic acid.

Deficiency

Folate deficiency may be due to dietary folate deficiency, malabsorption and other diseases of the small intestine or drug induced. Phenytoin, phenobarbitone, oral contraceptives, methotrexate and trimethoprim can induce folate deficiency. Increased requirement as in growing children, pregnancy and lactation can also cause deficiency. Manifestations include megaloblastic anaemia, glossitis, diarrhoea and weakness.

Uses

1. Megaloblastic anaemia due to folate as well as B_{12} deficiency—folic acid is given orally along with vitamin B_{12}.
2. In pregnancy lactation, infancy and other situations with increased requirement of folic acid.

HAEMATOPOIETIC GROWTH FACTORS

These are glycoprotein hormones that regulate erythropoiesis. Erythropoietin, granulocyte colony-stimulating factor (G-CSF), granulocyte macrophage colony-stimulating factor (GM-CSF) are the haematopoietic growth factors available for clinical use. They are useful in the prevention and treatment of anaemia and neutropenia in AIDs, aplastic anaemia, following cancer chemotherapy and bone marrow transplantation.

❑ DRUGS USED IN THE DISORDERS OF COAGULATION

Haemostasis is the spontaneous arrest of bleeding from the damaged blood vessels. In the process, complex interactions take place between the injured vessel wall, platelets and clotting factors.

When there is any injury, there is local vasoconstriction and platelets stick to one another. A clot forms on this with the help of fibrin forming a plug which temporarily stops bleeding.

DRUGS USED IN DISORDERS OF COAGULATION

Procoagulants
- Adrenaline
- Thrombin
- Fibrin
- Gelatin foam
- Astringents
- Vitamin K

Anticoagulants
- Heparin
- LMW heparin—
  enoxeparin, dalteparin
  oral anticoagulants
- Warfarin
- Nicoumalone
- Phenindione

Antiplatelet drugs
- Aspirin
- Dipyridamole
- Ticlopidine

Fibrinolytics (Thrombolytics)
- Streptokinase
- Urokinase
- Alteplase
- Retiplase

Antifibrinolytics
- Epsilon amino caproic acid (EACA)
- Tranexaemic acid

Clotting factors are proteins synthesized by the liver. Several proteins interact to form the clot (Fig. 9.1).

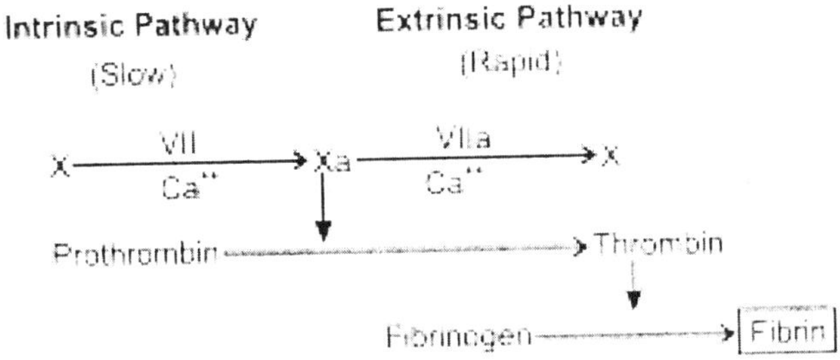

Fig. 9.1: Major reactions of blood coagulation

Anticoagulants

Anticoagulants are drugs that reduce the coagulability of the blood.

Classification

1. *Anticoagulants used in vivo*
   A. ***Fast acting*** Heparin, Heparinoids—Heparan sulphate, Dextran sulphate
   B. ***Slow acting***—oral anticoagulants
   Coumarin derivatives: Bishydroxycoumarin, Warfarin sodium, Nicoumalone
   Indandione derivatives: Phenindione, Diphenadione
2. *Anticoagulants used in vitro*
   Heparin, Citrates, Oxalates and Sodium edetate.

Heparin was discovered by McLean, a medical student in 1916. It was named 'heparin' as it was first extracted from the liver. It is found in the mast cells of the liver, lungs and intestinal mucosa. Heparin is the strongest acid in the body.

Actions Heparin is a powerful anticoagulant that acts instantaneously both *in vivo* and *in vitro*.

Mechanism of action Heparin activates plasma antithrombin III which binds to the clotting factors and inactivates them. Clotting time is prolonged.

Pharmacokinetics Heparin is not effective orally. It is given IV or SC. Treatment is monitored by the clotting time. Heparin is metabolised by heparinase in the liver.

Adverse reactions

1. *Bleeding* is the most common, major adverse effect of heparin. Careful monitoring and dose control will prevent this to a great extent.
2. *Hypersensitivity reactions* For commercial use heparin is obtained from bovine lung or porcine intestine. Because of its animal origin allergic reactions are quite common.
3. *Thrombocytopenia*
4. *Alopecia* is reversible.
5. *Osteoporosis*—on long-term use.

Contraindications to Heparin Therapy

Bleeding disorders, thrombocytopenia , haemophilia, severe hypertension, intracranial haemorrhage, cirrhosis, ulcers in the gut, renal failure and neurosurgery.

Low molecular weight (LMW) heparins e.g., Enoxaparin and dalteparin are LMW heparins which have longer action as well as lower risk of bleeding when compared to standard heparin preparations. They are used for the prevention and treatment of deep vein thrombosis.

Heparin antagonist **Protamine sulphate** is a protein obtained from the sperm of certain fish. Given intravenously, it neutralises heparin and act as heparin antagonist in heparin over dosage.

ORAL ANTICOAGULANTS

Bishydroxycoumarin was the first oral anticoagulant to be identified in North America. Many related compounds were then developed and are also being used as rat poison.

Mechanism of action Oral anticoagulants prevent the synthesis of vitamin K dependent clotting factors (factors II, III, IX and X) in the liver.

The onset of action is slow; it develops over 1-3 days because oral anticoagulants do not destroy the already circulating clotting factors. Prothrombin time (PT) is measured to monitor the treatment. It takes 5-7 days for PT to return to normal after stopping oral anticoagulants.

Pharmacokinetics Warfarin is completely absorbed orally and is 99% bound to plasma proteins.

Adverse effects

1. Haemorrhage is the main adverse effect. Bleeding in the intestines, brain, nose and gums can occur.

   Treatment—depends on the severity:

   a. Stop the anticoagulant.
   b. Fresh blood transfusion is given to supply the clotting factors.
   c. *Antidote* The specific antidote is **vitamin K_1 oxide** which allows synthesis of clotting factors. But the response to vitamin K_1 oxide needs several hours. Hence in emergency, **fresh whole blood** is necessary to counter the effects of oral anticoagulants.

2. Other adverse effects include allergic reactions, gastro-intestinal disturbances and teratogenicity.

Factors influencing oral anticoagulant activity

Factors enhancing activity	*Factors reducing activity*
Poor diet, bowel disease, liver disease and chronic alcoholism—result in vitamin K deficiency	Pregnancy—there is increased synthesis of clotting factors Hypothyroidism—there is reduced degradation of clotting factors.

Drug interactions

Many drugs increase warfarin action

1. Drugs that inhibit platelet function—NSAIDs like aspirin increase the risk of bleeding.
2. Drugs that inhibit hepatic drug metabolism like cimetidine, chloramphenicol and metronidazole enhance plasma levels of warfarin.
3. Drugs that displace warfarin from plasma protein binding sites like NSAIDs enhance plasma levels.
4. Drugs like broad spectrum antibiotics inhibit gut flora thus decreasing vitamin K synthesis.

Some drugs *reduce* the effect of oral anticoagulants.

1. Drugs that enhance the metabolism of oral anticoagulants—microsomal enzyme inducers like barbiturates, rifampicin,

griseofulvin enhance the metabolism of oral anticoagulants. When these drugs are suddenly withdrawn, excess anticoagulant activity may result in haemorrhages.
2. Drugs that increase the synthesis of clotting factors—oral contraceptives.

Uses of anticoagulants Anticoagulants can prevent extension of the thrombus but cannot destroy the existing clots. Heparin has rapid and short-action which makes it suitable for initiating treatment while warfarin is suitable for long-term maintenance due to its slow and prolonged action and convenience of oral use.

1. *Venous thrombosis and pulmonary embolism*—anticoagulants prevent extension of thrombus and recurrence of embolism.
2. *Postoperative, post-stroke patients; bedridden patients* due to leg fractures and other causes—who cannot be ambulant for several months—anticoagulants prevent venous thrombosis and pulmonary embolism in such patients.
3. *Rheumatic heart disease*—anticoagulants prevent embolism.
4. *Unstable angina*—heparin reduces the risk of myocardial infarction in patients with unstable angina.
5. *Vascular surgery, artificial heart valves and haemodialysis*—anticoagulants prevent thromboembolism.

Contraindications to anticoagulant therapy

- Bleeding disorders including thrombocytopenia
- Severe hypertension
- Malignancies
- Bacterial endocarditis
- Liver and kidney diseases.

THROMBOLYTICS (Fibrinolytics)

Thrombolytics lyse or dissolve the clot or thrombi by activating the natural fibrinolytic system.

$$\text{Plasminogen} \xrightarrow[\textit{activator}]{\textit{Tissue plasminogen}} \text{Plasmin} \longrightarrow \begin{array}{c}\text{Fibrin}\\ \downarrow \\ \text{Fibrin degradation products}\end{array}$$

Plasminogen circulates in the plasma and also some of it is bound to fibrin. Tissue plasminogen activator (tPA) activates plasminogen which is converted to plasmin. Plasmin degrades fibrin thereby dissolving the clot. Thrombolytic agents are **streptokinase, urokinase and alteplase.** All are expensive drugs.

Streptokinase obtained from β-haemolytic streptococci activates plasminogen. Antistreptococcal antibodies present in the blood due to previous streptococcal infections inactivate a large amount of streptokinase.

Urokinase is an enzyme prepared from cultures of human kidney cells (it was first isolated from human urine—hence the name). It activates plasminogen. It is more expensive than streptokinase.

Tissue plasminogen activator (tPA) preferentially activates plasminogen that is bound to fibrin which means circulating plasminogen is largely spared.

Alteplase is tPA produced by recombinant DNA technology. It is very expensive.

Reteplase is modified human tPA obtained by genetic engineering. It has less bleeding tendency when compared to other fibrinolytics.

Adverse effects of thrombolytics Bleeding is the major toxicity of all thrombolytics. Hypotension and fever can occur. Allergic reactions are common with streptokinase.

Uses

1. Acute myocardial infarction—Intravenous thrombolytics reduce the morality rate in acute MI.
2. Deep vein thrombosis and large pulmonary emboli are also treated with fibrinolytics.

Contraindications to thrombolytic therapy

- Recent surgery, injury, gastrointestinal bleeding, stroke
- Severe hypertension
- Bleeding disorders.

ANTIFIBRINOLYTICS

Antifibrinolytics inhibit plasminogen activation and thus prevent fibrinolysis.

Epsilon aminocaproic acid (EACA) and its analogue tranexaemic acid are antifibrinolytics. They are used in overdose of fibrinolytics, and to reduce bleeding after prostatic surgery or after tooth extraction in haemophiliacs—but the beneficial effect is uncertain.

ANTIPLATELET DRUGS

Platelets form the initial plug at the site of vascular injury and are also involved in the formation of atherosclerosis. By inhibiting the platelet function, thrombosis and atherosclerotic vascular disease can be largely prevented.

Antiplatelet drugs or drugs interfering with platelet function are aspirin, dipyridamole, sulphinpyrazone and ticlopidine.

Aspirin (see Chapter 5) Thromboxane A_2 promotes platelet aggregation. Aspirin inactivates cyclo-oxygenase (COX) and thereby inhibits the synthesis of thromboxane A_2 even in low doses (75 mg/day). The COX inhibition is irreversible and the effect lasts for 7 to 10 days—till fresh platelets are formed.

Uses of antiplatelet drugs

1. *Myocardial infarction* Aspirin is used in both acute MI and after MI to prevent further attack.
2. *Unstable angina* Aspirin reduces the risk of acute MI.
3. In, valvular heart disease and after coronary by-pass surgery—long-term use of low dose aspirin is recommended.
4. *Cerebral thrombosis* In patients with transient ischaemic attacks aspirin helps to prevents stroke.

COAGULANTS

Coagulants are drugs that promote coagulation (procoagulants) and control bleeding. They are also called *haemostatics.* They may be used locally or systemically. Local haemostatics are called *styptics.* Physical methods like application of pressure, tourniquet or ice can control bleeding.

Styptics are local haemostatics that are used on bleeding sites like tooth socket.

They are:

1. *Adrenaline* Sterile cotton soaked in 1:10,000 solution of adrenaline is commonly used in tooth sockets and as nasal packs for epistaxis. Adrenaline arrests bleeding by vasoconstriction.
2. *Thrombin* powder is dusted over the bleeding surface following skin grafting. It is obtained from bovine plasma.
3. *Fibrin* obtained from human plasma is available as sheets. It is used for covering or packing bleeding surfaces.
4. *Gelatin foam* is porous spongy gelatin used with thrombin to control bleeding from wounds. It gets completely absorbed in 4 to 6 weeks and can be left in place after suturing of the wound.
5. *Thromboplastin powder* is used in surgery as a styptic.
6. *Astringents* like tannic acid are used on bleeding gums.

COAGULANTS USED SYSTEMICALLY

Vitamin K

Vitamin K is a fat-soluble vitamin essential for the biosynthesis of clotting factors (factors II, VII, IX and X by the liver).

Uses

1. Vitamin K deficiency
2. *Newborn babies* lack intestinal flora and have low levels of prothrombin and other clotting factors. Routine administration of vitamin K—1 mg IM prevents haemorrhagic disease of the newborn.
3. Oral anticoagulant toxicity.

Other Coagulants

Fresh plasma or whole blood is useful in most coagulation disorders as it contains all the clotting factors. Other concentrated plasma fractions like fibrinogen, factors VIII, II, VII, IX and X are available for the treatment of specific deficiencies.

Snake venoms Some venoms like Russels viper venom stimulate thrombokinase and promote coagulation.

❑ HYPOLIPIDAEMIC DRUGS

Hyperlipoproteinaemias (HPL) are conditions in which the concentration of cholesterol or triglyceride (TG) carrying lipoproteins in the plasma is elevated above normal. When the lipoproteins increase, the development of atherosclerosis is faster and is a risk factor for myocardial infarction. LDL is the primary carrier of cholesterol while VLDL is the carrier of triglycerides. Along with reduction of body weight and low cholesterol diet, hypolipidaemic drugs may be given in patients with hyperlipoproteinaemias.

TABLE 9.2: Plasma lipid levels (mg/dl)

Grade	*Total cholesterol*	*Triglycerides*
Normal	< 200	< 200
Borderline	200-240	200-400
High	> 240	> 400

HYPOLIPIDAEMICS

1. ***HMG CoA reductase inhibitors***—Lovastatin, Simvastatin, Pravastatin
2. ***Fibric acids***—Gemfibrozil, Clofibrate, Fenofibrate
3. ***Bile acid binding resins***—Cholestyramine, Colestipol
4. ***Antioxidant***—Probucol
5. ***Miscellaneous***—Nicotinic acid, Neomycin.

HMG CoA Reductase Inhibitors

Hydroxymethylglutaryl-CoA (HMG-CoA) is the rate-controlling enzyme in the biosynthesis of cholesterol. HMG-CoA inhibitors lower plasma LDL cholesterol and triglycerides. The concentration of HDL-cholesterol (the protective lipoprotein) increases by 10%.

Adverse effects include GI symptoms, headache, rashes and rarely myopathy.

Fibric acids enhance the activity of the enzyme lipoprotein lipase which degrades VLDL resulting in lowering of triglycerides. They also increase HDL levels. Gemfibrozil is the drug of choice in patients with increased TG levels.

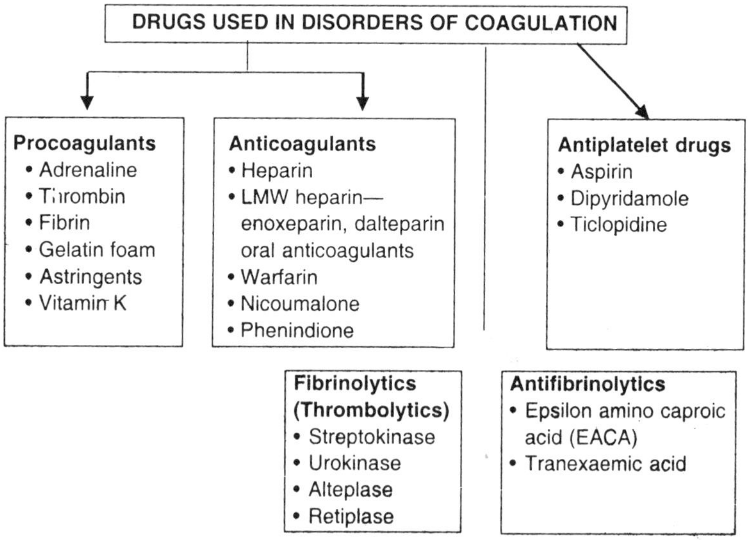

Adverse effects GI upset, skin rashes, headache, muscle cramps and blurred vision.

Bile acid binding resins bind bile acids in the intestine and increase their excretion. Bile acids are required for intestinal absorption of cholesterol. Plasma cholesterol and LDL levels fall. Bile acid binding resins are unpleasant to take; they may cause GI upset, constipation and piles. They also bind many drugs in the intestines thereby reducing their absorption.

Antioxidant

Probucol is a synthetic antioxidant which lowers plasma cholesterol, LDL and HDL levels. It is used with other hypolipidaemics.

TABLE 9.3: Choice of hypolipidaemics

Elevated TG levels	Gemfibrozil
Elevated LDL cholesterol	Lovastatin; adjuvant-binding resins/ nicotinic acid
Elevated TG + cholesterol	Lovastatin + Gemfibrozil

Miscellaneous

Nicotinic acid—a B group vitamin, inhibits lipolysis and increases lipoprotein lipase activity resulting in lowering of TGs and LDL levels. It reduces the synthesis of VLDL.

Neomycin forms insoluble complexes with bile acids in the intestines and thus lowers cholesterol levels.

10

Gastrointestinal Tract

- DRUGS USED IN PEPTIC ULCER
- PROKINETIC AGENTS
- EMETICS AND ANTIEMETICS
- DRUGS FOR CONSTIPATION AND DIARRHOEA

DRUGS USED IN PEPTIC ULCER

Acid-peptic disease is common in the present days that are full of tension and anxiety. Peptic ulcer results from an imbalance between acid-pepsin secretion and mucosal defense . The factors that protect the mucosa are its ability to secrete mucous, bicarbonate and prostaglandins. Gastric acid secretion is controlled by three pathways—vagus (ACh), gastrin and local release of histamine—each acting through its own receptors (Fig. 10.1). Histamine acts through H_2 receptors on parietal cells while acetylcholine through M_1 muscarinic and gastrin through G receptors on the parietal cells. These activate $H^+ K^+$ ATPase (proton pump) on the parietal cells resulting in the secretion of H^+ into the gastric lumen. This combines with Cl^- (drawn from plasma) and HCl is secreted.

CLASSIFICATION

1. *Drugs that neutralise gastric acid* Antacids—$MgOH_2$, $Al(OH)_3$
2. *Drugs that reduce gastric acid secretion*
   a. H_2 receptor blockers—Cimetidine, Ranitidine, Famotidine, Roxatidine, Nizatidine

   b. Proton pump inhibitors—Omeprazole, Lansoprazole
   c. Muscarinic antagonists—Pirenzepine
3. *Ulcer protectives* Sucralfate, Bismuth compounds
4. *Other drugs* Carbenoxolone, Cisapride, Prostaglandins.

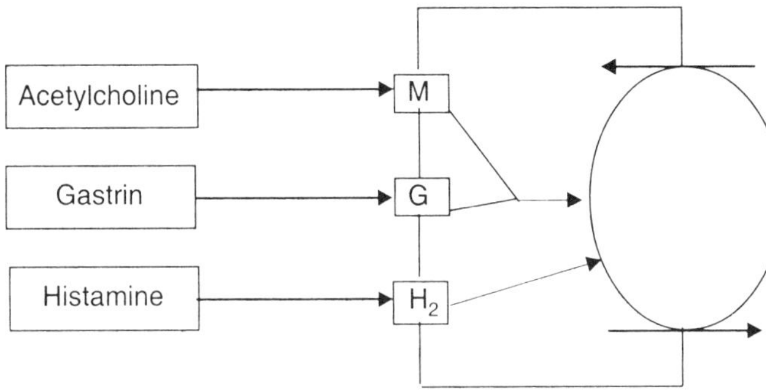

Fig. 10.1: Regulation of gastric secretion: M—Muscarinic receptor (M2/3); G—Gastrin receptors; H_2—Histamine H_2 receptor

ANTACIDS

Antacids are basic substances. Given orally they neutralize the gastric acid and raise the pH of gastric contents. Peptic activity is also reduced because, pepsin is active only above pH 4. Antacids are of 2 types:

1. *Systemic* Sodium bicarbonate
2. *Nonsystemic* Aluminium hydroxide, Magnesium trisilicate, Magnesium hydroxide, Calcium carbonate.

Systemic Antacids

Sodium bicarbonate is rapid but short-acting. CO_2 that is released in the stomach escapes as eructation. It gets absorbed from the intestines leading to systemic alkalosis. There is 'rebound' hyperacidity as gastrin levels increase due to raised gastric pH. Sodium load may increase. It is not preferred because of the above disadvantages.

Sodium bicarbonate is used with other antacids in peptic ulcer. Other uses are to alkalinise the urine in poisoning and to treat metabolic acidosis.

Non-systemic Antacids

Non-systemic antacids are insoluble compounds that react in the stomach with HCl to form a chloride salt and water. They are not absorbed.

Aluminium hydroxide is slow acting. Food further slows it's neutralizing capacity. It is also an astringent and demulcent—forms a protective coating over the ulcers. The aluminium ions relax the smooth muscles resulting in delayed gastric emptying and constipation. Aluminium hydroxide binds phosphate and prevents its absorption resulting in hypophosphataemia on prolonged use.

Magnesium salts The action is quick and prolonged. Rebound acidity is mild. Magnesium salts are osmotic purgatives and the dose used as antacids may cause mild diarrhoea.

Calcium carbonate acts quickly and has prolonged action but liberates CO_2 which may cause discomfort. It may also cause constipation and hypercalcaemia.

Antacids are given in combination to obtain maximum effects with least adverse effects as follows.

1. *Quick and prolonged effect*—Fast-acting [$Mg(OH)_2$] and slow acting [$Al(OH)_3$] are combined.
2. *Neutralising side effects*—Magnesium salts cause diarrhoea while aluminium salts are constipating—combination neutralizes each others side effects.
3. *Gastric emptying*—Magnesium salts hasten while aluminium salts delay gastric emptying.

All antacid tablets should be chewed and swallowed as they do not disintegrate well in the stomach. Gels are more effective than tablets. One dose given 1 hr after food neutralizes the acid for 2 hours.

TABLE 10.1: Some antacid combination preparations

Brand name	*Combination*
1. GELUSIL liquid, tablet	Aluminium hydroxide gel + Magnesium trisilicate
2. DIGENE gel, tablet	Magnesium hydroxide + Aluminium hydroxide gel + carboxymethyl cellulose sodium + Methylpolysiloxane

Uses

Antacids are used in hyperacidity, peptic ulcer and reflux oesophagitis.

Drug interactions Antacids form complexes with iron, tetracyclines, digoxin, ranitidine, fluoroquinolones, sulfonamides and antimuscarinic drugs. To avoid these, antacids should be taken 2 hours before or 2 hours after other drugs.

H_2 receptor blockers *Cimetidine, ranitidine, famotidine, roxatidine.*

These drugs bind to H_2 receptors and competitively inhibit the action of histamine on H_2 receptors and thereby reduce gastric secretion. Both volume and acidity of basal, nocturnal and food induced secretion are reduced. They can cause 90% reduction in gastric secretion by a single dose. Gastrin induced HCl secretion and pepsin is also reduced. Due to these actions, healing of peptic ulcers is faster.

Pharmacokinetics H_2 blockers are well-absorbed. Cimetidine acts for 5-8 hours, ranitidine and famotidine for 12 hours.

Adverse effects The H_2 blockers are well-tolerated.

Cimetidine has antiandrogenic actions, it increases plasma prolactin levels and inhibits oestrogen metabolism in the liver. On prolonged use it may result in gynaecomastia, impotence and loss of libido. CNS effects include confusion, delirium and hallucinations in the elderly. Headache, dizziness, rashes and diarrhoea can result. Cimetidine inhibits microsomal enzymes and interferes with the metabolism of many drugs.

Ranitidine is the preferred H_2 blocker as it has several advantages over cimetidine. Ranitidine is more potent, longer acting, has no antiandrogenic effects, no CNS effects as it does not cross BBB and does not inhibit microsomal enzymes significantly. Only adverse effects are headache and dizziness.

Famotidine is similar to but more potent than ranitidine. Headache and rashes can occur.

Roxatidine is similar to ranitidine but is more potent and longer-acting.

Uses of H_2 blockers
H_2 blockers are used in the treatment of peptic ulcer, gastritis, reflux oesophagitis, and as preanaesthetic medication—to prevent damage if aspiration pneumonia occurs during surgery. Ranitidine is the most preferred. It is given for 4-8 weeks (300 mg daily) in peptic ulcers. It may be continued for 6 months to prevent recurrence.

Proton Pump Inhibitors

Omeprazole The parietal cells of the stomach secrete H^+ with the help of an enzyme H^+K^+ ATPase (proton pump) present in the plasma membrane. This is the final step in gastric acid secretion. Proton pump inhibitors specifically inhibit this H^+ K^+ ATPase enzyme and thereby inhibit gastric secretion. Omeprazole is a prodrug, gets activated in the acidic environment of the stomach and a single dose can totally inhibit gastric secretion. Acid secretion starts only after new H^+K^+ATPase enzyme is synthesized. Ulcer heals rapidly even in resistant cases.

Adverse effects Omeprazole is well-tolerated. Prolonged acid suppression may allow bacterial over growth in the stomach. Dizziness, headache, nausea and rashes are rare.

Uses Omeprazole is used in peptic ulcers (20-40 mg daily) and severe gastroesophageal reflux that is not responding to H_2 blockers. Ulcers heal fast and pain is relieved. It is given for 4-8 weeks.

Lansoprazole is similar to omeprazole but is longer-acting.

Anticholinergics Though atropine reduces gastric secretion, the dose needed results in several adverse effects. A derivative of atropine—pirenzepine selectively blocks muscarinic (M_1) receptors present in the stomach and inhibits gastric secretion without much side effects. It also inhibits the secretion of gastrin, mucous and bicarbonate. It is used as an adjuvant.

Ulcer Protectives

Sucralfate In acidic medium (pH < 4), sucralfate polymerizes to form a sticky, viscid gel which firmly sticks to the base of the ulcers. It remains there for over 6 hours acting as a physical block and prevents contact with acid and pepsin. It also stimulates the PG synthesis in gastric mucosa. It thus promotes healing by protecting the ulcer. Sucralfate is not absorbed and is well-tolerated.

One tablet is given 1 hr before each meal and one at bed time for 4-8 weeks and then it is continued for 6 months to prevent recurrence.

Side effects are rare and include constipation and dryness of mouth.

Drug interactions

- Sucralfate needs acidic pH for activation. Hence antacids should not be given with it.
- Sucralfate absorbs and interferes with the absorption of tetracyclines, digoxin, phenytoin and cimetidine.

Bismuth salts Colloidal bismuth subcitrate on oral administration forms complexes with proteins in the ulcer base and forms a protective coating over the gastric mucosa. It also inhibits the growth of *H. pylori* on gastric mucosa and stimulates the mucous production and PG synthesis. By these actions it promotes ulcer healing in 4-8 weeks. It may cause constipation and black stools.

Other Drugs

Carbenoxolone On ingestion carbenoxolone alters the composition of mucous so that it sticks to gastric mucosa to protect the ulcer base. It also inhibits pepsin activity and prolongs the life of prostaglandins. Because of its steroid like effects, it causes salt and water retention. It is therefore not preferred.

Prostaglandins PGE_2 and PGI_2 synthesized by the gastric mucosa inhibits gastric secretion, enhances mucous production and exerts a protective effect. PG analogs misoprostol and enprostil are of special value in preventing drug induced (e.g. NSAIDs) gastric ulceration. Diarrhoea and muscle cramps are common.

Treatment of *H. pylori* Infection

Infection with *H. pylori* is associated with gastroduodenal disease including gastritis and peptic ulcer. It is also thought to be responsible for recurrence of peptic ulcer disease. Eradication of *H. pylori* along with drugs that reduce acid secretion has shown to reduce the relapse rate.

Various combination regimens are tried with clarithromycin, amoxicillin or tetracycline; metronidazole and omeprazole for 1-2 weeks.

One regimen: Clarithromycin 250 mg BD + metronidazole 400 mg BD + omeprazole 20 mg BD—for one week.

❑ PROKINETIC AGENTS

Drugs that enhance gastroduodenal motility and hasten gastric emptying are called **prokinetic agents.** Metoclopramide, domperidone and cisapride are some prokinetic agents.

Metoclopramide

Actions GIT—Metoclopramide promotes forward movement of contents of the upper GI tract, speeds up gastric emptying, prevents reflux oesophagitis and also slightly increases intestinal peristalsis.

CNS Metoclopramide acts as an antiemetic by its actions on the CTZ and by speeding up gastric emptying.

Mechanism of action Metoclopramide acts by blocking D_2 dopamine receptors.

Adverse effects are sedation, dystonia and diarrhoea; gynaecomastia, galactorrhoea and parkinsonism (extrapyramidal symptoms) can occur on long-term use.

Uses

1. Reflux oesophagitis—'heart burn' due to reflux of acid into the oesophagus is benefited by prokinetic agents.
2. As antiemetics—in postoperative period and vomiting due to anticancer drugs.
3. As preanaesthetic medication to promote gastric emptying before induction of general anaesthesia in emergency.
4. In endoscopy—to assist passage of tubes into the duodenum.

Domperidone is similar to metoclopramide except that it does not cross the blood-brain barrier and hence does not cause extrapyramidal side effects. Side effects include headache, dryness of mouth, diarrhoea and rashes.

Domperidone can be used in place of metoclopramide.

Cisapride enhances gastric motility by promoting the release of acetylcholine in the gut wall. It also promotes colonic motility which may result in diarrhoea. It was used in reflux oesophagitis but it is now a banned drug due to adverse effects.

Gastroesophageal reflux Reflux of acidic gastric contents into the oesophagus results in 'heart burn' due to oesophagitis. Based on severity, it may be treated with antacids, metoclopramide or drugs that reduce acid secretion. Omeprazole is the most effective agent. Avoiding—heavy meals, late night dinner, smoking and alcohol—all help.

❑ EMETICS AND ANTIEMETICS

Stimulation of the vomiting centre in the medulla oblongata results in vomiting. The vomiting centre receives afferents from the chemoreceptor trigger zone (CTZ), vestibular apparatus, GI tract and centres in the brain. CTZ is not protected by the blood-brain barrier and is stimulated by various drugs, chemicals and radiation.

Emetics are drugs that produce vomiting. When a noxious substance is swallowed, vomiting has to be induced. Mustard powder (1 teaspoon) with water or hypertonic salt solution can evoke vomiting.

Apomorphine is a derivative of morphine. Given SC/IM, it produces vomiting in 5-10 minutes. It acts by stimulating the CTZ.

Ipecacuanha contains an alkaloid emetine. Given as a syrup (15- 20 ml), it produces vomiting in 15 minutes. It is safe even in children.

Antiemetics Vomiting is a protective mechanism which tries to eliminate the unwanted harmful material from the stomach. But in some situations, vomiting may not serve any useful purpose and may only be troublesome. In such circumstances, vomiting needs to be suppressed.

CLASSIFICATION

1. *Dopamine D_2 antagonists—prokinetics* Metoclopramide, Domperidone.
2. *Antimuscarinics* Hyoscine, H_1 antihistamines like Cyclizine, Promethazine, Diphenhydramine.
3. *$5HT_3$ antagonists* Ondansetron, Granisetron.
4. *Neuroleptics* Chlorpromazine, Prochlorperazine, Haloperidol.
5. *Other agents* Cisapride, Corticosteroids.

Dopamine D_2 Antagonists

Metoclopramide acts centrally by blocking dopamine D_2 receptors in the CTZ. It increases the tone of the lower oesophageal sphincter and enhances gastric peristalsis. It is used in nausea and vomiting due to gastrointestinal disorders, migraine, in postoperative period and vomiting due to anticancer drugs and radiotherapy.

Domperidone acts like metoclopramide with fewer side effects.

Antimuscarinics

Hyosine (see Chapter 2) is very effective in motion sickness. Motion sickness or travelling sickness is due to over stimulation of the vestibular apparatus along with psychological and environmental factors. Taken 30 minutes before journey, hyoscine (0.4-0.6 mg oral) acts for 6 hours and the dose should be repeated if the journey is longer than that. A transdermal patch delivers hyoscine constantly over 3 days and is to be applied behind the ear. Sedation and dry mouth are common side effects.

H_1 antihistamines (see Chapter 6) like promethazine, diphenhydramine, cyclizine and cinnarizine have anticholinergic properties. They may act both centrally and on the GI tract. They are useful in motion sickness and postoperative vomiting.

5-HT3 Antagonists

Ondansetron 5-hydroxytryptamine released in the gut is an important transmitter of emesis. Ondansetron blocks 5 HT_3 receptors in the GI tract and CTZ and prevents vomiting. It is a powerful antiemetic and can be given orally or intravenously (4-8 mg). It is specially useful to control vomiting induced by anticancer drugs or radiotherapy. It is also useful in postoperative vomiting and other drug induced vomiting. Adverse effects include headache and gastrointestinal upset.

Granisetron is more potent than ondansetron as an antiemetic.

Neuroleptics (page 212) also block D_2-receptors in the CTZ and are useful in vomiting due to most causes except motion sickness. Sedation and extrapyramidal symptoms are the common side effects. Prochlorperazine is mainly used as an antiemetic in vomiting and is also effective in vertigo associated with vomiting.

Other Antiemetics

Corticosteroids are used as adjuvants along with other antiemetics like ondansetron or metoclopramide.

Dicyclomine is used to control vomiting in morning sickness and motion sickness (Table 10.2).

TABLE 10.2: Preferred drugs for vomiting due to various causes

Conditions	*Drugs*
Motion sickness	Hyoscine, Cyclizine, Promethazine, Cinnarizine
Vomiting due to cytotoxic drugs	Ondansetron + Dexamethasone
Vomiting due to other drugs	Chlorpromazine, Metoclopramide
Postoperative vomiting	Ondansetron, Metoclopramide
Vomiting in pregnancy	Dicyclomine, Pyridoxine, Cyclizine, Meclizine, Metoclopramide

❑ DRUGS FOR CONSTIPATION AND DIARRHOEA

Purgatives

Purgatives are drugs that promote defecation. They are also called *laxatives* and *cathartics*. Laxatives have milder action while cathartics or purgatives have more powerful action.

CLASSIFICATION

1. *Bulk laxatives* — Bran, Plantago seeds, Agar, Methylcellulose, Ispaghula husk
2. *Faecal softeners* — Docusate sodium, Liquid paraffin (emollients)
3. *Osmotic purgatives* — Magnesium sulphate, Magnesium hydroxide, Sodium sulphate, Lactulose
4. *Stimulant purgatives* — Phenolphthalein, Bisacodyl, Castor oil, Anthraquinones—Cascara sagrada, Senna

Bulk laxatives Bulk laxatives include vegetable fibre and other substances that are not digested but increase the volume of intestinal contents forming a large, soft, solid stool. Dietary fibre consists of cell walls and other parts of fruits and vegetables that are unabsorbable. Adding fibre to the diet is a safe and natural way of treating constipation in persons who are on low-fibre diet. ***Bran*** is the residue left when flour is made from cereals and contains 40% fibre—but is unpalatable. Ispaghula and plantago seeds contain natural mucilage which absorbs water to form a gelatinous mass and are more palatable than bran. Methylcellulose is a semisynthetic derivative of cellulose. Adequate water should be taken along with bulk laxatives.

Faecal softeners

Docusate sodium (dioctyl sodium sulphosuccinate) softens faeces by lowering the surface tension of the intestinal contents. This allows more water to be retained in the faeces which becomes soft.

Liquid paraffin is a mineral oil that is not digested. It lubricates and softens faeces. It is unpalatable; aspiration may cause lipoid pneumonia; it may leak out of the anus causing discomfort. Hence not preferred.

Osmotic purgatives are solutes that are not absorbed in the intestine, osmotically retain water and increase the bulk of intestinal contents. They increase peristalsis and expel a fluid stool. Magnesium hydroxide, magnesium sulphate, sodium potassium tartrate, sodium sulphate and phosphate are some inorganic salts used as osmotic or saline purgatives. They are used to prepare the bowel before surgery and in food poisoning.

Lactulose is a synthetic disaccharide that is not absorbed, holds water and acts as an osmotic purgative. Flatulence and cramps may be accompanied. In the colon, lactulose is fermented to lactic and acetic acids which inhibit the growth of ammonia-producing bacteria in the colon. It also inhibits the absorption of ammonia by lowering pH and thus lowers blood ammonia levels. It is used in hepatic coma for this effect (hepatic coma is worsened by ammonia).

Stimulant purgatives increase intestinal motility and increase the secretion of water and electrolytes by the mucosa. They may cause abdominal cramps.

When cascara sagrada and senna (source: plants) are given orally, active anthraquinones are liberated in the intestines which stimulate the myenteric plexus in the colon. Evacuation takes 6-8 hr. Long-term use causes melanotic pigmentation of the colon.

Phenolphthalein an indicator, acts on the colon after 6 to 8 hours to produce soft, semiliquid stools. It undergoes enterohepatic circulation which prolongs its actions. Allergic reactions including pink coloured skin eruptions and colic limit it's use.

Bisacodyl related to phenolphthalein is converted to the active metabolite in the intestines. It can be given orally (5 mg) but usually is used as rectal suppositories (10 mg) which results in defecation in 15-30 minutes. It is safe except that prolonged use may cause local inflammation.

Castor oil is hydrolysed in the upper small intestine to ricinoleic acid which is a local irritant and increases intestinal motility. It is a powerful and one of the oldest purgatives. Stool is semiliquid and is accompanied by gripping. It is not preferred.

Enema Enema produces defecation by softening stools and distending the bowel. Evacuant enema is used to prepare the gut for surgery, endoscopy and radiological examination (see Chapter 1).

TABLE 10.3: Choice of purgatives

Conditions	*Preferred laxative*
1. Functional constipation	Increasing dietary fibre and adequate fluid intake
2. Elderly patients	Increasing dietary fibre and adequate fluid intake
3. Pregnancy	Dietary fibre
4. To avoid straining at stools—as in hernia, piles, fissure, cardiovascular diseases like myocardial infarction	Bulk laxatives or faecal softeners
5. Irritable bowel syndrome—chronic constipation	Bulk laxatives
6. Food or drug poisoning	Osmotic purgatives
7. Bowel preparation before surgery, endoscopy and radiological examination	Bisacodyl, osmotic purgatives

Use of laxatives in constipation Fibre rich diet, adequate fluid intake and physical activity are the best measures to prevent and treat mild constipation. If these measures are inadequate, a laxative may be given (see Table 10.3).

Drug induced constipation Drugs like anticholinergics, NSAIDs, opioids, clonidine, iron, calcium channel blockers and antihistamines can cause constipation. When withdrawal of the causative drug is not possible, a laxative may be used.

Laxative abuse Habitual use of laxatives, especially stimulant laxatives may lead to various gastrointestinal disturbances like irritable bowel syndrome, loss of electrolytes, loss of calcium in the stool and malabsorption. Misconceptions regarding bowel habits should be cleared. The patient should be convinced that normal bowel habits may vary between 3 motions daily and 2 motions per week.

DRUGS USED IN THE TREATMENT OF DIARRHOEA

Diarrhoea is the frequent passage of liquid stools. It can be due to a variety of causes like infection, toxins, anxiety and drugs. Acute diarrhoea is one of the major causes of death in infants specially in the developing countries. Death is due to dehydration.

In diarrhoea, there is an increase in motility and secretions in the gut with absorption of water and electrolytes. Hence the approaches in the treatment of diarrhoea include:

1. replacement of fluid and electrolytes
2. treatment of the cause
3. antidiarrhoeal agents.

Correction of fluid and electrolyte disturbances can be life saving in most cases especially infants. Oral rehydration with sodium chloride, glucose and water is useful. In the ileum, glucose increases sodium absorption and water follows. Oral rehydration powders are available. They are to be mixed with water and given in small amounts every 15-20 minutes for mild to moderate cases. In severe degrees of dehydration, prompt intravenous rehydration is necessary (Table 10.4).

Treatment of the cause Acute diarrhoea could often be due to viral, bacterial or protozoal infection. The pathogen should be identified whenever possible and treated accordingly.

TABLE 10.4: Composition of oral rehydration salt/solution (ORS)

$NaCl^-$	—	3.5 gm
KCl^-	—	1.5 gm
Sodium citrate	—	2.9 gm
Glucose	—	20 gm
To be dissolved in 1 litre of boiled and cooled water		

Antidiarrhoeal drugs provide symptomatic relief and include ***adsorbents*** and ***antimotility drugs.***

Adsorbents include kaolin, pectin, chalk and activated charcoal. These adsorb intestinal toxins and microorganisms by coating them.

Antimotility Drugs (Table 10.5)

Codeine an opium alkaloid, stimulates the opioid receptors on the gastrointestinal smooth muscles to reduce peristalsis. This delays passage of intestinal contents and facilitates absorption of water. Nausea and vomiting may occur.

Diphenoxylate is an opioid related to pethidine. It is given with a small dose of atropine in order to discourage abuse. In therapeutic doses CNS effects are not prominent-hence no risk of abuse. It is used only in diarrhoeas. Nausea, drowsiness and abdominal pain may occur.

Loperamide is an opiate. It has selective action on GI tract with additional antisecretory action. CNS effects are negligible. It is less sedating, less addicting and is the most commonly used antimotility drug. It's low solubility in water discourages abuse by injection. Loperamide may cause nausea, vomiting and abdominal cramps.

TABLE 10.5: Antimotility drugs—some preparations and dosage

Drugs	*Trade names*	*Doses*
Diphenoxylate 2.5 mg + Atropine 0.025 mg	LOMOTIL	2-4 tablets stat; 1 every 6 hr
Loperamide	LOPESTAL	4 mg stat; 2 mg every 6 hr

Antimotility drugs are used for symptomatic treatment of non-infective diarrhoeas and traveller's diarrhoea (as adjuvant).

Other Drugs

Lactobacillus acidophilus is available as powders and tablets and is useful in some diarrhoeas. It promotes the growth of saccharolytic flora and alters the gut pH so that growth of pathogenic organisms is inhibited.

Antispasmodics Atropine derivatives like propantheline and dicyclomine relax gastrointestinal smooth muscles and relieve abdominal colics.

Traveller's diarrhoea Infection is the most common cause of traveller's diarrhoea and should be treated with suitable antimicrobials. Oral rehydration salts and loperamide may also be used.

11

Chemotherapy

GENERAL CONSIDERATIONS

Chemotherapy can be defined as the use of chemicals in infectious diseases to destroy microorganisms without damaging the host tissues. *Antibiotics* are substances produced by microorganisms which suppress the growth of or destroy other microorganisms.

Pasteur and Joubert were the first to identify that microorganisms could destroy *other* microorganisms. Paul Ehrlich 'The father of Modern Chemotherapy' coined the term 'chemotherapy'. He showed that certain dyes can destroy microbes and demonstrated that methylene blue can be used in malaria. He also synthesized some arsenical compounds for the treatment of syphilis and sleeping sickness. Domagk in 1936 demonstrated that prontosil, a sulfonamide dye is effective in some infections. The production of penicillin for clinical use in 1941 marked the beginning of the 'golden era' of antibiotics. In the last 60 years, several powerful antibiotics and their semi-synthetic derivatives have been produced.

Mechanism of action Based on their mechanisms of action, antimicrobials are classified (Fig. 11.1) as drugs that:

1. *Inhibit cell wall synthesis*—Penicillins, Cephalosporins, Vancomycins, Bacitracin, Cycloserine.
2. *Damage cell membrane* causing leakage of cell contents—Polymyxins, Amphotericin B, Nystatin.
3. *Bind to ribosomes and inhibit protein synthesis* Chloramphenicol, Tetracyclines, Erythromycin, Aminoglycosides, Clindamycin.

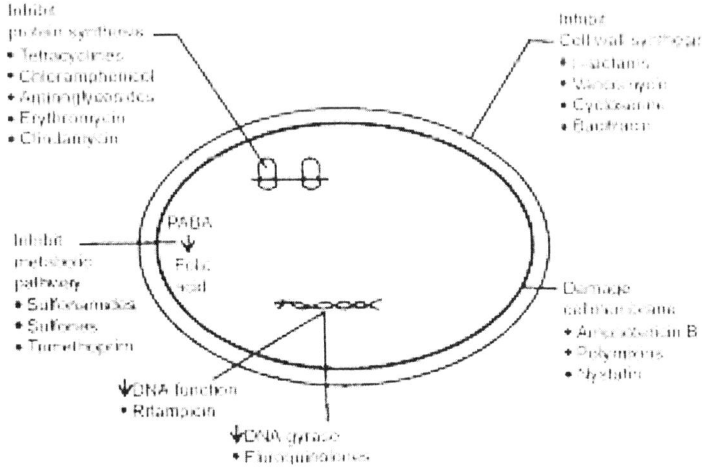

Fig. 11.1: Classification of antimicrobials based on their mechanisms of action

4. *Inhibit DNA gyrase* Fluoroquinolones like Ciprofloxacin, Norfloxacin
5. *Inhibit DNA function* (↓DNA dependant RNA polymerase)—Rifampicin
6. *Interfere with metabolic steps*—Sulfonamides, Sulfones, Trimethoprim, Pyrimethamine (antimetabolite action).

Resistance to Antimicrobial Agents

Resistance is the unresponsiveness of a microorganism to the antimicrobial agent. The resistance may be natural or acquired. In natural resistance, the organisms never respond to the antimicrobial—may be due to the absence of the particular enzyme or target site affected by the drug, e.g. gram-negative bacilli are not sensitive to PnG. But this type of resistance is clinically not a problem as alternate drugs are available.

Acquired resistance Here, the microbes which were previously sensitive to the antimicrobial agents become resistant to it. Clinically this poses a problem.

Bacteria acquire resistance by a change in their DNA. Such DNA changes may occur by: (i) Mutation or (ii) Transfer of genes.

Mutation is a genetic change that occurs spontaneously. In any population of bacteria, a few resistant mutants may be present. When the sensitive organisms are destroyed by the antibiotic, the resistant mutants freely multiply.

Transfer of genetic material Many bacteria contain genetic material called **plasmids** in the cytoplasm which carry genes coding for resistance. These plasmids are transferred to other bacteria and spread resistance (Fig. 11.2).

This spread may take place by:
1. *Transduction* Plasmid DNA is transferred through bacteriophage, i.e. virus which infects bacteria.
2. *Transformation* Resistant bacteria may release genetic material into the medium which is taken up by other bacteria.
3. *Conjugation* is the most important mode of spread of resistance. The plasmid is transferred from cell to cell by direct

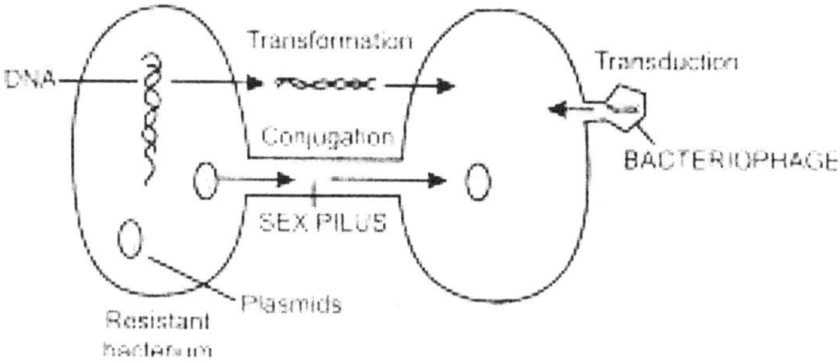

Fig. 11.2: Mechanisms of transfer of resistance

contact through a sex pilus or bridge and the process is known as conjugation.

The resistance acquired by the bacteria may result in the following:

- Production of enzymes that inactivate the drug, e.g. β-lactamase by staphylococci; aminoglycoside inactivating enzymes by *E.coli*.
- Decreased accumulation of the drug in the bacterium, e.g. resistance to tetracyclines by gram-positive and gram-negative bacteria.
- Altered target for the drug—the binding site may be altered, e.g. binding sites for aminoglycosides on the ribosomes may be altered.
- Altered metabolic pathway—bacteria may produce folic acid by an alternate pathway.

Cross resistance is the resistance seen among chemically related drugs. When a microorganism develops resistance to one drug, it is also resistant to other drugs of the same group, even when not exposed to it, e.g. resistance to one tetracycline means resistance to all other tetracyclines.

Prevention of Resistance to Antimicrobials

Development of resistance to drugs can be avoided to some extent by the following measures:

- antibiotics should be used only when necessary
- selection of the correct antibiotic is absolutely important
- correct dose and duration of treatment should be followed
- combination of drugs should be used as in tuberculosis to delay the development of resistance.

Combination of Antimicrobials

A combination of antimicrobial agents is indicated in certain specific situations. The combination serves one of the following purposes.

1. **To obtain synergism** Combination of antibiotics is recommended in conditions like
   - *Bacterial endocarditis*—Penicillin + streptomycin is synergistic.
   - *Amoxicillin + clavulinic acid*—β-lactamase producing organisms like *H. influenzae*.
2. **Treatment of mixed infections** In mixed infections with aerobic and anaerobic organisms, two or more antibiotics may be used.
3. **Initial treatment of severe infections** Drugs covering both gram-positive and gram-negative pathogens may be used initially till the culture report is available, e.g. penicillin + aminoglycoside.
4. **To prevent emergence of resistance** In the treatment of tuberculosis and leprosy, combination of drugs is used to prevent development of resistance.
5. **To reduce the adverse effects** The doses needed may be lower when a combination is used. This may reduce the incidence and severity of adverse effects, e.g. Amphotericin B + flucytosine in cryptococcal meningitis.

Disadvantages of Antimicrobial Combination

1. Risk of toxicity from each agent
   Vancomycin + aminoglycoside → more severe renal toxicity
2. Growth of resistant strains—The few resistant mutants that remain may multiply unchecked.
3. Emergence of organisms resistant to multiple drugs.
4. Increased cost of therapy.

Chemoprophylaxis

Chemoprophylaxis is the use of antimicrobial agents to prevent infection. This is recommended in the following situations:

1. **To protect healthy persons**
   - Penicillin G is given for prevention of gonorrhoea or syphilis in patients after contact with infected persons.
   - Malaria, leprosy, tuberculosis.
2. **To prevent infection in high risk patients**
   - In neutropenic patients—penicillin or fluoroquinolones or cotrimoxazole may reduce the incidence of bacterial infection.
   - In patients with valvular heart diseases even minor procedures like dental extraction, tonsillectomy or endoscopies may result in bacterial endocarditis (damage to mucosa results in bacteremia). Penicillin is used for prophylaxis.

3. **Surgical prophylaxis** Certain guidelines are to be followed: The drug should be started before surgery and should not be continued beyond 24 hours (risk of resistance) after surgery.

Superinfections

Superinfection/suprainfection is the appearance of a new infection resulting from the use of antimicrobials. Antibacterials alter the normal microbial flora of the intestinal, respiratory and genitourinary tracts. The normal flora help in host defence mechanisms by producing antibacterial substances called bacteriocins and by competing for nutrients. When the normal flora are destroyed by antibacterials, there can be dangerous infections due to various organisms especially the normal commensals. The broader the antibacterial spectrum of a drug, the more are the chances of superinfection, as the alteration of the normal flora is greater.

Candida, staphylococci and *E. coli* commonly cause superinfection.

Misuse of Antibiotics

Antibiotics are one of the most overused or misused drugs. Faulty practices like the use of antibacterials in viral infections, using too low doses or unnecessary prolonged treatment, using antibiotics in all fever cases—are all irrational and can do more harm than any benefit.

TABLE 11.1: Choice of antibiotics recommended in the treatment of some common infections

Microorganisms	*Clinical diagnosis*	*Drug of first choice*	*Alternate drugs*
Gram-positive organisms			
Group A Streptococcus	Pharyngitis, Otitis media, Sinusitis, Cellulitis, Erysipelas, Impetigo, Bacteraemia Dento-alveolar abscess	Penicillin or amoxicillin	Erythromycin, A first generation cephalosporin
Group B Streptococcus	Bacteraemia Endocarditis Meningitis	Ampicillin or penicillin + an aminoglycoside	A first generation cephalosporin
Staphylococcus aureus	Furuncle, Cellulitis, Bacteraemia, Osteomyelitis, Pneumonia		
• *Methicillin sensitive*		Cloxacillin or dicloxacillin	A first generation cephalosporin or vancomycin
• *Methicillin resistant*		Vancomycin	Ciprofloxacin + rifampicin
Pneumococcus	Pneumonia, Sinusitis, Otitis, Endocarditis, Meningitis	Penicillin Amoxicillin	A first generation cephalosporin
Penicillin resistant	—	Ceftriaxone Cefotaxime Vancomycin	Clindamycin Cotrimoxazole
Enterococcus	Endocarditis,	Penicillin G + gentamicin	Vancomycin + gentamicin
Gonococcus	Gonorrhoea, Pelvic inflammatory disease	Ceftriaxone	Ampicillin Amoxicillin Doxycycline Erythromycin
Meningococcus	Meningitis	Ceftriaxone Cefotaxime	Penicillin G Chloramphenicol
	Carrier state	Rifampicin	Minocycline
Corynebacterium diphtheriae	Diphtheria	Erythromycin	A first generation cephalosporin Clindamycin
Clostridium tetani	Tetanus	Penicillin G	Clindamycin Doxycycline
Clostridium difficile	Pseudomembranous colitis	Metronidazole	Vancomycin

Contd...

Contd...

Microorganisms	*Clinical diagnosis*	*Drug of first choice*	*Alternate drugs*
Clostridium perfringens	Gas gangrene	Penicillin G	Ceftizoxime Cefoxitine Chloramphenicol Doxycycline
Bacillus anthracis	Malignant pustule, pneumonia	Penicillin G	Erythromycin Doxycycline A first generation cephalosporin
Gram-negative organisms			
Escherichia coli	Urinary tract infection	Norfloxacin Ciprofloxacin Cotrimoxazole	Ampicillin + gentamicin; Amoxicillin + clavulinic acid; Aztreonam
Proteus mirabilis	Urinary tract infection Bacteraemia and other infections	Ampicillin or Amoxicillin	Ciprofloxacin A cephalosporin Gentamicin
Pseudomonas aeruginosa	Urinary tract infection	Amoxicillin Ciprofloxacin	Gentamicin A cephalosporin Imipenem
Klebsiella pneumoniae	Urinary tract infection	A cephalosporin	Mezlocillin An aminoglycoside
	Pneumonia	A cephalosporin + gentamicin	Mezlocillin Aztreonam Amoxicillin + clavulinic acid
Salmonella	Typhoid fever Bacteraemia	Ciprofloxacin Ceftriaxone	Chloramphenicol Ampicillin Cotrimoxazole
Shigella	Gastroenteritis	Ciprofloxacin or norfloxacin	Cotrimoxazole Ampicillin
Haemophillus influenzae	Sinusitis Pneumonia Otitis media	Amoxicillin + clavulinic acid Cotrimoxazole	Amoxicillin Ciprofloxacin Azithromycin A cephalosporin
	Meningitis	Ceftriaxone	Chloramphenicol Ampicillin + sulbactam

Contd...

Contd...

Microorganisms	*Clinical diagnosis*	*Drug of first choice*	*Alternate drugs*
Haemophillus ducreyi	Chancroid	Ceftriaxone Cotrimoxazole	Ciprofloxacin Erythromycin Doxycycline
Brucella	Brucellosis	Doxycycline + rifampicin	Cotrimoxazole Gentamicin
Yersenia pestis	Plague	A tetracycline + streptomycin	Doxycycline Chloramphenicol Ciprofloxacin
Vibrio cholerae	Cholera	Doxycycline	Cotrimoxazole
		Ciprofloxacin	Chloramphenicol
Campylobacter jejuni	Enteritis	Ciprofloxacin	Erythromycin
Treponema palladium	Syphilis	Penicillin G	Ceftriaxone Doxycycline
Leptospira	Weil's disease Meningitis	Penicillin G	Doxycycline
Other agents			
Mycoplasma pneumoniae	Atypical pneumonia	Erythromycin Doxycycline	Azithromycin
Rickettsia	Typhus fever, Q fever Rocky mountain spotted fever	Doxycycline	Chloramphenicol
Chlamydia trachomatis	Lymphogranuloma venereum Trachoma Inclusion conjunctivitis, Urethritis	Doxycycline	Erythromycin Azithromycin
Chlamydia psittaci	Psittacosis	Doxycycline	Chloramphenicol
Chlamydia pneumoniae	Pneumonia	Doxycycline	Erythromycin Azithromycin
Pneumocystis carinii	Pneumonia	Cotrimoxazole	Trimethoprim + dapsone

❑ SULFONAMIDES

Sulfonamides were the first effective antibacterial agents to be used systemically in man. They contain a sulfonamide group.

Classification

1. *Short-acting*—Sulfisoxazole, Sulfadiazine
2. *Intermediate-acting*—Sulfamethoxazole
3. *Long-acting*—Sulfamethoxypyridazine, Sulfadoxine
4. *Poorly absorbed*—Sulfasalazine
5. *Topical*—Sulfacetamide, Mefenide, Silver sulfadiazine.

Antibacterial spectrum Sulfonamides inhibit gram-positive and some gram-negative bacteria, nocardia, chlamydiae and some protozoa.

Mechanism of action Bacteria synthesize their own folic acid from p-amino benzoic acid (PABA) with the help of the enzyme folic acid synthetase (Fig. 11.3). Sulfonamides are structurally similar to PABA and competitively inhibit the enzyme folic acid synthetase. This results in folic acid deficiency and injury to the bacterial cell.

Sulfonamides are **bacteriostatic.**

Presence of pus, blood and tissue breakdown products make sulfonamides ineffective as these are rich in PABA.

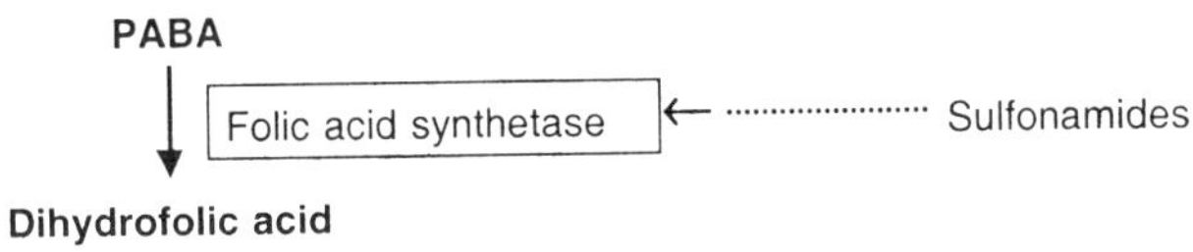

Fig. 11.3: Inhibition of folic acid synthesis by sulfonamides

Resistance Bacteria acquire resistance to sulfonamides by:

1. Mutations—resulting in over production of PABA.
2. Using alternate metabolic pathway for folic acid synthesis.
3. Low permeability to sulfonamides.

Pharmacokinetics Sulfonamides are well-absorbed, extensively bound to plasma proteins and are well distributed to all tissues. They are metabolized in the liver by acetylation.

Adverse effects

1. Renal irritation, haematuria, albuminuria and crystalluria—due to precipitation of the drug in acidic urine. This can be avoided by intake of large volumes of fluids and by alkalinising the urine.

2. Hypersensitivity reactions like rashes, fever, Steven-Johnsons syndrome and rarely exfoliative dermatitis.
3. Anorexia, nausea and abdominal pain.
4. Haemolytic anaemia in patients with G6PD deficiency.
5. Kernicterus—sulfonamides displace bilirubin from binding sites which crosses BBB and may cause kernicterus in the newborn. Hence contraindicated in pregnancy and in infants.

Uses Because of the development of resistance and availability of better antimicrobials, sulfonamides are not commonly used now except in a few cases.

1. *Urinary tract infections* Sulfonamides may be used in areas where resistance is not high.
2. *Nocardiosis* High doses of sulfonamides can be used.
3. *Toxoplasmosis* Sulfonamides with pyrimethamine is the treatment of choice.
4. *Trachoma and inclusion conjunctivitis* Tetracylines are the drug of choice, sulfonamides are used as alternative.
5. *Lymphogranuloma venereum and chancroid* Sulfonamides are used as alternative to tetracyclines.
6. *Malaria* Sulfadoxine is used with pyrimethamine in chloroquine resistant malaria.
7. *Prophylactic use* In patients allergic to penicillins, sulfonamides may be used for prophylaxis of streptococcal pharyngitis in rheumatic fever.
8. *Topical* Sulfacetamide eye drops are used in bacterial conjunctivitis; mafenide and silver sulfadiazine are used in burns to prevent infection.
9. *Ulcerative colitis* Sulfasalazine is useful in ulcerative colitis and rheumatoid arthritis.

❑ COTRIMOXAZOLE

The combination of trimethoprim and sulfamethoxazole is cotrimoxazole. Trimethoprim is effective against several gram-positive and gram-negative organisms. But when used alone, resistance develops rapidly.

Mechanism of action Sulfonamides inhibit the conversion of PABA to dihydrofolic acid (DHF) and trimethoprim inhibits dihydrofolate reductase (DHFR) and thus prevents the reduction of DHF to tetrahydrofolic acid (THF). The two drugs thus block sequential steps in folic acid synthesis and the combination in bactericidal.

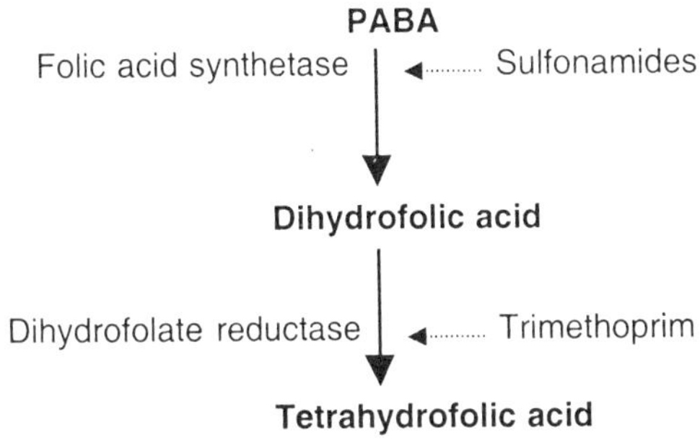

Fig. 11.4: Sequential blockade in folic acid synthesis

The ratio of 'trimethoprim : sulfamethoxazole' used is 1 : 5 to attain the right plasma concentration. Among sulfonamides, sulfamethoxazole is chosen since its pharmacokinetic properties closely match with that of trimethoprim.

Antibacterial spectrum Cotrimoxazole is effective against several gram-positive and gram-negative organisms like *Staph. aureus*, streptococci, meningococci, *C. diphtheriae, E. coli, Proteus, H. influenzae, Salmonella and Shigella.*

Resistance Development of resistance to the combination is slower when compared to either drugs given alone. Bacteria may acquire resistance by mutation or by acquisition of a plasmid coding for an altered DHFR.

Adverse effects

- Nausea, vomiting, headache, glossitis, stomatitis and allergic skin rashes are relatively common.
- In patients with folate deficiency, cotrimoxazole may precipitate megaloblastic anaemia.
- Haematological reactions like anaemia and granulocytopenia are rare.

- AIDs patients are more likely to develop adverse effects to cotrimoxazole.

Preparations

Trimethoprim	Sulfamethoxazole (SEPTRAN, CIPLIN)
80 mg	400 mg
160 mg	800 mg—double strength (DS)

Uses

1. *Urinary tract infection* Uncomplicated acute UTI is treated for 7-10 days with cotrimoxazole.
   Chronic and recurrent UTI—small doses are given for prophylaxis.
   Bacterial prostatitis—Trimethoprim attains high concentration in prostatic fluid.
2. *Respiratory tract infections* Upper and lower respiratory infections including bronchitis, sinusitis and otitis media respond.
3. *Bacterial gastroenteritis* due to *Shigella* and *E. coli* respond to cotrimoxazole.
4. *Typhoid* Cotrimoxazole is used as an alternative to fluoroquinolones.
5. *Pneumocystis carinii infection* Cotrimoxazole is used for prophylaxis and treatment (high doses) of *Pneumocystis carinii* pneumonia in neutropenic and AIDS patients. It also protects against infection with other gram-negative bacteria.
6. *Chancroid* Cotrimoxazole is the drug of choice.

❑ QUINOLONES

The quinolones are a group of synthetic antimicrobial agents. Nalidixic acid is the older agent in the group.

NALIDIXIC ACID

Nalidixic acid is bactericidal against various gram-positive organisms like *E. coli, Shigella, Proteus and Klebsiella.* It is excreted too rapidly to have systemic effects but attains high concentration in the urine. Mechanism of action is similar to fluoroquinolones.

Allergic reactions including haemolytic anaemia and CNS effects like headache, myalgia and drowsiness may be encountered.

Uses Nalidixic acid is used in uncomplicated UTI and diarrhoea due to *E.coli, Shigella* and *Proteus.*

FLUOROQUINOLONES

The fluorinated quinolones were derived with wider spectrum of activity, fewer side effects, less chance of resistance and better tissue penetration when compared to quinolones. The fluoroquinolones include *norfloxacin, ciprofloxacin, pefloxacin, ofloxacin, lomefloxacin and sparfloxacin*—many more are being added. The newer agents include trovafloxacin, gatifloxacin, moxifloxacin and clinafloxacin

Mechanism of action Fluoroquinolones are bactericidal. They inhibit the bacterial enzyme DNA gyrase which is required for DNA replication and transcription.

Resistance is not very common because of its unique mechanism of action. Resistance is due to mutations in the DNA gyrase enzyme or a change in the permeability of the organism. Several strains of *E.coli, Staphylococci, Pseudomonas* and *Serratia* have now developed resistance.

Antibacterial spectrum Gram-negative organisms like *gonococci, meningococci, H. influenzae, E. coli, Salmonella, Shigella, enterobacteria; H pylori,* gram-positive organisms like staphylococci; *Chlamydiae, Mycoplasma, Myobacterium* are susceptible. Some of the newer agents are effective against some anaerobic organisms.

Pharmacokinetics On oral administration, fluoroquinolones are well-absorbed and widely distributed. Food and antacids interfere with absorption; these are excreted by kidneys.

Adverse reactions Fluoroquinolones are well-tolerated. Nausea, vomiting, abdominal discomfort, diarrhoea and rashes may be seen. Tendinitis with associated risk of tendon rupture has been reported. Fluoroquinolones damage the growing cartilage resulting in arthropathy and are therefore contraindicated up to 18 years of age.

Uses (Table 11.2)

1. *Urinary tract infections* Very effective in UTI even when caused by multi-drug resistant bacteria—norfloxacin is generally used.
2. *Typhoid* Ciprofloxacin is the drug of choice (500 mg BD—10 days)—also eradicates carrier state.
3. *Diarrhoea* due to *Shigella, E.coli* and Campylobacter respond.
4. *Gonorrhoea* Single dose 250 mg ciprofloxacin is curative.
5. *Chancroid* As an alternative to cotrimoxazole
6. *Respiratory tract infection*—due to *H. influenzae, Legionella and Mycoplasma* can be treated with fluoroquinolones.
7. *Bone, joint, soft tissue and intra-abdominal infections*—osteomyelitis and joint infections require prolonged treatment. Soft tissue infections due to sensitive bacteria can be treated with fluoroquinolones.
8. *Tuberculosis* Ciprofloxacin is one of the drugs in multi-drug regimens used for resistant tuberculosis. It is also useful in atypical mycobacterial infections.
9. *Eye infections:* Ciprofloxacin and ofloxacin may be used topically in the treatment of eye infections.

TABLE 11.2: Dose and route of administration of some fluoroquinolones

Drug	*Dose and route*
Norfloxacin (NORFLOX)	Oral: 400 mg BD
Ciprofloxacin (CIPLOX)	Oral: 250-750 mg BD
Pefloxacin (PEFLOX)	Oral: 400 mg BD
Ofloxacin (TARIVID)	Oral: 200-400 mg OD
Lomefloxacin (LOMEF)	Oral: 400 mg OD
Sparfloxacin (SPARLOX)	Oral: 200-400 mg OD

❑ BETA-LACTAM ANTIBIOTICS

The β-lactam antibiotics have a β-lactam ring. Penicillins, cephalosporins, monobactams and carbapenems are β-lactams.

PENICILLINS

Sir Alexander Fleming discovered penicillin in 1928. Penicillins are one of the most important groups of antibiotics. Penicillin is now obtained from the fungus *Penicillium chrysogenum.*

Mechanism of action The rigid cell wall of the bacteria protects it from lysis. Peptidoglycan, is an important component which gives strength to the cell wall. β-lactam antibiotics inhibit the synthesis of this peptidoglycan, resulting in the formation of cell wall deficient bacteria. These undergo lysis. Thus, penicillins are bactericidal.

Classification of Penicillins

A. *Natural* Penicillin G
B. *Semisynthetic*
   1. *Acid resistant* Penicillin V
   2. *Penicillinase resistant*—Methicillin, Oxacillin, Cloxacillin, Nafcillin
   3. *Aminopenicillins*—Ampicillin, Bacampicillin, Amoxicillin
   4. *Antipseudomonal penicillins*
      a. Carboxypenicillins—Carbenicillin, Carbenicillin-indanyl, Ticarcillin
      b. Ureidopenicillins—Mezlocillin, Piperacillin.

NATURAL PENICILLINS

Penicillin G (Benzyl Penicillin)

Antibacterial spectrum Penicillin G (PnG) has a narrow antibacterial spectrum and is effective against gram-positive cocci and bacilli and a few gram-negative cocci. Thus streptococci, pneumococci, gonococci, meningococci, B. anthracis, C. diphtheriae, clostridia, listeria and spirochetes are highly sensitive.

Resistance Many organisms like staphylococci produce a penicillinase which is a beta-lactamase—which opens the β-lactam ring and inactivates penicillins.

Pharmacokinetics PnG is destroyed by gastric juice; food interferes with its absorption —hence it is to be given 2 hr after food. Has a short t½ of 30 min. Though it does not readily cross the BBB, in presence of inflammation, therapeutic concentration is attained in the CSF. It is excreted by the kidneys. Probenecid blocks the renal tubular secretion of penicillin and thereby prolongs its duration of action.

Preparations PnG is mainly given parenterally. Orally effective form is potassium PnG. Oral penicillin is used only in minor infections. Since benzyl penicillin is short-acting, repository forms like procaine penicillin and benzathine penicillin—which are longer-acting are made available. Given deep IM they release penicillin slowly from the site. Procaine penicillin is given 12-24 hourly while a single injection of benzathine penicillin is effective for 3-4 weeks. For preparation and dose see Table 11.3.

Adverse effects

Hypersensitivity PnG is the most common cause of drug allergy. It can cause skin rashes, urticaria, fever, bronchospasm, serum sickness and rarely exfoliative dermatitis and anaphylaxis. Though all forms of penicillins can cause allergy, anaphylaxis is more common with parenteral than oral preparations. The highest incidence is with procaine penicillin where allergy is most often due to the procaine component. There is cross-sensitivity among different penicillins. Topical penicillins are highly sensitizing and their use is banned.

History of allergy to penicillins should be taken before prescribing. A scratch test or intradermal sensitivity test with 2-10 units should be done. Even if this is negative, it does not completely rule out allergy. Penicillin should be given cautiously and a syringe loaded with adrenaline to treat anaphylaxis should be kept ready.

Other adverse effects

Local Pain at the site of injection, thrombophlebitis on IV injection.

CNS Large doses of PnG may produce confusion, muscle twitchings, convulsions and coma.

Suprainfections are rare due to its narrow spectrum of activity.

Jarisch-Herxheimer reaction When penicillin is injected in a patient with syphilis, there is sudden destruction of spirochetes and release of its products. This triggers a reaction with fever, myalgia, shivering, exacerbation of syphilitic lesions and vascular collapse.

TABLE 11.3: Preparations, dose and route of administration of penicillins

Drug	*Dose*	*Route*	*Trade name*
NATURAL PENICILLINS			
Sodium penicillin G (Crystalline penicillin)	0.5-5 MU 4-6 hr	IM/IV	CRYSTAPEN
Procaine penicillin G	0.5-1 MU 12-24 hr	IM	PROCAINE-PENICILLIN G
Benzathine penicillin G	1.2-2.4 MU every 3-4 weeks	Deep IM	PENIDURE LA
SEMISYNTHETIC PENICILLINS			
Penicillin	250-500 mg QID	Oral	CRYSTAPEN-V
Cloxacillin	250-500 mg QID	Oral	KLOX
Dicloxacillin	250-500 mg QID	Oral	BIOCLOX
Nafcillin	1-2 gm 4-6 hr	IV	UNIPEN
Ampicillin	250 mg or 1 gm QID	Oral IM/IV	AMPILLIN ROSCILLIN
Ampicillin + sulbactum	1 gm Ampi + 0.5 gm sulb 6-8 hr	IV	SULBACIN
Amoxicillin	250-500 mg TID	Oral	NOVAMOX SYNAMOX
Amoxicillin + clavulanic acid	250 mg Amox + 125 mg Clav TID	Oral	AUGMENTIN
Piperacillin	3-4 gm 4-6 hr	IV	PIPRAPEN
Ticarcillin	3 gm 4-6 hr	IV	TICAR

Uses Penicillin G is the antibiotic of choice for several infections unless the patient is allergic to it.

1. ***Pneumococcal infections*** For infections due to penicillin-sensitive pneumococci, like pneumonia, meningitis and osteomyelitis, PnG is the ***drug of choice***.
2. ***Streptococcal infections*** Pharyngitis, sinusitis, pneumonia, meningitis and endocarditis are all treated with penicillin. Infective endocarditis due to *Strep. viridans* is treated with high dose PnG ± an aminoglycoside.
3. ***Meningococcal infections*** PnG is the drug of choice for all meningococcal infections.

4. ***Staphylococcal infections*** Since most staphylococci produce penicillinase, a penicillinase resistant penicillin should be used.
5. ***Syphilis*** is treated with procaine penicillin for 10 days or with benzathine penicillin.
6. ***Diphtheria*** Antitoxin is the only effective treatment. PnG eliminates carrier state.
7. ***Anaerobic infections*** Pulmonary, periodontal and brain abscesses due to anaerobes respond to PnG.
8. ***Actinomycosis*** PnG is the drug of choice for all forms of actinomycosis.
9. ***Tetanus and gas gangrene*** Antitoxin is the treatment for tetanus—but PnG kills the bacteria.
   Gas gangrene— PnG is the **drug of choice**.
10. ***Other infections*** PnG is the **agent of choice** for infections like anthrax, trench mouth and listeria infections.
11. ***Prophylactic uses***:
    - *Rheumatic fever* Benzathine penicillin 1.2 MU every month prevents colonisation by streptococci and thereby decreases the recurrences of rheumatic fever. It is to be continued for several years.
    - *Gonorrhoea and syphilis* Sexual contacts are effectively protected against these diseases when treated with penicillin within 12 hours of exposure.
    - *Valvular heart diseases*—25% cases of bacterial endocarditis are seen following dental extractions. Such patients undergoing dental extractions, endoscopies and other minor surgical procedures that may cause bacteraemia should be given penicillin prophylaxis.

SEMISYNTHETIC PENICILLINS

Acid resistant penicillins *Penicillin V* (Phenoxymethyl penicillin) is acid stable and can be given orally. It is used only in mild streptococcal pharyngitis, sinusitis and trench mouth.

Penicillinase resistant penicillins like methicillin and cloxacillin are resistant to hydrolysis by penicillinase produced by bacteria. However, against other microorganisms—they are less effective than PnG.

Methicillin is destroyed by gastric juice—hence given parenterally. Cloxacillin is given orally.

Uses Penicillinase resistant penicillins are the drugs of choice for infections with penicillinase producing staphylococci. Methicillin resistant strains have now emerged and are treated with vancomycin.

Extended Spectrum Penicillins

Aminopenicillins These agents have a wider antibacterial spectrum including many gram-negative bacilli. They are orally effective but are sensitive to beta-lactamases.

Antibacterial spectrum Both gram-positive and gram-negative organisms including streptococci, meningococci, pneumococci, *H. influenzae, E. Coli, Proteus, Salmonella, Shigella* and *Klebsiella* are sensitive. Many strains are now resistant.

Ampicillin is well-absorbed orally; food interferes with absorption. It is excreted mainly through kidneys.

Adverse effects Diarrhoea due to irritation of the gut by the unabsorbed drug is the most common adverse effect with ampicillin. Skin rashes are also fairly frequent.

Uses

1. *Respiratory tract infections* like bronchitis, sinusitis and otitis media respond to ampicillin.
2. *Urinary tract infections* Though ampicillin was the drug of choice earlier, many organisms have now become resistant.
3. *Meningitis* Ampicillin is given with a cephalosporin.
4. *Typhoid* Ampicillin is an alternative to ciprofloxacin.
5. *Septicaemia due to gram-negative organisms* Ampicillin may be used, with an aminoglycoside.

Bacampicillin is an ester of ampicillin. It is a prodrug that is better absorbed (hence diarrhoea is less common) and longer-acting than ampicillin.

Amoxicillin Amoxicillin is used in similar infections as ampicillin like respiratory infection, salmonella gastroenteritis and urinary tract infection. Amoxicillin is a component of the various regimens to eradicate H. pylori. Amoxicillin is preferred over ampicillin by many

Amoxicillin differs from ampicillin in the following:

1. Amoxicillin is better absorbed orally
2. Food does not interfere with its absorption
3. Diarrhoea is rare
4. Given thrice daily

ANTIPSEUDOMONAL PENICILLINS

Carboxypenicillins Carbenicillin is effective in *Pseudomonas aeruginosa* and *Proteus* infections. It is given parenterally while carbenicillin indanyl is effective orally. Both are susceptible to penicillinase.

Adverse effects Carbenicillin is used as a sodium salt and in higher doses this excess sodium may cause oedema and CCF; may also cause bleeding due to abnormal platelet aggregation.

Ureidopenicillins are effective against *Pseudomonas* and *Klebsiella* infections.

Beta-Lactamase inhibitors β-lactamases are enzymes produced by bacteria that open up the β-lactam ring and inactivate the β-lactam antibiotics. β-lactamase inhibitors bind to and inactivate β-lactamases preventing the destruction of the β-lactam antibiotics. Examples are clavulanic acid sulbactam and tazobactam.

Clavulanic acid is combined with amoxicillin for both oral and parenteral administration. It extends the antibacterial spectrum of amoxicillin. The combination is used for mixed nosocomial infections.

Sulbactam is combined with ampicillin. It is given parenterally for mixed pelvic and other infections. Tazobactam is combined with piperacillin.

CEPHALOSPORINS

Cephalosporins are semisynthetic antibiotics with a beta-lactam ring related to penicillins. They are derived from cephalosporin-C and have a wider spectrum of activity than penicillins (Table 11.4).

Mechanism of action Cephalosporins inhibit the bacterial cell wall synthesis similar to penicillins.

CLASSIFICATION

Cephalosporins are classified into 4 generations.

	Parenteral	**Oral**
First generation	Cephalothin Cefazolin	Cephalexin Cefadroxil
Second generation	Cefamandole Cefuroxime	Cefachlor Cefuroxime axetil
Third generation	Cefotaxime Ceftrioxone Cefoperazone Ceftizoxime Ceftazidime	Cefixime
Fourth generation	Cefepime Cefpirome	

Resistance As in the case of penicillins, beta-lactamases determine resistance to cephalosporins.

First Generation Cephalosporins

First generation cephalosporins are very effective against gram-positive organisms. Cephalothin is resistant to penicillinase, hence can be used in staphylococcal infections. Cefazolin has a longer t½ and its tissue penetrability is good—therefore used for surgical prophylaxis. Cephalexin is used orally for minor infections like abscesses or cellulitis.

Second Generation Cephalosporins

Second generation cephalosporins are more active against some gram-negative organisms compared to first generation ones. *H. influenzae, E. coli, Proteus and Klebsiella* are inhibited. Cefuroxime is resistant to β-lactamases; attains good CSF concentration and is useful in meningitis.

Third Generation Cephalosporins

Third generation cephalosporins are highly resistant to β-lactamases; have good activity against gram-negative organisms.

Many cross BBB and are useful in meningitis. Ceftrioxone has a long t½ and can be given once daily. It is excreted mainly through biliary tract and no dosage adjustment is needed in renal failure.

Fourth Generation Cephalosporins

Cefepime, a fourth generation agent has activity similar to III generation ones except that it is more resistant to β-lactamases and is effective against organisms resistant to other cephalosporins. It attains very good CSF levels. It is used in serious gram-negative infections including nosocomial infections.

Adverse reactions

Cephalosporins are generally well-tolerated.

1. *Hypersensitivity reactions* like skin rashes, fever, serum sickness and rarely anaphylaxis are seen. 20% of patients allergic to penicillin show cross-reactivity to cephalosporins. There are no reliable skin tests for testing allergy.
2. *Nephrotoxicity* Mild nephrotoxicity is noted with some cephalosporins. Combination with other nephrotoxic drugs should be avoided.
3. *Diarrhoea* can result from some of the cephalosporins.
4. *Bleeding* is due to hypoprothrombinaemia which is more common in malnourished patients.
5. *Low* WBC count may be seen though rarely.
6. *Pain* at the injection site may occur.
7. *Disulfiram-like reaction* with alcohol is reported with some cephalosporins.

Uses of cephalosporins

1. *Gram-negative infections* Urinary, respiratory and soft tissue infections due to gram-negative organisms respond.
2. *Surgical prophylaxis* Cefazolin is preferred.
3. *Gonorrhoea* Ceftriaxone (single dose 250 mg) is the drug of choice.
4. *Meningitis* Due to *H. influenzae, N. meningitidis and S. Pneumoniae*—3rd generation agents are used.

5. *Mixed aerobic-anaerobic infections*—common following pelvic surgeries—a 3rd generation agent is used.

6. *Typhoid* As alternative to ciprofloxacin.

7. *Nosocomial infections* can be treated with 3rd generation cephalosporins.

TABLE 11.4: Preparation, doses and route of administration of some cephalosporins

Drugs	*Doses*	*Routes*
Cephalothin (KAFLIN)	1-2 gm q 6 h	IV
Cefazolin (ALCIZON)	0.5-1 gm q 6 h	IM/IV
Cephalexin (SPORIDEX)	0.25-1 gm QID	Oral
Cefadroxil (DROXYL)	0.5-1 gm BID	Oral
Cefamandole (KEFADOL)	0.5-2 gm q 4-8 h	IM/IV
Cefuroxine (SUPACEF)	0.75-1.5 gm q 8 h	IM/IV
Cefuroxime axetil (CEFTUM)	0.25 -0.5 gm BD	Oral
Cefachlor (KEFLOR)	0.25-0.5 gm q 8 h	Oral
Cefotaxime (OMNATAX)	1-2 gm q 8 h	IM/IV
Ceftriaxone (OFRAMAX)	1-2 gm q 12-24 h	IM/IV
Cefoperazone (CEFOBID)	1-2 gm q 8-12 h	IM/IV
Cefixime (CEFSPAN)	0.2-0.4 gm q 12 h	Oral
Cefpirome (CEFROM)	1-2 gm q 12 h	IV

CARBAPENEMS

Carbapenems contain a β-lactam ring fused with a five-membered penem ring. Carbapenems include imipenem and meropenem.

Antibacterial spectrum Carbapenems have a wide antibacterial spectrum and inhibit various gram positive, gram negative organisms and anaerobes including streptococci, staphylococci, enterococci, *Listeria, enterobacteriaeceae, Pseudomonas* and *B. fragilis.*

Mechanism of action Carbapenems inhibit bacterial cell wall synthesis similar to penicillins.

Imipenem is not absorbed orally and is administered intravenously (250-500 mg every 6-8 hours); it has good tissue penetrability. Imipenem is inactivated quickly by an enzyme in the renal tubules. Hence it is always combined with cilastatin which inhibits the renal enzyme and prolongs the plasma half-life of imipenem.

Adverse effects to imipenem include nausea, vomiting and diarrhoea. Allergic reactions are seen especially in patients allergic to other β-lactam antibiotics. High doses can occasionally cause seizures.

Imipenem-cilastatin is used in UTI, respiratory, skin, bone, soft tissue, intra abdominal and gynaecological infections due to susceptible microorganisms. It is particularly useful in nosocomial infections resistant to other antibiotics.

Meropenem has the following advantages over imipenem.

- It isot destroyed by renal dipeptidase and therefore does not require to be combined with cilastatin.
- Seizures risk is less than with imipenem.

Indications are similar to imipenem.

MONOBACTAMS are monocyclic beta lactams, i.e. they contain a single ring—the beta lactam ring.

Aztreonam is the monobactam available. It is active against gram-negative bacilli including Pseudomonas aerugenosa but is *not* effective against gram-positive organisms and anaerobes. Aztreonam acts by inhibiting cell wall synthesis like penicillins. It is given parenterally.

Aztreonam can be used in patients allergic to penicillins as there is no cross allergenicity with other β-lactams . The only reported adverse effects are occasional skin rashes. Aztreonam is used in pseudomonas infections especially nosocomial and in other gram-negative infections

❑ BROAD SPECTRUM ANTIBIOTICS

TETRACYCLINES

Tetracyclines are antibiotics with four cyclic rings (hence the name) obtained from the soil actinomycetes. In addition to gram-positive and gram-negative bacteria, tetracyclines also inhibit the growth of other microorganisms like rickettsiae, chlamydiae, *Mycoplasma* and some protozoa. Therefore they are called **broad spectrum antibiotics.**

Tetracyclines	**Semisynthetic tetracyclines**
Chlortetracyline	Demeclocycline
Tetracycline	Methacycline
Oxytetracycline	Doxycycline
	Minocycline

Mechanism of action Tetracyclines are bacteriostatic. They bind to 30S ribosomes and inhibit protein synthesis.

Antibacterial spectrum is broad including gram-positive and gram-negative organisms like *Streptococci, Staphylococci, Gonococci, Meningococci, H. influenza, Brucella, V. cholerae, Campylobacter, Y.pestis* and many anaerobes. They also inhibit rickettsiae, chlamydiae, *Mycoplasma, Actinomyces, E. histolytica* and *Plasmodia.* Many organisms have now become resistant.

Pharmacokinetics Older tetracyclines are incompletely absorbed from the gut; food interferes with their absorption. Doxycycline and minocycline are 100% absorbed and food does not affect the absorption of these two agents. Tetracyclines chelate calcium and other metals which reduce their absorption. Hence tetracyclines should not be given with milk, iron preparations and antacids.

Tetracyclines except doxycycline and minocycline are excreted through kidneys. Doxycycline and minocycline are excreted through gut and are therefore safe in renal insufficiency.

Adverse effects

1. *GIT* Gastrointestinal irritation, nausea, vomiting and diarrhoea—tetracyclines are to be given with food to minimize these effects.
2. *Hepatotoxicity* may result in jaundice. Acute hepatic necrosis may occur in pregnant women but is rare.
3. *Renal toxicity* Renal failure may be aggravated. Outdated tetracyclines cause a syndrome like Fanconi's syndrome with vomiting, polyuria, proteinuria, glycosuria and acidosis due to metabolites of the outdated tetracyclines.

4. *Phototoxicity* Skin reactions and dermatitis on exposure to sun are more likely with doxycycline and demeclocycline.
5. *Effect on teeth and bones* Tetracyclines chelate calcium. The calcium-tetracycline-orthophasphate tetracycline—orthophosphate complexes get deposited in the developing teeth and bones. The deformities depend on the time of tetracycline administration. Brownish discolouration and pigmentation of the teeth occur. The growth of skeleton is also depressed when given up to 8 years of age. Hence tetracyclines are teratogenic.
6. *Suprainfections* Since the intestinal flora are extensively suppressed by tetracyclines, these are the most common antibiotics to cause suprainfections.
7. *Hypersensitivity reactions* are not very common.

Uses

A. *Tetracyclines are the **drugs of choice** in*

1. *Rickettsial infections* All rickettsial infections respond to tetracyclines.
2. *Chlamydial infections:*
   — lymphogranuloma venereum
   — trachoma—both topical and oral
   — inclusion conjunctivitis.
3. *Atypical pneumonia* Due to *Mycoplasma pneumoniae.*
4. *Cholera* Tetracyclines reduce the duration of illness and are of adjuvant value.
5. *Brucellosis* Doxycycline 200 mg + Rifampicin 600 mg daily for 6 weeks is the treatment of choice.
6. *Plague* Tetracyclines may be combined with an aminoglycoside.

B. *Tetracyclines are useful in other conditions like*

1. Traveller's diarrhoea—Doxycycline reduces the incidence of traveller's diarrhoea.
2. Sexually transmitted diseases like syphilis, gonorrhea and chancroid also respond to tetracyclines—but are not preferred.
3. Acne—The propioni bacteria in the sebaceous follicles metabolize lipids into irritating free fatty acids which trigger the

development of acne. Tetracyclines inhibit these bacteria. Low doses are given for a long time (250 mg BD for 4 weeks).

4. Protozoal infections:
   - Amoebiasis—Tetracyclines are useful in chronic intestinal amoebiasis (page 335).
   - Malaria—Doxycycline is given with quinine in multi-drug resistant malaria.

Contraindications Tetracyclines are contraindicated in pregnancy, lactation and in children up to 8 years of age.

Dosage of some tetracyclines	
Tetracyclines	*Doses*
Chlortetracycline (AUREOMYCIN)	250-500 mg QID
Tetracycline (HOSTACYCLINE)	250-500 mg QID
Doxycycline (DOXYCAPS)	200 mg initially then 100 mg OD
Minocycline (CYANOMYCIN)	200 mg initially then 100 mg OD

Doxycycline and minocycline are semisynthetic tetracyclines.

- Given orally they are 100% absorbed.
- Food does not interfere with their absorption
- Have long t½—can be given once daily
- Excreted through gut hence can be given in renal impairment
- Minocycline causes vestibular toxicity.

CHLORAMPHENICOL

Chloramphenicol is a broad spectrum antibiotic first obtained from *Streptomyces venezuelae* in 1947.

Mechanism of action Chloramphenicol is bacteriostatic but to some organisms it is bactericidal. It binds to 50S ribosomal subunit and inhibits protein synthesis.

Antibacterial spectrum is broad and includes gram-negative organisms, some gram-positive organisms, anaerobic bacteria, rickettsiae, chlamydiae and *Mycoplasma*. Thus *H. influenzae, Salmonella, Shigella, Bordatella, Brucella,* gonococci, meningococci, streptococci, staphylococci, *Clostridium, E.coli and Klebsiella*—are inhibited apart from rickettsiae, Chlamydia and *Mycoplasma*.

Resistance is plasmid mediated and may be due to:

1. Inactivating enzymes
2. ↓ permeability of the microorganisms

Pharmacokinetics Chloramphenicol is rapidly absorbed from the gut; penetration into tissues is excellent; attains high concentration in CSF. It is metabolised in the liver by conjugation.

Adverse reactions

1. *Gastrointestinal disturbances* Nausea, vomiting, diarrhoea.
2. *Bone marrow depression* Chloramphenicol may cause bone marrow depression by an idiosyncratic response—resulting in aplastic anaemia which may be fatal. It may be due to a toxic metabolite.
3. *Gray baby syndrome* Newborn babies given high doses of chloramphenicol may develop vomiting, refusal of feeds, hypotonia, hypothermia, abdominal distension and ashen gray cyanosis—described as gray baby syndrome. It may be fatal. As the newborn cannot metabolize and excrete chloramphenicol adequately, toxicity results.
4. *Hypersensitivity reactions* like rashes and fever are uncommon.
5. *Superinfection* can occur.

Drug interactions Chloramphenicol inhibits hepatic microsomal enzymes and thereby prolongs the duration of action of drugs metabolised by this system. This may result in toxicity of some drugs like phenytoin, tolbutamide and dicumarol.

Uses Because of the risk of bone marrow toxicity and availability of safer drugs, chloramphenicol is not generally preferred. The indications are:

1. *Typhoid fever* Very effective in typhoid
2. *Bacterial meningitis* Chloramphenicol is an alternative to penicillin.
3. *Anaerobic infections* Chloramphenicol + penicillin + an aminoglycoside can be used in severe anaerobic infections as an alternative to metronidazole and clindamycin.
4. *Rickettsial infections* As an alternative when tetracyclines are contraindicated.
5. *Eye infections* Chloramphenicol is used as eye drops because of the good penetration into aqueous humour.

❑ AMINOGLYCOSIDES

Aminoglycosides are antibiotics with amino sugars in glycosidic linkages. They are derived from the soil actinomycetes. Aminoglycosides are streptomycin, gentamicin, kanamycin, tobramycin, amikacin, neomycin and netilmicin.

Common Properties of Aminoglycosides

1. Aminoglycosides are not absorbed orally, remain extracellularly and penetration into CSF is very poor.
2. They are all bactericidal.
3. They act by inhibiting bacterial protein synthesis.
4. They are mainly effective against gram-negative organisms.
5. They produce variable degrees of ototoxicity and nephrotoxicity as adverse effects.
6. They are excreted unchanged by the kidneys.

Antibacterial spectrum Aminoglycosides have a narrow spectrum and are effective mainly against aerobic gram-negative bacilli like *E. coli, Proteus, Pseudomonas, Brucella, Salmonella, Shigella* and *Klebsiella.*

Mechanism of action Aminoglycosides bind to 30S ribosomes and inhibit bacterial protein synthesis. They are *bactericidal.* Aminoglycosides have a postantibiotic effect, i.e. the antibacterial activity remains even after the drug in excreted.

Resistance to aminoglycosides is acquired by

1. Aminoglycoside inactivating enzymes.
2. Low affinity of ribosomes—acquired by mutation.
3. Decrease in permeability to the antibiotic.

There is partial cross-resistance among various aminoglycosides.

Adverse effects

1. *Ototoxicity* is the most important toxicity. Both vestibular and auditory dysfunction can occur depending on the dose and duration. The aminoglycosides get concentrated in the inner ear and damage both cochlear hair cells and vestibular sensory cells. As the cochlear cells cannot regenerate, there

is progressive, *permanent deafness*. Elderly people are more susceptible. Stopping the drug can prevent further damage. Vestibular dysfunction results in headache, nausea, vomiting, dizziness, vertigo, nystagmus and ataxia. Recovery is slow over 1-2 years.

2. *Nephrotoxicity* Aminoglycosides attain high concentration in the kidney and cause damage to the renal tubules. These effects are reversible.
3. *Neuromuscular blockade* Aminoglycosides have curare-like effects and block neuromuscular transmission.

Precautions in using aminoglycosides

1. Avoid simultaneous use of other ototoxic drugs like loop diuretics.
2. Avoid simultaneous use of other nephrotoxic drugs like amphotericin B, cephalothin and cisplatin.
3. To be used cautiously in elderly, in renal damage and in combination with skeletal muscle relaxants.
4. Contraindicated in pregnancy.
5. Do not mix aminoglycosides with any other drug in the same syringe.
6. Determination of plasma levels of aminoglycosides may be needed in severe infections and in patients with renal dysfunction.

Streptomycin obtained from *Streptomyces griseus* is mainly effective against aerobic gram-negative bacilli. When used alone, bacteria, especially the tubercle bacillus rapidly develops resistance to it. Streptomycin is the least nephrotoxic among aminoglycosides.

Uses

1. *Tuberculosis* (page 317).
2. *Subacute bacterial endocarditis (SBE)*—Combination of streptomycin and penicillin is synergistic in this condition.
3. *Plague, tularaemia and brucellosis*—streptomycin is given with a tetracycline.

Gentamicin obtained from *micromonospora purpurea* is more potent and has a broader spectrum of action compared to streptomycin. Development of resistance has limited its use.

Uses

1. *UTI* Gentamicin is effective in uncomplicated UTI as it is released for a long time from the renal cortex.
2. *Pneumonia* due to gram-negative organisms may be treated with gentamicin + penicillin.
3. *Osteomyelitis, peritonitis, septicaemia* caused by gram-negative organisms can be treated with gentamicin.
4. *Meningitis due to gram-negative bacilli*—gentamicin is used with a III generation cephalosporin.
5. Gentamicin may be used in place of streptomycin.

Topical Gentamicin cream is used topically in burns and other infected wounds. Gentamicin eye drops is used in bacterial conjunctivitis.

Tobramycin has better activity against *Pseudomonas* and is used with an antipseudomonal penicillin in such infections.

Kanamycin Due to its toxicity, its use is limited to multi-drug resistant tuberculosis.

Amikacin has widest antibacterial spectrum among the aminoglycosides. It is resistant to aminoglycoside inactivating enzymes.

Uses

1. Nosocomial infections due to gram-negative organisms
2. Tuberculosis—Amikacin is useful in multidrug resistant tuberculosis in combination with other drugs. It is also used in infections due to *atypical mycobacteria* in patients with AIDS.

Netilmicin Like amikacin, netilmicin is resistant to aminoglycoside inactivating enzymes. It is used in serious infections due to gram-negative bacilli.

Sisomicin has actions, toxicity and uses similar to gentamicin.

Neomycin has a wide antibacterial spectrum. As it is highly ototoxic, it is not given systemically. It is used topically as ointments, creams and powder.

Adverse effects Neomycin can cause skin rashes on topical use. Oral use can cause diarrhoea, steatorrhoea and malabsorption due to damage to the intestinal villi. Superinfection with *Candida* can also occur.

Uses

1. Neomycin is used topically in skin infections, burns, ulcers and wounds; eye and ear infections.
2. Orally—Neomycin is not absorbed when given orally. But it is used to prepare the bowel for surgery, i.e. for preoperative gut sterilization.
3. Hepatic coma—Normally ammonia produced by colonic bacteria is absorbed and converted to urea by the liver. But in severe hepatic failure, liver is unable to handle this NH_3, and blood NH_3 levels rise resulting in encephalopathy. Neomycin inhibits intestinal flora and decreases NH_3 production.

❑ MACROLIDES AND OTHER ANTIBACTERIAL AGENTS

Macrolides are antibiotics with a macrocyclic lactone ring.

Macrolides are: Erythromycin, Roxithromycin, Azithromycin, Clarithromycin.

ERYTHROMYCIN

Erythromycin is obtained from *Streptomyces erythreus.*

Antibacterial spectrum Erythromycin has a narrow spectrum and is effective against aerobic gram-positive bacteria and a few gram-negative organisms.

Streptococci, pneumococci, staphylococci, gonococci, *C. diphtheriae, C. jejuni, Mycoplasma, Chlamydiae* and some atypical mycobacteria are sensitive.

Mechanism of action Erythromycin is bacteriostatic at low and bactericidal at high concentrations. It binds to 50S ribosomes and inhibits bacterial protein synthesis.

Resistance Resistance to macrolides is acquired through plasmids. The mechanism involved may be:

- Low permeability of the bacteria to the antibiotic
- Production of inactivating enzymes
- Ribosomes may not bind to macrolides.

Pharmacokinetics Erythromycin is destroyed by gastric acid and is therefore given as enteric coated tablets. It is mainly excreted through bile; dose adjustment is not needed in renal failure.

Adverse effects Hepatitis with cholestatic jaundice starts after 2-3 weeks of treatment and is more common with the estolate salt. The symptoms—nausea, vomiting and abdominal cramps mimic acute cholecystitis and may be wrongly treated. These are followed by jaundice and fever. It may be an allergic response to the estolate salt. The patient recovers on stopping the drug.

Erythromycin can also cause epigastric pain, nausea, difficulty in hearing diarrhoea and hypersensitivity reactions. Patients with cardiac disease may develop cardiac arrhythmias while on erythermycin.

Drug interactions Erythromycin inhibits the hepatic metabolism of many drugs like carbamazepine, terfenadine, valproate, and warfarin resulting in toxicity due to these drugs.

TABLE 11.5: Dose of macrolide antibiotics

Drug	*Dose (oral)*
Erythromycin stearate (ERYTHROCIN)	250-500 mg q 6 h
Erythromycin estolate (ALTHROCIN)	250-500 mg q 6 h
Roxithromycin (ROXID)	150 mg q 12 h (to be taken 30 minutes before food)
Clarithromycin (CLARIBID)	250-500 mg q 12 h
Azithromycin (AZITHRAL)	Ist day 500 mg OD 250 mg OD for next 3-4 days

Uses Erythromycin can be used as an alternative to penicillin in patients allergic to penicillin.

1. *Atypical pneumonia* due to *Mycoplasma pneumoniae*—erythromycin is the **drug of choice.**
2. *Legionnaire's pneumonia*—is treated with erythromycin.

3. *Whooping cough*—erythromycin is the drug of choice for treatment and prophylaxis.
4. *Streptococcal infections*—pharyngitis and tonsillitis respond to erythromycin.
5. *Staphylococcal infections*—minor infections may be treated. But now resistant strains are common.
6. *Diphtheria*—erythromycin is very effective in acute stage though antitoxin is life saving. Erythromycin also eradicates carrier state.
7. *Syphilis and gonorrhoea*—erythromycin is used as an alternative.
8. *Campylobacter gastroenteritis* and anthrax—erythromycin is used as an alternative
9. *Tetanus*—erythromycin eradicates carrier state.
10. *Topical*—erythromycin ointment is used for skin infections and boils.

Roxithromycin is longer-acting, acid stable, more potent, better absorbed and has better tissue penetrability compared to erythromycin. It does not inhibit the metabolism of other drugs—hence drug interactions are avoided. It should be taken 30 min before food.

It can be used as an alternative to erythromycin but is more expensive.

Clarithromycin Compared to erythromycin, clarithromycin is longer-acting, acid stable and better absorbed; it is more effective against atypical mycobacteria, *H. pylori* and some protozoa.

Clarithromycin is used:

1. As a component of triple regimen for *H. pylori* infections in peptic ulcer patients.
2. Atypical mycobacterial infections.

Though clarithromycin is effective in other indications of erythromycin, its higher cost makes it less preferable.

Azithromycin is a derivative of erythromycin with activity similar to clarithromycin. It is acid stable, rapidly absorbed, has better tissue penetrability, is longer acting and better tolerated than erythromycin. It is given as a single loading dose of 500 mg followed by 250 mg for the next 4 days. Azithromycin is free of drug interactions as it does not suppress hepatic metabolism of other drugs.

It is used in the prophylaxis and treatment of atypical mycobacterial infections in AIDS patients. Like erythromycin it can also be used in respiratory, genital and skin infections and in pneumonias.

MISCELLANEOUS ANTIBIOTICS

Lincosamides

Clindamycin is a congener of lincomycin. It binds to 50S ribosomal subunit and suppresses protein synthesis. Streptococci, staphylococci, pneumococci and many anaerobes are inhibited by clindamycin. Clindamycin is well-absorbed on oral administration. It attains good concentration in the bone and many other tissues.

Adverse effects include diarrhoea due to pseudomembranous colitis, skin rashes and neuromuscular blockade. Intravenous use can cause thrombophlebitis.

Uses Anaerobic infections—abdominal, pelvic, bone and joints infections due to anaerobes are treated with clindamycin.

Clindamycin is also useful in *Pneumocystis carinii* pneumonia and toxoplasmosis in AIDS patients.

Glycopeptides Vancomycin and Teicoplanin.

Vancomycin produced by *Streptococcus orientalis* is active against gram-positive bacteria particularly staphylococci including those resistant to methicillin. It acts by inhibiting cell wall synthesis and is bactericidal. Vancomycin is not absorbed orally—given IV. It is widely distributed and excreted through kidneys.

Adverse effects are skin rashes, pain at the site of injection, thrombophlebitis, ototoxicity and nephrotoxicity.

Uses

1. Pseudomembranous colitis—oral vancomycin is used.

2. Methicillin resistant staphylococcal infection—vancomycin is given IV for serious infections like osteomyelitis, endocarditis and soft-tissue abscesses.
3. Enterococcal endocarditis—as an alternative to penicillin.
4. Penicillin resistant pneumococcal infections—vancomycin is recommended with a cephalosporin.

Teicoplanin has mechanism of action and antibacterial spectrum similar to vancomycin, but teicoplanin can be safely given intramuscularly. It is also less toxic. Occasionally causes allergic reactions. It is used in osteomyelitis and endocarditis due to methicillin resistant staphylococci and enterococci.

POLYPEPTIDE ANTIBIOTICS

Polymyxin and Colistin

Polymyxin and colistin are used topically. Polymyxin obtained from *Bacillus polymyxa* and colistin from *Bacillus colistinus* are effective against gram-negative bacteria.

Mechanism of action Polymyxin and colistin alter the permeability of the cell membrane resulting in leakage of the cell contents. They are bactericidal.

Polypeptide antibiotics are not absorbed orally; applied topically, they may rarely cause skin rashes.

Uses

1. Used topically for skin infections, ear and eye infections.
2. Oral colistin is used in children for diarrhoea due to gram-negative bacilli.

Others

Bacitracin produced by *Bacillus subtilis* is effective against gram-positive bacteria. It inhibits the cell wall synthesis and is bactericidal. It is too toxic to be given systemically and is therefore used only for topical application—in skin infections, surgical wounds, ulcers and ocular infections (NEOSPORIN powder is bacitracin + neomycin).

Spectinomycin is related to aminoglycosides and is effective against gram-negative bacteria. It can be used only in gonorrhoea.

Sodium fusidate (fusidic acid) is effective against gram-positive organisms particularly staphylococci. It is bactericidal. It is mainly used topically as a 2% ointment (FUCIDIN). It may be given orally for resistant staphylococcal infections.

Mupirocin is bactericidal against gram-positive and some gram-negative organisms. It is used as an ointment (BACTROBAN) for skin infections.

NEWER AGENTS

Streptogramins A combination of **quinupristin** and **dalfopristin** in the ratio 30:70 is bactericidal against gram-positive cocci including methicillin-resistant staphylococci. Streptogramins are given intravenously; they are rapidly metabolised and excreted largely through faeces. Hence adjustment of dose is not required in renal insufficiency. Adverse effects include myalgia and pain at the site of injection. The combination is used in the treatment of serious infections due to streptococci and methicillin-resistant staphylococci.

Linezolid is a recently developed antimicrobial effective against gram-positive anaerobic organisms. It acts by inhibiting protein synthesis. It is orally effective. Linezolid is useful in the treatment of nosocomial infections resistant to other drugs.

❑ CHEMOTHERAPY OF URINARY TRACT INFECTIONS

Infection of the urinary tract is quite common and may be acute or chronic. *Urinary antiseptics* are drugs which exert antibacterial activity only in the urinary tract (and no systemic activity). They include nitrofurantoin and methenamine mandelate.

Nitrofurantoin is effective against many gram-positive and gram-negative bacteria. It attains high concentration in urine and is used in acute UTI, long-term suppression of chronic UTI and for prophylaxis of UTI.

Methenamine mandelate—a salt of mandelic acid and methenamine, releases formaldehyde in acidic urine below pH 5.5. Formaldehyde is bactericidal and resistance does not develop to it. It is used orally in chronic UTI that is resistant to other drugs.

Other drugs used in UTI are sulfonamides, cotrimoxazole, nalidixic acid, fluoroquinolones, ampicillin, cloxacillin, carbenicillin, aminoglycosides, tetracyclines and cephalosporins.

Urinary analgesic—phenazopyridine has analgesic actions on the urinary tract and relieves burning symptoms of dysuria and urgency.

❑ CHEMOTHERAPY OF TUBERCULOSIS

Tuberculosis is a chronic granulomatous disease caused by *Mycobacterium tuberculosis*. In developing countries, it is a major public health problem; 5 lakh people die in India every year due to this disease. After the spread of AIDS, the problem has become more complex, as tuberculosis and *Mycobacterium avium* complex (MAC) infections are more common and rapidly progress in patients with AIDS.

Drugs used in tuberculosis may be classified as:

First line drugs Isoniazid, Rifampicin, Pyrazinamide, Ethambutol, Streptomycin.

Second line drugs Ethionamide, Thiacetazone, Para-aminosalicylic acid (PAS), Amikacin, Ciprofloxacin, Capreomycin, Cycloserine, Rifabutin, Kanamycin.

Based on antitubercular activity, drugs may be grouped as:

1. **Tuberculocidal agents**—Isoniazid, Rifampicin, Streptomycin, Pyrazinamide, Capreomycin, Kanamycin, Ciprofloxacin.
2. **Tuberculostatic agents**—Ethambutol, Ethionamide, Thiacetazone, Cycloserine and PAS.

Isoniazid (INH) is the most effective and cheapest primary antitubercular drug. It is tuberculocidal for rapidly multiplying bacilli but static for resting bacilli. INH destroys: (i) intracellular bacilli as it penetrates into the cells, i.e. tubercle bacilli in the macrophages, and (ii) bacilli multiplying in the walls of the cavities. Thus it is effective against both intra- and extracellular organisms. If used alone, mycobacteria develop resistance to it. Hence it should be used in combination with other drugs.

Mechanism of action INH inhibits the synthesis of mycolic acids which is an important component of the mycobacterial cell wall.

Pharmacokinetics INH is completely absorbed orally, penetrates all tissues, tubercular cavities, necrotic tissues and CSF. It is metabolised by acetylation and excreted in urine.

Adverse effects Peripheral neuritis (which is due to interference with utilization and increased excretion of pyridoxine) can be avoided by giving prophylactic pyridoxine with INH. Hepatitis is another major adverse effect, more common in alcoholics. It can cause CNS toxicity including psychosis and seizures but are rare. Other minor effects like anorexia, GI discomfort and allergic reactions can occur.

Rifampicin is a semisynthetic derivative of rifamycin, an antibiotic obtained from *Streptomyces mediterranei*. It is bactericidal to *M. tuberculosis*, *M. leprae* and atypical mycobacteria. It also inhibits most gram-positive and gram-negative bacteria like *Staph. aureus*, *N. meningitidis*, *E.coli*, *Proteus* and *Pseudomonas*.

Antitubercular action Rifampicin is highly effective, tuberculocidal and is the only drug that acts on persisters; acts on both intra- and extracellular organisms and is effective against tubercle bacilli resistant to other drugs. If used alone resistance develops.

Mechanism of action Rifampicin binds to DNA dependent RNA polymerase and inhibits RNA synthesis in bacteria.

Pharmacokinetics Rifampicin is well-absorbed and has good tissue penetrability—reaches caseous material, cavities and CSF. It is a microsomal enzyme inducer.

Adverse effects Rifampicin is well-tolerated. Skin rashes, diarrhoea, nephritis and hepatotoxicity can occur. In intermittent dosing regimen, a flu-like syndrome can occur.

The urine turns orange yellow colour.

Uses (Table 11.6)

1. Tuberculosis and atypical mycobacterial infections.
2. Leprosy (see page 320).
3. Prophylaxis of *H. influenzae* meningitis in close contacts.

4. Resistant staphylococcal infections—as an alternative.
5. Brucellosis—Rifampicin + doxycycline—drug of choice.
6. To eradicate meningococcal carrier state.

TABLE 11.6: Recommended doses of antitubercular drugs

Drugs	*Doses*
Isoniazid (INH)	300-400 mg
Ethambutol (E)	800-1000 mg
Rifampicin (R)	450-600 mg
Streptomycin (S)	750-1000 mg
Pyrazinamide (Z)	1200-1500 mg
Thiacetazone (T)	150 mg

Pyrazinamide is tuberculocidal, and is more active in acidic pH. Mechanism of action is not known. It is effective against intracellular bacilli. If used alone resistance develops. It is well-absorbed and reaches good concentration in the CSF. Hepatotoxicity is the most common adverse effect. Hyperuricaemia (due to ↓ excretion of uric acid), arthralgia, anorexia, vomiting and rashes are the adverse effects.

Streptomycin (page 306) is tuberculocidal, acts only against extracellular organisms due to poor penetrating power. It has to be given IM. When used alone resistance develops. Because of these disadvantages and its toxicity (oto and nephrotoxicity), streptomycin is not preferred now.

Ethambutol is tuberculostatic and acts on fast multiplying bacilli in the cavities. It is also effective against atypical mycobacteria. It inhibits the incorporation of mycolic acids into the mycobacterial cell wall.

Optic neuritis resulting in ↓ visual acuity and inability to differentiate red from green is an important adverse effect which needs stopping of the drug. Other adverse effects include nausea, anorexia, headache, fever and allergic reactions.

Thiacetazone is tuberculostatic with low efficacy; it delays the development of resistance to other drugs and its low cost makes it a suitable drug in combination regimens. Hepatotoxicity, dermatitis, allergic reactions and GI side effects may occur.

Ethionamide This tuberculostatic drug is effective against both intra and extracellular organisms. It is also effective in atypical mycobacteria.

Anorexia, nausea, vomiting and metallic taste in the mouth are the most common adverse effects. It can also cause hepatitis, skin rashes and peripheral neuritis (needs prophylactic pyridoxine).

Ethionamide is a secondary agent used only when primary drugs are ineffective.

Para-aminosalicylic acid (PAS) related to sulfonamides is tuberculostatic. Gastrointestinal effects like nausea, anorexia, epigastric pain and diarrhoea make it a poorly tolerated drug. Allergic reactions and hepatitis are also seen. It is rarely used.

Other Second Line Drugs

Amikacin, kanamycin and capreomycin are second line drugs that need parenteral administration. They are oto and nephrotoxic and are used only in resistant cases. Amikacin is also effective against atypical mycobacteria.

Cycloserine is an antibiotic that inhibits cell wall synthesis, is tuberculostatic and is also effective against some gram-positive organisms. It causes CNS toxicity including psychosis. It is used only in resistant tuberculosis.

Fluoroquinolones Ciprofloxacin, ofloxacin and sparfloxacin inhibit tubercle bacilli and atypical mycobacteria. They are useful in multi-drug resistant tuberculosis in combination with other drugs.

Treatment of Tuberculosis

Tuberculosis is one of the most difficult infections to cure. The need for long-term treatment, drug toxicity, cost of treatment and poor patient compliance have all made the problem more complex. AIDs patients have more severe disease due to depressed immunity. But, with the availability of effective drugs, most patients can now be treated as outpatients.

A combination of drugs is used in tuberculosis to:

1. delay the development of resistance
2. reduce toxicity
3. shorten the course of treatment.

Short-term regimen

INH + R + Z + E/S daily for 2 months followed by INH + R daily for 4 months.

Short-term therapy has rapid response, less chances of resistance and better patient compliance.

Conventional regimen

- INH + S + T daily for 2 months
- INH + T daily for 10 months

Failure rates are high and compliance is poor.

Resistant tuberculosis should be treated with 4-5 drugs, of which 3 are first line drugs and treatment is continued for at least 1 year after the sputum becomes negative.

Role of glucocorticoids As steroids depress host defense mechanisms, they should be used only in conditions like tubercular meningitis, miliary tuberculosis, pleural effusion, renal tuberculosis and rapidly progressing pulmonary tuberculosis. Steroids suppress inflammatory reaction which can lead to fibrosis and damage.

TABLE 11.7: Antitubercular actions and characteristic adverse effects of some antitubercular drugs

Drug	*Antitubercular action*	*Serious toxicity*
Isoniazid	Tuberculocidal; acts on intra and extracellular organisms	Peripheral neuritis, seizures, psychosis
Rifampicin	Tuberculocidal; Acts on intra and extracellular organisms, persisters and drug resistant organisms	Hepatotoxicity, flu-like syndrome, nephritis; urine and secretions are coloured orange-red
Pyrazinamide	Tuberculocidal, kills intracellular organisms; more active in acidic pH	Hepatotoxicity, arthralgia, hyperuricaemia
Streptomycin	Tuberculocidal, acts on extracellular organisms	Ototoxicity, nephrotoxicity
Ethambutol	Tuberculostatic; inhibits tubercle bacilli in the walls of cavities	Optic neuritis with ↓ visual acuity and red-green colour blindness
Thiacetazone	Tuberculostatic low efficacy. Delays development of resistance to other drugs	Hepatotoxicity dermatitis

Chemoprophylaxis is given INH for 6-12 months only in:

i. Close contacts of open cases especially children
ii. Patients with old inactive disease who have not been adequately treated.

Drugs for *Mycobacterium avium* complex (MAC) Infection with MAC is more common in HIV patients. The drugs effective are rifabutin, clarithromycin, azithromycin, fluoroquinolones, ethambutol, clofazimine, amikacin and ethionamide. Clarithromycin + ethambutol is the preferred regimen for MAC infection and needs life long treatment. Rifabutin is used for prophylaxis.

❑ CHEMOTHERAPY OF LEPROSY

Leprosy caused by *Mycobacterium leprae* is a chronic infectious disease affecting skin, mucous membranes and nerves. Hansen discovered lepra bacillus in 1873.

In India leprosy *(kusta roga)* is a major public health problem affecting millions of people.

Drugs used in leprosy

- Sulfones: Dapsone
- Rifampicin
- Clofazimine
- Ethionamide.

Dapsone is diaminodiphenylsulfone (DDS) and is related to sulfonamides.

Mechanism of action Like sulfonamides, it inhibits the incorporation of PABA into folic acid.

Actions Dapsone is leprostatic. Though it inhibits growth of many other bacteria, the dose needed is high and is therefore not used. The lepra bacillus develops resistance to dapsone on prolonged use.

Dapsone is completely absorbed on oral administration and reaches high concentrations in skin. It is metabolised in the liver and excreted in bile.

Adverse effects Dapsone is well-tolerated—anorexia, nausea and vomiting are common and allergic reactions can occur. Hepatitis and agranulocytosis can occur. Patients with lepromatous leprosy may develop lepra reactions.

Rifampicin is rapidly bactericidal to *M. leprae* and is highly effective. It can be conveniently given once monthly. Used in combination with dapsone, it shortens the duration of treatment. Given alone—resistance develops.

Clofazimine a dye, has weak bactericidal actions against *M. leprae*. It also has anti-inflammatory properties which is useful in suppressing lepra reactions. It is used orally in multi-drug regimens.

Clofazimine causes reddish-black discolouration of the skin specially on the exposed parts which remains for several months. It can also cause dryness of skin, itching and phototoxicity.

TREATMENT OF LEPROSY

For the sake of treatment, leprosy is divided into paucibacillary (non-infectious) and multibacillary (infectious) leprosy.

WHO has recommended a combination of drugs in leprosy to:

1. eliminate persisters
2. prevent drug resistance
3. reduce the duration of therapy.

Multi-drug regimen

Drugs	*Multibacillary leprosy (for 24 months)*	*Paucibacillary leprosy (for 6 months)*
Rifampicin	600 mg once a month supervised	600 mg once a month supervised
Dapsone	100 mg daily self-administered	100 mg daily self-administered
Clofazimine	300 mg once monthly supervised	—
	50 mg daily self-administered	—

All drugs are given orally

Lepra reactions are the acute exacerbations that occur in leprosy. They are triggered by acute infections, stress, anxiety and treatment with dapsone.

Type I reactions seen in tuberculoid leprosy is a delayed hypersensitivity reaction to the antigens of *M. leprae*. Skin ulcerations occur and existing lesions become red. It is treated with corticosteroids or clofazimine.

Type II reactions are seen in lepromatous leprosy (are known as *erythema nodosum leprosum* ENL). New lesions appear and the existing lesions become worse. Fever, lymphadenitis and neuralgia may occur. It is a hypersensitivity reaction to the antigens of *M. leprae.* Type II reactions can be treated with clofazimine which is effective due to its anti-inflammatory properties. Chloroquine, corticosteroids or thalidomide are also effective. Dapsone should be continued throughout.

❑ ANTIFUNGAL DRUGS

Fungal infections may be systemic or superficial. There has been an increase in the incidence and severity of fungal infections in the recent years. Several unusual and drug-resistant organisms have emerged. These may be due to the use of broad spectrum antibiotics, anticancer drugs and HIV infection. Antifungal drugs may be classified into:

CLASSIFICATION

1. *Antifungal antibiotics*
   — Amphotericin B, Griseofulvin, Nystatin, Hamycin
2. *Antimetabolites*
   — Flucytosine (5-FC)
3. *Azoles*
   — *Imidazoles* Clotrimazole, Econazole, Miconazole, Ketoconazole
   — *Triazoles* Fluconazole, Itraconazole
4. *Miscellaneous*
   - Terbinafine
5. *Other topical agents*
   - Tolnaftate, Undecylenic acid, Benzoic acid, Salicyclic acid, Selenium sulfide, Ciclopirox olamine.

Antifungal Antibiotics

Amphotericin B obtained from *Streptomyces nodosus* is a polyene antibiotic containing many double bonds.

Antifungal spectrum Amphotericin B has a wide antifungal spectrum. It inhibits the growth of *Candida albicans, Histoplasma capsulatum, Cryptococcus neoformans, Coccidioides, Aspergillus* and *Blastomyces dermatitidis.* It is fungistatic at low and fungicidal at high concentrations.

Mechanism of action Amphotericin B binds to ergosterol present in fungal cell membrane and forms pores in the cell membrane. Through these pores, cell contents leak out resulting in cell death.

Pharmacokinetics Amphotericin B is not absorbed orally and hence given IV. It has a long t½ of 15 days.

Adverse effects Fever, chills, muscle spasms, vomiting, headache and hypotension can be encountered on IV infusion. Renal impairment and anaemia due to bone marrow depression can also occur.

Uses Amphotericin B is the drug of choice for all life-threatening mycotic infections. It is used topically in candidiasis.

Leishmaniasis: In kala-azar and mucocutaneous leishmaniasis, amphotericin is used as an alternative.

Nystatin obtained from *Streptomyces noursei* has actions similar to amphotericin B. But as it is too toxic for systemic use. It is used topically for local candidial infections like oral thrush and vaginal candidiasis.

Hamycin is similar to nystatin. It is used topically for cutaneous candidiasis and otomycosis.

Griseofulvin is derived from *Penicillium griseofulvum.* It is effective in superficial dermatophytosis (caused by *Trichophyton, Microsporum* and *Epidermophyton*). Griseofulvin is the antifungal given orally for superficial dermatophytes. It gets deposited in the newly forming skin, binds to keratin and protects the skin from getting newly infected.

Adverse effects include allergic reactions, hepatitis and neurotoxicity.

Antimetabolites

Flucytosine is effective against *Cryptococcus neoformans* and some strains of *Candida*. It is taken up by the fungal cells and converted to 5-fluorouracil which inhibits DNA synthesis.

Bone marrow depression and gastrointestinal disturbances are the most common adverse effects. It is used with amphotericin B (used alone, resistance develops rapidly) in cryptococcal meningitis and systemic candidiasis.

Azoles

Imidazoles and Triazoles The older antifungals need to be given intravenously and are quite toxic. Azoles are newer antifungals that are effective orally and are less toxic.

Antifungal spectrum Azoles have a broad spectrum antifungal activity. They inhibit *dermatophytes, candida, cryptococcus neoformans* and other *deep mycoses.*

Mechanism of action Azoles inhibit the synthesis of ergosterol, an important component of the fungal cell membrane.

Ketaconazole (KTZ) is the first oral azole to be available. It is well-absorbed from the gut. Food and low gastric pH enhance absorption. In large doses it inhibits the biosynthesis of adrenal and gonadal steroids in humans—resulting in gynaecomastia, infertility and menstrual irregularities.

Adverse reactions include gastric irritation, headache, allergic reactions, gynaecomastia and rarely hepatotoxicity.

Drug interactions

Rifampicin and phenytoin induce KTZ metabolism and decrease its efficacy.

Uses Mucocutaneous candidiasis and dermatophytosis can be treated with ketoconazole. It is also useful in Cushing's syndrome.

Fluconazole is well-absorbed orally and attains good CSF concentration.

Adverse effects are mild gastrointestinal disturbances, headache and rashes. Since it has very little effect on hepatic microsomal enzymes, drug interactions are less common.

Uses Fluconazole is used in cryptococcal meningitis, systemic candidiasis and other systemic fungal infections. Though it is also effective in tinea infections and mucocutaneous candidiasis, its higher cost makes it less preferable.

Itraconazole is the most potent azole. Given orally, its absorption is increased by food and gastric acid. Its effect on hepatic microsomal enzymes is less; does not affect steroid synthesis. Thus it is preferred over ketoconazole. It is useful in dermatophytosis, candidiasis, aspergillosis and onychomycosis (ITASPOR, SPORANOX 100 mg cap).

Clotrimazole and Miconazole are used topically in dermatophytic infections (ringworm) and mucocutaneous candidiasis. Clotrimazole troche is available for oral thrush. Miconazole has better efficacy. Both can cause mild irritation at the site of application.

- Clotrimazole (CANDID, CLODERM) } Lotion, cream,
- Miconazole (DAKTARIN, ZOLE) } vaginal pessary

Terbinafine is a synthetic antifungal that is effective against dermatophytes and *Candida*. It is orally effective and is fungicidal. It gets concentrated in the keratin like griseofulvin. It inhibits an enzyme needed for biosynthesis of ergosterol by fungi.

Adverse effects are rare—gastrointestinal disturbances, rashes and headache. Terbinafine is used in dermatophytosis, pityriasis, onychomycosis and candidiasis. SEBIFIN—250 mg tab, 1% cream.

Other Topical Antifungal Agents

Apart from nystatin, clotrimazole, miconazole and terbinafine, some drugs like salicyclic acid, benzoic acid, tolnaftate, cyclopirox olamine are used topically for dermatophytosis and pityriasis versicolor.

Selenium sulfide is useful in tinea versicolor caused by *Malassezia furfur*, and also in dandruff. SELSUN is 2.5% suspension of selenium sulfide in a shampoo base. It is irritant to the eyes and the odour is unpleasant.

❑ ANTIVIRAL DRUGS

Viruses are intracellular parasites and depend on the host cells for their food, growth and multiplication. The virus attaches itself to the host cell membrane, penetrates it and DNA/RNA is released in the host cell. The viral components are assembled and the mature viral particle is then released from the host cell. Chemotherapy can interfere with any of these steps. But drugs that interfere with viral replication may also interfere with host cell function.

CLASSIFICATION

1. *Anti-herpes virus agents:* Acyclovir, Ganciclovir, Idoxuridine, Trifluridine, Vidarabine, Foscarnet.
2. *Anti-influenza virus agents:* Amantadine, Rimantadine.
3. *Others:* Ribavirin, Interferons.
4. Antiretroviral agents:

Nuclease Reverse transcriptase inhibitors: Zidovudine, didanosine, stavudine, zalcitabine, lamivudine, abacavir

Non-nuclease Reverse transcriptase inhibitors—Nevirapine, efavirenz, delavirdine

Protease inhibitors Saquinavir, indinavir, ritonavir, nelfinavir, amprenavir, lopinavir

ANTI-HERPES VIRUS AGENTS

Acyclovir is effective against Herpes simplex virus (HSV) type 1 and type 2, Varicella zoster virus (VZV) and Epstein-Barr virus (EBV).

Mechanism of action Acyclovir inhibits viral DNA synthesis by inhibiting viral DNA polymerases.

Adverse effects Acyclovir is well-tolerated; nausea, diarrhoea, headache and rashes may occur occasionally. Topical acyclovir can cause burning and irritation. Given IV, it may cause renal and neurotoxicity but are uncommon.

Uses (Table 11.8)

1. *HSV infections* Infection with HSV-1 causes diseases of the mouth, face, skin, oesophagus or brain. HSV-2 usually

causes infections of the genitals, rectum, skin, hands or meninges.

- Oral acyclovir is effective in primary and recurrent genital and labial herpes. In mild cases, topical acyclovir can be tried. In recurring genital herpes—oral acyclovir is given for 1 year.
- *HSV encephalitis* and other severe HSV infections—IV acyclovir is the drug of choice.
- *HSV keratoconjunctivitis* Acyclovir eye drops are effective.

2. *Herper zoster* Acyclovir shortens the duration of illness.
3. *Chickenpox* In adults and in immunodeficient patients, acyclovir reduces duration and severity of illness. In children, routine use is not recommended.

Valacyclovir is a prodrug of acyclovir. Famciclovir is a prodrug of penciclovir—used in HSV and VZV infections.

Ganciclovir is effective against herpes viruses especially cytomegalovirus (CMV). Toxicity includes myelosuppression and gonadal toxicity. It is used in immunocompromised patients with CMV retinitis.

Idoxuridine is effective in DNA viruses. It acts by inhibiting viral DNA synthesis. Idoxuridin is used topically in HSV keratitis (it is too toxic for systemic use). Eyelid oedema, itching and allergic reactions may occur.

Trifluridine is used topically in HSV eye infections.

Foscarnet is given intravenously to treat CMV retinitis as an alternative to ganciclovir.

Vidarabine was used earlier for HSV and VZV infections but is now replaced by acyclovir.

ANTI-INFLUENZA VIRUS AGENTS

Amantadine and Rimantadine inhibit the replication of influenza A viruses. Generally well-tolerated, nausea, vomiting, diarrhoea, dizziness, insomnia and ankle oedema are reported. Rimantadine is longer-acting and has fewer adverse effects.

Uses

1. Treatment of influenza A during an epidemic—reduces duration and severity—dose: 200 mg/day for 5 days.

2. Prophylaxis of influenza A during an epidemic especially in high-risk patients. Also for seasonal prophylaxis in high-risk patients.
3. Parkinsonism—amantadine enhances the release of dopamine and is beneficial in parkinsonism.

OTHER ANTIVIRAL AGENTS

Ribavirin has broad spectrum antiviral activity. It is effective against influenza A and B, respiratory syncytial virus (RSV) and many DNA and RNA viruses. It is used as an aerosol in RSV bronchiolitis in children. Also it can be used in severe influenza and measles in immunocompromised patients.

Interferons are cytokines produced by host cells in response to viral infections. There are three types α, β, γ interferons in man. They also have immunomodulating and antiproliferative properties. They inhibit the multiplication of many DNA and RNA viruses.

Adverse effects include myelosuppression, hypotension, arrhythmias, alopecia, headache and arthralgia. It can also cause neurotoxicity resulting in confusion, sedation and rarely seizures.

Uses

1. Chronic hepatitis B and C.
2. Kaposi's sarcoma in AIDS patients.
3. Genital warts caused by Papilloma virus—interferons are injected into the lesion.
4. Hairy cell leukaemia.
5. HSV, herpes zoster and CMV infections in immunocompromised patients.
6. Rhinovirus cold—interferon α is given intranasally for prophylaxis.

ANTI-RETROVIRAL AGENTS

Nuclease reverse transcriptase (NRT) inhibitors.

Zidovudine (Azidothymidine, AZT) is a thymidine analog, active against HIV infections and other retroviruses.

TABLE 11.8: Indications of some commonly used antiviral drugs

Drugs	*Routes*	*Indications*
Acyclovir	Topical	Herpes genitalis, HSV eye infections
	Oral	Herpes genitalis/mucocutaneous HSV chickenpox
	IV	HSV encephalitis, severe herpes genitalis, chickenpox/herpes zoster in immunocompromised patients
Idoxuridine Trifluridine	Topical	HSV keratitis
Ganciclovir	IV/oral	CMV infections
Foscarnet	IV	CMV retinitis, acyclovir resistant HSV infections
Amantadine Rimantadine	Oral	Influenza A
Ribavirin	Aerosol oral/IV	RSV bronchiolitis, severe influenza and measles
Interferon α	IV	Chronic hepatitis B and C, genital warts, Kaposi's sarcoma
Zidovudine	Oral	HIV infection

Mechanism of action NRT inhibitors are converted to their triphosphate derivatives by cellular enzymes which inhibit reverse transcriptase.

Adverse effects Bone marrow suppression, headache, nausea, vomiting and insomnia can occur. High doses cause myopathy and neurotoxicity.

Uses AZT is the drug of choice in HIV infections. Treatment with AZT results in prolonged survival, decreased opportunistic infections, weight gain and in early cases it delays disease progression.

Given during pregnancy and continued in new borns for 6 weeks, AZT reduces the risk of transmission to the baby. But it has **no** prophylactic value in those who are accidentally exposed to HIV infection (e.g. following blood transfusion). Combination therapy of AZT with didanosine or zalcitabine gives better results.

Didanosine, Zalcitabine, Stavudine Lamivudine and **abacavir** are other NRT inhibitors effective against AZT resistant HIV infections. They are used as alternative to AZT in patients with advanced HIV who are intolerant to AZT or are not responding to AZT.

Peripheral neuropathy, pancreatitis, rash, fever and headache can occur.

Non-nucleoside reverse transcriptase (NNRT) inhibitors like nevirapine, delavirdine and efavirenz inactivate the enzyme reverse transcriptase. They are useful in HIV-1 infections.

Protease inhibitors like saquinavir indinavir and others bind to HIV protease and block viral maturation. They are well tolerated with mild adverse effects like gastrointestinal disturbances. They are used in combination with other drugs in HIV infections.

❑ CHEMOTHERAPY OF MALARIA

Malaria is caused by protozoa of the genus *Plasmodium,* transmitted through the bite of a female Anopheles mosquito. It is a major public health problem in most of the developing countries including India.

Antimalarial drugs can be classified as:

1. ***Causal Prophylactics*** Primaquine, Pyrimethamine

These destroy the tissue forms of the parasite in liver cells and prevent invasion of the erythrocytes. They are also called primary tissue schizontocides.

2. ***Blood schizontocides (suppressives)*** Chloroquine, quinine, melfloquine, halofantrine, pyrimethamine, chloroguanide and artemisinin.

Suppressives destroy the protozoa in the RBCs and terminate clinical attacks of malaria.

3. ***Tissue schizontocides used to prevent relapse***— Primaquine They act on hepatic forms of *P. vivax* and *P. ovale* that produce relapses. Given with a blood schizontocide, they bring about **radical cure** and eradicate the parasite from the body in these relapsing malarial infections.

4. ***Gametocidal drugs*** Primaquine, chloroquine and quinine. These destroy gametocytes and prevent the transmission of malaria.

Chloroquine is a synthetic 4-aminoquinoline. It is a highly effective blood schizontocide with activity against all 4 species of plasmodia. It also destroys gametocytes of *P. vivax, P. ovale* and *P. malaria* and completely cures falciparum malaria. Patients become afebrile in 24-48 hr.

Chloroquine is safe in pregnancy. It also has anti-inflammatory properties.

Mechanism of action is not clear. Chloroquine is a base. It concentrates in acidic food vacuoles of the parasite and interferes with the degradation of haemoglobin.

Adverse effects Nausea, vomiting, pruritus, headache, visual disturbances, insomnia and skin rashes may occur. Prolonged treatment with high doses can cause irreversible retinopathy. High doses can also cause cardiomyopathy and psychiatric problems.

Uses (Table 11.9)

1. *Malaria* Chloroquine is highly effective in the treatment of malaria due to sensitive strains of all 4 species (600 mg base stat, 300 mg after 6 hours and 300 mg for the next 2 days). It is also used for prophylaxis—300 mg/week.
2. Extraintestinal amoebiasis (page 335)
3. Rheumatoid arthritis
4. Photogenic reactions
5. Lepra reactions

} Chloroquine is effective in these (3–5) because of its anti-inflammatory property

Quinine is an alkaloid obtained from the bark of the cinchona tree. It destroys erythrocytic forms of the parasite similar to chloroquine and is useful as a suppressive. It is also gametocidal (except for *P. falciparum).*

Quinine also has mild analgesic and antipyretic activity; myocardiac depressant and local anaesthetic properties.

Adverse effects are high. Quinine is a gastric irritant and causes nausea, vomiting and epigastric pain. Cinchonism with ringing in the ears, headache, nausea, visual disturbances and vertigo may be encountered. In more severe poisoning, hypoglycaemia, fever, delirium, confusion, hypotension, cardiac arrhythmias and coma may develop. Death is due to respiratory arrest.

Uses Quinine is used in the treatment of resistant falciparum malaria and cerebral malaria.

Mefloquine in a single dose is highly effective against erythrocytic forms of vivax and falciparum malaria—even the multi-

TABLE 11.9: Preferred antimalarials in the treatment and prophylaxis of malaria

Malaria	*Drug*	*Dose, route and duration*
Chloroquine sensitive strains		
Treatment	Chloroquine	Oral 600 mg base stat, 300 mg after 6 hr 300 mg/day for next 2 days
Prophylaxis	Chloroquine	2 tabs/week; start 1 week before and continue for 4 weeks after leaving the endemic area
Chloroquine resistant strains		
Treatment	Choices are: 1. Quinine followed by	Oral 600 mg TDS for 3 days Severe cases IV 10 mg/kg 8 hourly followed by
	A. Doxycycline or Quinine	100 mg BD for 7 days or Dose as above
	B. Pyrimethamine + sulfadoxine	Pyrimethamine 25 mg + Sulfadoxine 500 mg 3 tab
	2. Mefloquine	15 mg/kg single dose (Max 1000 mg)
	3. Artemisinin	100 mg BD on first day, 50 mg BD for next 5 days
Prophylaxis	1. Mefloquine	250 mg weekly; start 1 week before and continue for 4 weeks after leaving the area
	2. Doxycycline	100 mg daily; start 2 days before and continue for 4 weeks after leaving the area

For all cases of *P. vivax* and *P. ovale*, Primaquine 15 mg/day should be given for 2 weeks

drug resistant (MDR) strains of *P. falciparum*. It is well-tolerated. Nausea, vomiting, dizziness, confusion, abdominal pain and bradycardia are common.

Mefloquine is indicated only in MDR strains of falciparum malaria.

Halofantrine is schizonticidal against erythrocytic forms of all *Plasmodium* species including MDR strains of *P. falciparum*.

It is used as an alternative in MDR strains of falciparum malaria.

Primaquine is effective against persistent tissue forms of *P. vivax* and *P. ovale* and prevents relapse in these cases. It is also a causal prophylactic and gametocidal agent.

Primaquine is used for *radical cure* along with a blood schizontocide in *P. vivax* and ovale and as a gametocidal agent in *P. falciparum* malaria.

Pyrimethamine is effective against the erythrocytic forms of all 4 species of plasmodia. When given with sulfadoxin (a sulfonamide), the combination is synergistic and the development of resistance is slower.

Uses

1. *Malaria*
   i. *acute attacks*—Pyrimethamine + sulfadoxine combination is used as an alternative to chloroquine.
   ii. *Prophylaxis*—1-2 tablets once weekly for prophylaxis against MDR falciparum malaria—when a person is visiting an endemic area.
2. *Toxoplasmosis*—Pyrimethamine + sulfadoxine combination is the treatment of choice for toxoplasmosis.

Chloroguanide (Proguanil) is a schizontocide with causal prophylactic activity against *P. falciparum*. It is used for causal prophylaxis of falciparum malaria and as an alternative to pyrimethamine-sulfadoxine for the prophylaxis of MDR falciparum malaria.

Artemisinin obtained from the plant *Artemisia annua* has been used in chinese traditional medicine 'Quinghaosu' for almost 2000 years.

It is a potent, rapidly acting, blood schizontocide effective against all the 4 plasmodial species, including MDR *P. falciparum*. Mechanism of action is not known. It is useful in cerebral malaria.

Artemisinin is the best tolerated antimalarial—mild GI symptoms, fever, itching and bradycardia are reported.

Artemisinin is contraindicated in pregnancy.

Uses Acute attacks of MDR falciparum malaria as an alternative to quinine.

❑ ANTIAMOEBIC DRUGS

Amoebiasis caused by the protozoan *Entamoeba histolytia* is a tropical disease common in developing countries. It spreads by faecal contamination of food and water. Though it primarily affects colon, other organs like liver, lungs and brain are the secondary sites. Acute amoebiasis is characterised by bloody mucoid stools and abdominal pain. Chronic amoebiasis manifests as anorexia, abdominal pain, intermittent diarrhoea and constipation. Cyst passers or carriers are symptom free.

CLASSIFICATION

1. *Drugs effective in both intestinal and extraintestinal amoebiasis* Metronidazole, Tinidazole, Secnidazole, Emetine, Dehydro-emetine.
2. *Drugs effective only in intestinal amoebiasis (Luminal amoebicides)* Diloxanide furoate, Quiniodochlor, Iodoquinol, Tetracylines.
3. *Drugs effective only in extraintestinal amoebiasis* Chloroquine

Metronidazole a nitroimidazole, is a powerful amoebicide. Apart from this it also inhibits *Trichomonas vaginalis, Giardia lamblia* and *Balantidium coli.* Anaerobic bacteria are also sensitive.

Mechanism of action In the microorganisms, metronidazole is reduced to a derivative which is toxic to the DNA.

Metronidazole is well-absorbed and reaches adequate concentrations in the CSF.

Adverse effects Gastrointestinal effects like nausea, anorexia, abdominal pain and metallic taste in the mouth are the most frequent. Headache, stomatitis, dizziness, insomnia, skin rashes and rarely peripheral neuropathy can occur. High doses can cause convulsions.

Metronidazole has a disulfiram like effect; on alcohol intake, antabuse like reaction can follow.

Uses

1. *Amoebiasis*—Metronidazole is the drug of choice in all forms of amoebiasis in the dose of 400-800 mg TDS for 7-10 days. But it does not eradicate the cysts.
2. *Trichomonas vaginitis*—Metronidazole 200 TDS for 7 days is the drug of choice.
3. *Giardiasis*—Metronidazole given 200 mg TDS for 7 days is the treatment of choice.
4. *Anaerobic infections*—Metronidazole is given intravenously for serious anaerobic infections. It is also useful for surgical prophylaxis of abdominal and pelvic infections.
5. *H. pylori infections* in peptic ulcer patients can be treated with a combination of metronidazole, clarithromycin and omeprazole/ranitidine.
6. *Pseudomembranous colitis* due to *Clostridium difficile*—responds to metronidazole.
7. *Acute ulcerative gingivitis* As an alternative to penicillin G.
8. *Dracunculosis* Metronidazole facilitates extraction of the guinea worm.

Tinidazole is longer-acting and is better tolerated than metronidazole due to lesser side effects. It can be given 2 gm once daily for 3 days in amoebiasis and as a single dose for other indications.

Secnidazole is longer-acting and can be given as a single 2 gm dose for most indications of metronidazole.

Emetine and dehydroemetine directly affects the trophozoites but not the cysts. They can be used only in severe amoebiasis but are not preferred due to toxicity.

Diloxanide furoate is directly amoebicidal. Flatulence, nausea and occasionally abdominal cramps and rashes can occur. It is used alone in asymptomatic cyst passers, mild intestinal amoebiasis and along with a nitroimidazole—for the cure of amoebiasis, because diloxanide eradicates cysts.

Chloroquine attains high concentration in the liver, is directly toxic against trophozoites and is therefore useful in hepatic amoebiasis. As chloroquine is completely absorbed from the small intestines, it is not effective against amoebae in the colon. It is used as an alternative to metronidazole in hepatic amoebiasis.

Tetracyclines The older tetracyclines are not well-absorbed and large amounts reach the colon—hence these are useful in intestinal amoebiasis. They inhibit the intestinal flora and break the symbiosis between them and the amoebae. Tetracyclines are used as adjuvants in chronic cases.

❑ DRUGS USED LEISHMANIASIS AND TRYPANOSOMIASIS

LEISHMANIASIS

Leishmaniasis is caused by protozoa of the genus leishmania—kala-azar or visceral leishmanias is caused by *Leishmania donavani*; oriental sore by *L. tropica* and mucocutaneous leishmaniasis by *L. braziliensis*. The infection is transmitted by the bite of the female sandfly phlebotomus. It is endemic in Bihar.

Drugs used in leishmaniasis include:

Sodium stibogluconate is an antimony compound which is effective in kala-azar and in mucocutaneous and cutaneous leishmaniasis.

Adverse effects include a metallic taste in the mouth, nausea, vomiting, diarrhoea, headache, myalgia, arthralgia, pain at the injection site, bradycardia, skin rashes, haematuria and jaundice. Some cases of sudden death due to shock have occurred. ECG should be monitored as arrhythmias can occur during the later days of therapy.

Meglumine antimonate and **ethyl stibamine** can also be used in all forms of leishmaniasis.

Pentamidine is effective against *Leishmania donovani*, trypanosomes, *Pneumocystis carinii* and some fungi.

Adverse effects Pentamidine liberates histamine which is responsible for vomiting, diarrhoea, flushing, pruritis, rashes, tachycardia and hypotension apart from pain at the injection site.

Pentamidine is useful in visceral *leishmaniasis, trypanosomiasis* and in *pneumocystis carinii* infections.

Other Drugs

Amphotericin B (page 321) has been tried in leishmaniasis in the endemic areas where antimonials may be ineffective.

Ketoconazole inhibits ergosterol synthesis in the leishmania and is effective in cutaneous leishmaniasis.

Allopurinol In leishmania, allopurinol is converted to a metabolite which inhibits protein synthesis. It may be used along with antimonials.

Dose: 300 mg 3-4 times a day for 2-4 weeks.

Paramomycin (aminosidine) is an amoebicidal drug which is also found to be effective in leishmaniasis. It is useful in all forms of leishmaniasis. It can be used alone or in combination with antimonials.

TRYPANOSOMIASIS

Trypanosomiasis is caused by protozoa of the genus *Trypanosoma*. African trypanosomiasis or sleeping sickness is caused by *T. gambiense* and *T. rhodesiense* while South American trypanosomiasis is caused by *T. Cruzi*. Drugs used in trypanosomiasis are suramin, pentamidine, melarsoprol, eflornithine, nifurtimox and benznidazole. **Suramin sodium** is the drug of choice for early stage of trypanosomiasis but it does not cross the BBB and therefore cannot be used in later stages of the disease. It is also used for the prophylaxis but pentamidine is preferable. Suramin is also effective in eradicating adult forms of onchocerca volvulus.

Toxicity is high; vomiting, shock and loss of consciousness may follow IV injections. Rash, neuropathies, haemolytic anaemia and agranulocytosis may also occur.

Melarsoprol is the preferred drug in later stages of trypanosomiasis which is associated with encephalitis and meningitis.

Eflornithine is used as an alternative in CNS trypanosomiasis. **Nifurtimox** and **benznidazole** are useful in Chaga's disease (American trypanosomiasis).

❑ ANTHELMINTICS

Worm infestations are more common in the developing countries. It is seen in people with poor hygiene. Anthelmintics are deworming agents. A *vermicidal* kills while a *vermifuge* promotes expulsion of worms.

Mebendazole a broad spectrum anthelmintic cures roundworm, hookworm, pinworm and strongyloides infestations. The eggs and larvae are also destroyed. It blocks the glucose uptake in the parasite. It is well-tolerated; nausea, abdominal pain and diarrhoea are seen in heavy infestations.

Uses Mebendazole is used in the treatment of roundworm, hookworm, pinworm, tapeworm, trichuriasis and hydatid disease. It is of special value in multiple worm infestations.

Albendazole a congener of mebendazole, has actions similar to mebendazole but is *better tolerated* and is effective in a *single dose.* Adverse effects are similar to mebendazole but milder.

Uses

1. Albendazole is the drug of choice in roundworm, hookworm, pinworm, trichuriasis infestations in a single 400 mg dose. Dose to be repeated after 2 weeks in pinworm infestation to prevent reinfection from ova that have matured later.
2. Trichinosis, tapeworms and strongyloidosis require 3 days treatment.
3. Neurocysticercosis—Albendazole is the drug of choice.
4. Hydatid disease—Albendazole is the drug of choice ; given for 4 weeks.

Thiabendazole a benzimidazole, acts like mebendazole. But due to frequent side effects, it is not preferred. It is used as an alternative to albendazole in strongyloidosis and cutaneous larva migrans.

Pyrantel pamoate is effective against roundworm, hookworm and pinworms. It stimulates the nicotinic cholinergic receptor in the worm leading to persistant depolarisation and spastic paralysis (depolarising neuromuscular blocker). The paralysed worms are expelled.

Uses In the treatment of roundworm, hookworm and pinworm infestations.

Piperazine citrate is effective in roundworm and pinworm infestations. It competitively blocks the action of acetylcholine and thereby contractions in the worms. Flaccid paralysis results and the worms are expelled.

Levamisole is effective against roundworms and hookworms and can be used as an alternative drug in these infestations. It is well-tolerated and is effective in a single dose. It is also an immunomodulator.

Niclosamide is effective against most tapeworms. The segments of the dead tapeworms are partly digested and in case of *T. solium,* may result in visceral cysticercosis. A purgative may be given 2 hours after niclosamide to wash off the worms and avoid cysticercosis.

Uses Niclosamide is the drug of choice in infestations by tapeworms like *T. solium, T. saginata, H. nana* and *D. latum.* It is also an alternative drug in intestinal fluke infestation.

Praziquantel is effective against schistosomes of all species, most other trematodes and cestodes including cysticercosis.

Adverse effects are mild and include GI disturbances, headache, dizziness, drowsiness, rashes and myalgia.

Uses

1. *Schistosomiasis* Praziquantel is the drug of choice in all forms of schistosomiasis.
2. *Tapeworms* Single dose (10 mg/kg) of praziquantel is effective in all tapeworm infestations. In *T. solium* it has the advantage that it kills the larvae and therefore visceral cysticercosis is avoided.
3. *Neurocysticercosis* Praziquantel is an alternative to albendazole.

TABLE 11.10: Preferred drugs for helminthiasis infection

Worms	*Drugs of choice*	*Alternative drugs*
1. Roundworm *(Ascaris lumbricoides)*	Mebendazole/ albendazole/pyrantel	Piperazine
2. Hookworms *(Ancylostoma duodenale, Necator americanus)*	Mebendazole/ albendazole	Pyrantel
3. Pinworm *(Enterobius vermicularis)*	Mebendazole/ albendazole/pyrantel	Piperazine
4. Whipworm *(Trichuris trichura)*	Mebendazole	Albendazole
5. Strongyloides stercoralis	Albendazole	Thiabendazole
6. Guineaworm *(Dracunculous medinensis)*	Metronidazole	Mebendazole
7. Tapeworms *(Taenia saginata, Taenia solium, H. nana, D. latum)*	Niclosamide/ praziquantel	Albendazole
Neurocysticercosis	Albendazole	Praziquantel
8. Hydatid disease *(E. granulosus, E. multilocularis)*	Albendazole	Mebendazole
9. Filaria *(Wuchareria bancrofti, Brugia malayi)*	Diethylcarbamazine	—
10. Schistosomes	Praziquantel	—

Diethylcarbamazine (DEC) is the drug of choice in filariasis. It immobilizes the microfilariae resulting in their displacement in the tissues.

Adverse effects are mild; anorexia, nausea, vomiting, dizziness and headache; an allergic reaction with itching, rashes and fever due to release of antigens from the dying worms may occur. Antihistamines are given with DEC to minimize these reactions. DEC can be given during pregnancy.

Uses

- *Filariasis* DEC is the drug of choice (2 mg/kg TDS for 21 days). In 7 days patients are rendered non-infective to mosquitoes as microfilariae rapidly disappear. But adult worms may need repeated courses.
- *Tropical eosinophilia* (2 mg/kg TDS for 7 days). Symptoms rapidly disappear.

❑ CANCER CHEMOTHERAPY

Cancer is one of the major causes of death. The treatment of cancers is still unsatisfactory due to certain characteristics of the cancer cells—like capacity for uncontrolled proliferation, invasiveness and metastasis. Moreover the cancer cells are our own cells unlike microbes which means that, drugs which, destroy these cells also can affect normal cells. The host defence mechanisms which help us in infections is not doing so in cancers as these cancer cells are also host cells. Moreover, the cancer cells can be in a resting phase during which they are not sensitive to anticancer drugs but can start multiplying later—resulting in recurrence. These features have made cancer chemotherapy more difficult.

CLASSIFICATION

1. ***Alkylating agents***	
Nitrogen mustards	Mechlorethamine Cyclophosphamide, Ifosfamide, Chlorambucil, Melphalan
Ethylenimines	Thio-TEPA
Alkyl sulfonate	Busulfan
Nitrosoureas	Carmustine, Streptazocin
Triazine	Dacarbazine
2. ***Antimetabolites***	
Folate antagonist	Methotrexate
Purine antagonist	6-Mercaptopurine
Pyrimidine antagonist	5-Fluorouracil, Floxuridine, Cytarabine (Cytosine arabinoside), Thioguanine, Pentastatin, Fludarabin, Cladribin
3. ***Antibiotics***	Actinomycin-D (Dactinomycin), Daunorubicin, Doxorubicin, Bleomycin, Mitomycin-C, Mithramycin (Plicamycin)
4. ***Epipodophylotoxins***	Etoposide teniposide
5. ***Camphothecins***	Topotecan, Irinotecan

6. ***Taxanes***	Paclitaxel, Docetaxel
7. ***Vinca alkaloids***	Vincristine, Vinblastine
8. ***Hormones***	Glucocorticoids, Androgens, Antiandrogens, Oestrogens, Antioestrogens and Progestins
9. ***Miscellaneous***	Procarbazine, Mitotane, L-asparaginase, Cisplatin, Interferon-α, Imatinib

General adverse effects to anticancer drugs Since most anticancer drugs act on the rapidly multiplying cells, they are also toxic to the normal rapidly multiplying cells in the bone marrow, epithelial cells, lymphoid organs and gonads. Thus the common adverse effects are:

1. *Bone marrow depression* resulting in leukopenia, anaemia, thrombocytopenia and in higher doses—aplastic anaemia. In such patients, infections and bleeding are common.
2. *Other proliferating cells* GIT—stomatitis and ulcers; alopecia (loss of hair), reduced spermatogenesis in men and amenorrhoea in women (due to damage to the germinal epithelium).
3. *Immediate adverse effects* Nausea and vomiting are very common with most cytotoxic drugs. Prior treatment with powerful antiemetics is required.
4. *Teratogenicity* All cytotoxic drugs are teratogenic and are therefore contraindicated in pregnancy.
5. *Carcinogenicity* Cytotoxic drugs themselves may cause secondary cancers,e.g. leukaemias are common after treatment of Hodgkin's lymphoma.

Apart from the above, the adverse effects unique to some drugs are discussed under individual drugs (Table 11.11).

TABLE 11.11: Specific adverse effects of some anticancer drugs

Drugs	*Specific adverse effects*	*Other prominent adverse effects*
Cyclo-phosphamide	Cystitis	Bone marrow depression, alopecia, stomatitis, vomiting, amenorrhoea, teratogenicity
Busulfan	Pulmonary fibrosis	Bone marrow depression, alopecia, stomatitis, vomiting, amenorrhoea, teratogenicity
Cisplatin	Ototoxicity	Renal dysfunction
Bleomycin	Pulmonary fibrosis, oedema of hands	Stomatitis, alopecia
Daunorubicin	Cardiotoxicity, red coloured urine	Bone marrow depression, alopecia
Doxorubicin	Cardiotoxicity	Bone marrow depression, alopecia
Mithramycin (Plicamycin)	Hepatotoxicity	Thrombocytopenia
Vincristine	Neurotoxicity, Peripheral neuritis	Muscle weakness, alopecia
Asparaginase	Pancreatitis, hepatotoxicity, mental depression	Allergic reactions
Mitotane	Dermatitis, mental depression	Diarrhoea

ALKYLATING AGENTS

Actions Alkylating agents exert cytotoxic, immunosuppressant and radiomimetic effects (similar to radiotherapy).

Mechanism of action These drugs form highly reactive derivatives which transfer alkyl groups to various cellular consistents and bind them with covalent bonds. Alkylation of DNA results in breakage of DNA strand.

Mechlorethamine is given IV as it is a highly irritant compound. It is used in Hodgkin's (MOPP regime) and other lymphomas.

Cyclophosphamide is converted to its active metabolite aldophosphamide in the body. It can be given orally. It causes cystitis due to a metabolite acrolein. This can be prevented by giving IV *Mesna*, irrigating the bladder with acetylcysteine, and by taking in large amounts of fluids. Mesna and acetylcystine contain—SH groups which bind the toxic metabolites and inactivate them.

Cyclophosphamide is used in Hodgkin's lymphoma, leukaemias in children and as an immunosuppressive agent.

Ifosfamide has actions and toxicities similar to cyclophosphamide.

Chlorambucil (LEUKERAN) is very effective against lymphoid series. It is the drug of choice in chronic lymphocytic leukaemia.

Melphalan is given orally in multiple myeloma.

Busulfan (MYLERAN) has selective activity against cells of the myeloid series and is the drug of choice in chronic myeloid leukaemia.

Nitrosoureas are effective in meningeal leukaemias and brain tumours because they cross the blood-brain barrier.

Dacarbazine is useful in malignant melanoma.

ANTIMETABOLITES

Methotrexate is a folic acid antagonist. It binds to dihydrofolate reductase and prevents the formation of tetrahydrofolate (THF). This THF is a coenzyme essential in several reactions in protein synthesis. The deficiency results in inhibition of protein synthesis. Thus rapidly multiplying cells are the most affected.

Dihydrofolate

DHFR ↓ ←--- Methotrexate

Tetrahydrofolate

Actions Cytotoxic actions—methotrexate mainly affects bone marrow, skin and gastrointestinal mucosa.

It also has immunosuppresant and anti-inflammatory properties.

Methotrexate toxicity can be largely prevented by administering folinic acid. This folinic acid gets converted to a form of THF that can be utilised by the cells.

Uses Methotrexate is curative in choriocarcinoma and is useful in acute leukaemias, breast cancer and soft tissue sarcomas. It is also used in rheumatoid arthritis and psoriasis.

6-Mercaptopurine (6-MP) is converted to a metabolite which inhibits purine synthesis.

Drug interaction 6-MP is metabolised by xanthine oxidase. Allopurinol inhibits xanthine oxidase and thus prolongs the action of 6-MP.

Uses 6-MP is used in acute leukaemias in children, choriocarcinoma and some solid tumours.

5-Fluorouracil inhibits the synthesis of thymidylate and thereby inhibits DNA synthesis. It is used in carcinoma of the stomach, colon, rectum, breast and ovaries.

Cytosine arabinoside is the drug of choice in acute myeloid leukaemia in adults.

ANTIBIOTICS

Actinomycin D (Dactinomycin) acts by inhibiting DNA—dependent RNA synthesis. It is one of the most potent anticancer drug and is used in Wilms' tumour, rhabdomyosarcoma, choriocarcinoma and some soft tissue sarcomas.

Daunorubicin and doxorubicin act by inhibiting DNA synthesis. Cardiotoxicity with hypotension, arrhythmias and CCF, is unique to both these drugs. They also cause vomiting, stomatitis, alopecia and bone marrow depression.

Daunorubicin is used in acute leukaemias while doxorubicn is useful in solid tumours and in acute leukaemias.

Epirubicin and mitoxantrone are analogs of doxorubicin which are less cardiotoxic.

Mitomycin C is converted to an alkylating agent in the body. It is used in cancers of the stomach, lungs and cervix.

Bleomycin forms free radicals and causes breakage in DNA strand. It has the advantage of the unique mechanism of action and is less toxic to the bone marrow—this is advantageous in combination regimens.

It is used in solid tumours—testicular tumours, squamous cell carcinoma of the head, neck and oesophagus.

It's most serious toxicity is pulmonary fibrosis and cutaneous toxicity but does not cause significant bone marrow depression.

Mithramycin (Plicamycin) is highly toxic, used in disseminated testicular tumours and in severe hypercalcaemia due to bone cancers. It reduces plasma calcium levels by its action on osteoclasts.

VINCA ALKALOIDS

Vincristine and vinblastine are obtained from *vinca rosea,* the periwinkle plant. They bind to microtubules in the mitotic apparatus and arrest cell division in metaphase. They are spindle poisons. The alkaloids differ in toxicity.

Vincristine (ONCOVIN) Vincristine is neurotoxic while bone marrow depression is less. It is used in leukaemias, Hodgkin's lymphoma, Wilms' tumour and brain tumour.

Vinblastine causes bone marrow depression, alopecia and vomiting. It is used with bleomycin and cisplatin (VBC) in testicular tumours; it is also useful in Hodgkin's lymphoma.

HORMONES IN CANCER CHEMOTHERAPY

Glucocorticoids Due to their lympholytic action, glucocorticoids are used in acute leukaemias and lymphomas. Rapid clinical improvement is seen but duration can vary from 2 weeks to 9 months. They are used for initiation of therapy due to their rapid action.

Glucocorticoids are also of value in the following.

1. with radiation therapy to reduce radiation oedema
2. in intracranial tumours to reduce cerebral oedema and
3. for symptomatic relief in critically ill patients.

Prednisolone or dexamethasone are commonly used.

Oestrogens are useful in (i) prostatic carcinoma as it is an androgen dependent tumour, (ii) breast cancer in males and in postmenopausal women—oestrogens are used in advanced cases where surgery or radiotherapy cannot be employed.

Antioestrogens Tamoxifen is an oestrogen receptor antagonist used in oestrogen receptor containing breast cancer (page 384).

Progestins are useful in the palliative management of endometrial carcinoma.

Androgens are used in the palliative treatment of breast cancer in postmenopausal women along with oophorectomy.

Antiandrogen Flutamide is used in prostatic cancer.

Drugs which cause least/no bone marrow depression
- Hormones
- Vincristine
- Bleomycin
- L-asparaginase
- Cisplatin

Curable cancers
- Hodgkin's disease
- Choriocarcinoma
- Burkitt's lymphoma
- Testicular tumours
- Wilms' tumour
- Acute leukaemias in children
- Ewing's sarcoma

MISCELLANEOUS

Procarbazine is effective orally in Hodgkin's lymphoma (MOPP regimen component). It damages DNA. This may make it carcinogenic.

Cisplatin gets converted to its active form in the cell, inhibits DNA synthesis and causes cytotoxicity. It causes ototoxicity, nephrotoxicity, peripheral neuropathy, nausea, vomiting and anaemia. Anaphylactoid reactions can follow its use. It is relatively less toxic to bone marrow. Cisplatin is used in ovarian and testicular tumours and cancers of the head and neck.

L-asparaginase The amino acid asparagine is synthesized by normal cells but malignant cells are unable to synthesize asparaginase and depend on the supply from the host. Asparaginase is an enzyme that converts asparagine to aspartic acid and deprives the malignant cells of asparagine supplies resulting in inhibition of protein synthesis. It is used in acute leukaemias.

General Principles in the Treatment of Cancers (Table 11.12)

Chemotherapy in cancers is generally palliative and suppressive. Chemotherapy is just one of the modes in the treatment of cancer. Other modes like radiotherapy and surgery are also employed. Combination of drugs is preferred for synergistic effect, to reduce adverse effects and to prevent rapid development of resistance. Drugs which do not depress bone marrow are useful in combination regimens to avoid overlapping of adverse effects. With appropriate treatment, cure can now be achieved in a few cancers. Maintenance of good nutrition, treatment of anemia, protection against infections, adequate relief of pain and anxiety and good emotional support—all go a long way in the appropriate management of this dreaded disease.

TABLE 11.12: Choice of drugs in some malignancies

Malignancy	*Preferred drugs*
Acute lymphatic leukaemia	Vincristine + prednisolone
Acute myeloid leukaemia	Cytosine arabinoside + daunorubicin
Chronic lymphatic leukaemia	Chlorambucil
Chronic myeloid leukaemia	Busulfan
Hodgkin's disease	M-Mechlorethamine O-Oncovin (Vincristine) P-Procarbazine P-Prednisolone
Multiple myeloma	Melphalan
Choriocarcinoma	Methotrexate
Carcinoma of testis	Etoposide + bleomycin + cisplatin
Osteogenic sarcoma	Methotrexate, vincristine
Wilms' tumour	Vincristine + actinomycin-D
Carcinoma of the head and neck	Fluorouracil + cisplatin

❑ IMMUNOSUPPRESSANTS AND IMMUNOSTIMULANTS

Immunosuppressants are drugs which inhibit immunity. They may suppress cell mediated or humoural immunity or both. They are:

1. **T-cell inhibitors** Cyclosporine, Tacrolimus, Sirolimus, Mycophenolate mofetil.
2. **Cytotoxic drugs** Azathioprine, Methotrexate, Cyclophosphamide, Chlorambucil
3. **Adrenocorticosteroids**
4. **Antibodies**

Cyclosporine is a cyclic peptide produced by a fungus.

Actions Cyclosporine acts at an early stage and selectively inhibits T cell-proliferation. It also inhibits interleukin-2 production. Thus cyclosporine selectively suppresses cell mediated immunity but not humoural immunity.

Adverse effects include nephrotoxicity, hepatotoxicity, anorexia, gum hypertrophy and increased susceptibility to infections.

Uses

- *In organ transplantation* Cyclosporine is very effective for the prophylaxis and treatment of graft rejection in organ transplantation surgeries—like kidney, liver, bone marrow and other transplants.
- *Autoimmune disorders* Cyclosporine is also useful in some autoimmune disorders like rheumatoid arthritis.

Tacrolimus is a macrolide antibiotic obtained from Streptomyces tsukubaensis. Its mechanism of action is similar to cyclosporine. Tacrolimus can be given both orally and parenterally but absorption from the gut is incomplete. It is extensively bound to plasma proteins.

Adverse effects include nephrotoxicity, gastrointestinal disturbances, hypertension, hyperglycaemia, tremors and seizures.

Sirolimus obtained from Streptomyces hygroscopicus acts by inhibiting the activation of T-cells. Sirolimus may be used in combination with other drugs for the prophylaxis of organ transplant rejection and in psoriasis and uveoretinitis.

Toxicity includes hyperlipidaemia, gastrointestinal disturbances and an increased risk of infections and lymphomas.

Mycophenolate mofetil a prodrug is converted to mycophenolic acid, which inhibits guanine nucleotide synthesis and inhibits the proliferation and functions of lymphocytes.

Mycophenolate mofetil is indicated as an adjunct to other immunosuppressive drugs in the prophylaxis of transplant rejection.

Cytotoxic drugs like azathioprine, cyclophosphamide and methotrexate inhibit cell mediated immunity (while cyclophosphamide predominantly suppresses humoural immunity).

They are used in the prevention of graft rejection and in autoimmune disorders.

Glucocorticoids have potent immunosuppressant activity and are used in the prevention of organ transplant rejection and in autoimmune disorders.

ANTIBODIES AS IMMUNOSUPPRESSANTS

Muromonab CD3 is a monoclonal antibody to CD3 antigens on T lympholytes. On intravenous administration, T cells disappear from the circulation within minutes. It is used with other immunosuppressants in organ transplantation. Fever, chills and pulmonary oedema may occur.

Antithymocyte globulin (ATG) binds to T lymphocytes and deplete them thereby suppressing immune response. It is used in the management of organ transplantation.

Infliximab is a monoclonal antibody and **etanercept** is a protein that block TNFα. They are useful in rheumatoid arthritis and Crohn's disease.

IMMUNOSTIMULANTS

Immunostimulating or immunomodulating agents are drugs that modulate the immune response and can be used to increase the immune responsiveness of patients with immunodeficiency as in AIDS, chronic illness and cancers. This is still a developing field of pharmacology. The drugs currently used for this purpose are BCG, levamisole and interferons. BCG has been tried in cancers. Levamisole used in helminthiasis is also found to enhance cell-mediated immunity in humans. It has been tried in some cancers.

Immunisation vaccines are used for active immunisation and antisera are used for passive immunization. Both of them impart immunity.

Interferons

Interferons are cytokines with antiviral and immunomodulatory properties. Recombinant interferons α, β and γ are avilable for clinical use. They bind to specific receptors and bring about immune activation and increase host defenses. There is an increase in the number and activity of cytotoxic and helper T cells and killer cells.

Interferons α, and β are mainly used for antiviral effects while interferon γ is used for its immunomodulating actions.

Interferons are indicated in several tumors including malignant melanoma, hairy cell leukemia, lymphomas, Kaposi's sarcoma, condylomata acuminata and in viral infections.

❑ VACCINES AND ANTISERA

Active immunisation is the administration of antigen to the host in order to induce antibody production. Vaccines are used for active immunisation. Vaccines are suspensions of microorganisms (dead or live attenuated) which stimulate the immunological defence of the host by developing antibodies. They impart active immunity, which takes sometime to develop and are therefore used prophylactically. The antibodies so developed destroy the specific microorganism when it enters the body (Table 11.13).

Toxoids Bacterial exotoxins modified to remove toxicity but retain antigenicity are toxoids.

Passive immunisation is imparting immunity to a host passively by the transfer of antibodies, e.g. antisera and immunoglobulins (Ig). This affords immediate protection as readymade antibodies are available. Antisera like tetanus antitoxin, gas gangrene antitoxin, diphtheria and antirabies serum are obtained from serum of horses which are actively immunised against the specific organism. Sensitivity tests should be done before giving antisera.

Immunoglobulins (Ig) are human gammaglobulins that carry the antibodies—like normal human gammaglobulin, tetanus Ig, rabies Ig, anti-diphtheria Ig and hepatitis-B Ig. Allergic reactions including serum sickness and anaphylaxis can occur with antiserum, while it is uncommon with Igs.

TABLE 11.13: Vaccines in common use and their recommended schedules

Vaccine	*Type of agent*	*Route of administration*	*Primary immunisation*	*Booster*	*Indication*
Bacterial vaccines					
BCG	Live attenuated	ID/SC	At Birth	7 and 14 years	In all children
Cholera	Inactivated	SC/IM	Adults: two doses 1 month apart	Every 6 months	People living in endemic areas
Diphtheria TRIPLE ANTIGEN	Toxoid	IM of age	6, 10,14 weeks at 4-6 years	18 months and	For all children
Pertussis	Inactivated	IM	6, 10,14 weeks of age	18 months and at 4-6 years	For all children
Tetanus	Toxoid	IM	6, 10,14 weeks of age	18 months and at 4-6 years	For all children; Adults: Post-exposure prophylaxis if > 5 yrs has passed since last dose
Typhoid/ Parathyroid	Inactivated	SC	After 3 years at any age: two doses 4 weeks apart	Every 3 years	Risk of exposure to typhoid fever
Typhoid (TYPHORAL)	Live inactivated	Oral (capsules)	Above 6 years at any age: 3 doses on alternate days 1 hr before food	Every 3 years	Risk of exposure to typhoid fever

Contd...

Contd...

Vaccine	*Type of agent*	*Route of administration*	*Primary immunisation*	*Booster*	*Indication*
Meningococcal	Bacterial poly-saccharides	SC	One dose	--	1. Travellers to areas with meningococcal epidemics 2. Control of out-break in closed population
Plague	Inactivated	IM	One dose	--	In an epidemic
Viral Vaccines					
Poliomyelitis (OPV)	Live virus	Oral	6, 10 and 14 weeks of age	18 months; again at 4-6 years	For all children
Measles, mumps, rubella (MMR) (MORUPAR)	Live virus	SC	12-15 months	11-12 years	For all children
Hepatitis A	Inactivated virus	IM	1 dose (2-4 weeks before travelling to endemic areas)	After 6-12 months	1. Travellers to endemic areas 2. Homosexual men 3. Persons at occupational risk
Hepatitis B	Inactive viral antigen	IM	At birth, 1 month, 6-18 months	After 5 yrs but not routinely recommended	1. For all children 2. Persons at occupational risk 3. Haemophiliacs 4. Postexposure prophylaxis
Influenza	Inactivated virus	IM	One dose	Yearly	1. High risk people like elderly, asthmatics

Contd...

Contd...

Vaccine	*Type of agent*	*Route of administration*	*Primary immunisation*	*Booster*	*Indication*
Rabies (RABTPUR)	Inactivated virus	IM/ID	**Pre-exposure** 3 doses at days 0,7 and 21 **Postexposure:** 6 doses IM 0,3,7,14,30 and 90	After 1 year then at 2-5 years	1. Postexposure treatment 2. Pre-exposure prophylaxis in persons at risk for contact with rabies virus
Varicella	Live virus	SC	2 doses 4-8 weeks apart at 18 months	--	All children from 18 months to 13 years with no history of varicella infection
Yellow fever	Live virus	SC	1 dose	every 10 years	1. Travellers to areas where yellow fever is seen 2. Laboratory personnel at risk of exposure

ID—intradermal, SC—subcutaneous, IM—intramuscular

Primary immunisation provides primary immunity and is usually given in children, e.g. DPT (triple antigen given to infants) (Table 11.14).

Secondary immunisation is done to reinforce the primary immunity by giving booster doses.

TABLE 11.14: Passive immunisation

Preparation with source	*Dose and Route*	*Indication*
Diphtheria anti-toxin (horse)	IV or IM 20,000-1,20,000 units	*Diphtheria* Clinical diphtheria to be given immediately
Tetanus immune globulin (human)	IM Prophylaxis: 2500 U Treatment : 3000-6000 U	*Tetanus* Treatment and postexposure prophylaxis of unclean wounds in inadequately immunised persons
Tetanus antitoxin (ATS) (horse) (If tetanus Ig is not available)	IM/SC Prophylaxis 1500-3000 IU Treatment: 50,000-1,00,000 IU	*Tetanus* Treatment and Postexposure prophylaxis of unclean wounds in inadequately immunised persons
Rabies immuno-globulin (human)	20 IU/kg half the dose infiltrated around the wound; remaining IM	*Rabies* Postexposure prophylaxis combined with rabies vaccine
Antirabies serum (horse)	IM 40 IU/ kg	Used if rabies Ig is not available but is inferior to it
Gas gangrene antitoxin (AGS) (horse)	IM/SC/IV Prophylaxis: 10,000 IU Treatment: 30,000-75,000 IU	*Gas gangrene* Postexposure prophylaxis and treatment
Hepatitis B immuno-globulin (HBIG)	IM 0.06 ml/kg	Postexposure prophylaxis in nonimmune persons; Hepatitis B vaccine shall also be given
Antisnake venom polyvalent (horse)	IV 20-30 ml to be given within 4 hr after the bite; additional doses may be required	Snake bite— Cobra, vipers, krait
Human gamma-globulin		Gammaglobulin deficiency; prophylaxis of hepatitis A, measles, mumps, rubella

12

Hormones

❑ HYPOTHALAMUS AND ANTERIOR PITUITARY HORMONES

The pituitary gland, under the influence of the hypothalamus secretes many hormones which either control the secretion of other glands or directly act on the target tissues. These are peptides and act by binding to specific receptors present on the target cells.

TABLE 12.1: Hormones secreted by the hypothalamus and anterior pituitary and their chief functions

Hypothalamic hormone	*Anterior pituitary hormone*	*Chief actions*
1. a. Growth hormone releasing hormone (GHRH)	Growth hormone (GH)	Regulates growth
b. Growth hormone release-inhibiting hormone (somatostatin) (GHRIH)	Inhibits GH release	

Contd...

Contd...

Hypothalamic hormone	*Anterior pituitary hormone*	*Chief actions*
2. Corticotropin releasing factor (CRF)	Corticotrophin (ACTH)	Stimulates adrenal cortex to secrete glucocorticoids, mineralocorticoids and androgens
3. Thyrotropin–releasing hormone (TRH)	Thyroid-stimulating hormone (TSH) (Thyrotrophin)	Stimulates release of T_3 and T_4
4. Gonadotrophin releasing hormone (GnRH, gonadorelin)	• Follicle stimulating hormone (FSH) • Luteinising hormone (LH) or (ICSH)	Stimulates growth of ovum and grafian follicle in the female and gametogenesis in the male; stimulates ovulation in females and regulates testosterone secretion in males
5. Prolactin–releasing factor	Prolactin (PRL)	Development of breast and lactation
6. Prolactin-release inhibiting factor	—	Inhibits prolactin-release

HYPOTHALAMIC HORMONES

Growth hormone releasing hormone stimulates anterior pituitary to secrete growth hormone. ***Sermorelin*** is an analogue of GHRH used in diagnostic tests of growth hormone deficiency.

Somatostatin is growth hormone release-inhibiting hormone present in the hypothalamus, parts of the CNS, pancreas and in gastrointestinal tract. It inhibits secretion of GH, TSH, PRL, insulin, glucagon and gastrointestinal secretions. But it is very short-acting. Octreotide is the synthetic analog of somatostatin which is longer-acting and useful in acromegaly and some hormone secreting tumours.

Thyrotrophin releasing hormone (TRH) secreted by the hypothalamus stimulates the release of TSH from the anterior pituitary.

HORMONES AND RELATED DRUGS

HYPOTHALAMIC

Releasing hormones
- TRH
- CRH (CRF)
- GnRH ***Analog—Leuprolide***
- PRIH
- MSH-RH

Inhibiting hormones
- PIH
- Somatostatin, (GHRIH)
- MSH-IH

PITUITARY

Anterior Pituitary
- Growth hormone
  - ***Antagonist***
  - Octreotide
- TSH
- ACTH
- FSH
- LH
- PL
- MSH

Posterior Pituitary
- Oxytocin
- ADH

THYROID

Hormones
- T_3
- T_4

Antithyoid drugs
Propylthiouracil
Carbimazole
Methimazole
Iodides
I^{131}

- ***Calcitonin***

PARATHYROID

Paratharmone

PANCREAS

Insulin
Glucagon

ADRENAL

Cortex

Glucocorticoids
- Hydrocortisone
- Prednisolone
- Beclomethasone

Mineralocorticoids
- Aldosterone

Sex hormones

Medulla

Adrenaline, Noradrenaline

GONADS

Sex hormones	***Antagonists***
• Oestrogens –	• Tamoxifen • Clomiphene
• Progestins –	• Mifepristone
• Androgens –	• Flutamide

Few examples have been given for each group

Corticotrophin releasing factor (CRF) releases ACTH and β-endorphins from the anterior pituitary. It is used in diagnostic tests in Cushing's disease.

Gonadotrophin-releasing hormone (GnRH, LHRH, Gonadorelin)—secreted in a pulsatile manner, regulates the secretion of gonadotrophins—FSH and LH. It is used in diagnostic tests in hypogonadism. Pulsatile administration of GnRH is used in infertility and delayed puberty. Continuous administration inhibits gonadotrophin secretion and is used in prostatic cancers. GnRH analogue **leuprolide** is used in prostatic cancer and some gynaecological conditions like uterine fibroids and endometriosis.

ANTERIOR PITUITARY HORMONES

Growth hormone (GH) a peptide, stimulates the growth of all organs except brain and eye. It increases the uptake of amino acids by the tissues, promotes protein synthesis and positive nitrogen balance. It causes lipolysis and reduces glucose uptake by skeletal muscles. It brings about linear growth. These anabolic actions are mediated by *somatomedins or insulin-like growth factors* (IGF) produced in the liver.

The secretion of growth hormone is regulated by GHRH and somatostatin (GHRIH).

GH deficiency in children results in *dwarfism* while excessive production results in *gigantism* in children and *acromegaly* in adults.

Uses

- *GH deficiency* Replacement therapy with GH in deficient children brings about normal growth. It can also be used in GH deficient adults.
- *Other conditions* GH has been tried in chronic renal failure and in catabolic states like severe burns and AIDS. It is liable for abuse in athletes to promote growth.

Corticotrophin (Adrenocorticotrophic hormone, ACTH) controls the synthesis and release of glucocorticoids, mineralo-corticoids, and androgens from the adrenal cortex (Fig. 12.1). It is used in the diagnosis of adrenocortical insufficiency.

TABLE 12.2: Uses of hypothalamic and anterior pituitary hormones and their analogues

Hypothalamic hormone	*Uses*
Sermorelin	Diagnosis of GH deficiency
Octreotide	Acromegaly, Hormone secreting tumors
TRH	Diagnosis of thyroid disorders
CRF	Diagnostic tests in Cushing's disease and hypothalamic-pituitary function
GnRH (gonadorelin)	Diagnostic tests of hypogonadism
Leuprolide	Prostatic cancer, uterine fibroids
Anterior pituitary hormone	
Growth hormone	GH deficiency, chronic renal failure, burns
Corticotrophin	Diagnosis of adrenocortical insufficiency
Thyrotrophin	Test for thyroid functions
Gonadotrophins	FSH-LH deficiency, undescended tests, amenorrhoea, infertility

Thyroid-stimulating hormone (TSH, Thyrotropin) Thyrotropin stimulates the production and secretion of thyroid hormones and thus regulates thyroid function. It is used to increase the uptake of radioactive iodine in thyroid carcinoma.

Gonadotrophins Follicle stimulating hormone (FSH) and luteinising hormone (LH)—produced by the anterior pituitary regulate gonadal function. They stimulate follicular development in women and also stimulate ovarian steroidogenesis (oestrogens and progesterone synthesis). In men they promote spermatogenesis.

Uses 'Menotropins' is the combination of FSH and LH obtained from urine of postmenopausal women. It is used in:

1. Gonadotrophin deficiency in males.
2. Undescended testes.
3. Amenorrhoea and infertility.
4. *In vitro* fertilization—to time the ovulation.

Prolactin This peptide hormone promotes the growth and development of breast during pregnancy. It stimulates milk production along with other hormones like oestrogens and progestins. Deficiency results in lactation failure while excess prolactin results in galactorrhoea.

Regulation of secretion—suckling is the principal stimulus for prolactin secretion. Suckling stimulates the release of prolactin-releasing factor from hypothalamus. Oestrogens and dopamine antagonists also stimulate prolactin-release. Prolactin is not used clinically.

Dopamine agonists like bromocriptine inhibit prolactin-release.

Bromocriptine is an ergot derivative with dopamine agonistic properties.

Bromocriptine is used

1. To suppress lactation and breast engorgement after delivery (like in still birth) and following abortion.
2. In galactorrhea—due to excess prolactin.
3. Prolactin secreting tumours.
4. Parkinsonism—bromocriptine is used with levodopa.

❑ THYROID HORMONES AND ANTITHYROID DRUGS

Thyroxine (T_4) and triiodothyronine (T_3) are the hormones secreted by the thyroid gland (for calcitonin see page 399). T_4 is a less active precursor of T_3.

Synthesis, storage and secretion The thyroid hormones are synthesized and stored in the thyroid follicles. The principle source of iodine is diet. The main steps involved in the synthesis of thyroid hormones are as follows:

1. *Uptake* of plasma iodide by thyroid cells by an active transport process.
2. *Oxidation* of iodide to I^+ (iodinium ions) by a peroxidase enzyme with the help of hydrogen peroxide. These combine with tyrosine residues of thyroglobulin (TG) to form monoiodotyrosine (MIT) and diiodotyrosine (DIT).
3. *Coupling* Pairs of MIT and DIT are coupled to form T_3 and T_4 catalysed by the same peroxidase enzyme.
4. *Storage* TG containing iodinated tyrosine residues are stored in the follicles.

The hormones T_4 and T_3 are released into the circulation and the secretion is regulated by TSH secreted by the anterior pituitary and TRH from the hypothalamus. In the peripheral tissues, most of the secreted T_4 is converted to T_3 which is the active hormone. Both T_4 and T_3 are extensively bound to plasma proteins. The free hormone is metabolised in the liver and excreted in the bile. The t½ of T_4 is 6-7 days and that of T_3 is 1-2 days. T_3 is 3-5 times more potent than T_4 and acts faster.

Actions Thyroid hormones are essential for normal growth, development, function and maintenance of all body tissues. Congenital deficiency results in cretinism. Thyroid hormones have important metabolic functions—they increase metabolic rate, enhance carbohydrate and protein metabolism and stimulate lipolysis. They facilitate erythropoiesis, are essential for normal functioning of the CNS (mental retardation is seen in cretinism), skeletal muscles, cardiovascular system, reproductive system and gastrointestinal system (hypothyroid patients are constipated while hyperthyroid have diarrhoea).

Uses Both thyroxine and triiodothyronine (leothyronine) are available and are given orally.

1. *Replacement therapy*
   - *In cretinism,* treatment should be started immediately to avoid mental retardation. Replacement should be continued lifelong.
   - *Hypothyroidism in adults* can be reversed by appropriate treatment.
   - *Myxoedema coma* is a medical emergency. IV thyroxine or liothyronine should be given with prophylactic corticosteroids to avoid adrenal insufficiency.
2. *Non-toxic goitre* T_4 suppresses TSH production and the goitre regresses.
3. *Thyroid carcinoma* T_4 induces temporary remission. It is used after surgery.
4. *Miscellaneous* Thyroxine is tried in refractory anaemias, infertility and non-healing ulcers.

Hyperthyroidism and Antithyroid Drugs

Hyperthyroidism is due to an excess of circulating thyroid hormones and could be due to various causes. Graves' disease, an autoimmune disorder, is the most common cause. It is characterised by hyperthyroidism, diffuse goitre and IgG antibodies that activate TSH receptors. Antithyroid drugs may act by interfering with the synthesis, release or actions of thyroid hormones.

Drugs used in hyperthyroidism

1. *Antithyroid drugs* Thionamides—Propylthiouracil, Methimazole, Carbimazole.
2. *Iodine* Iodides and Radioactive iodine.

Thionamides act by inhibiting the synthesis of thyroid hormones. Propylthiouracil also inhibits peripheral conversion of T_4 to T_3. T_3 and T_4 levels fall. Large doses may stimulate release of TSH resulting in thyroid enlargement. Carbimazole is commonly used as it is more potent and long-acting. Adverse effects are allergic reactions, jaundice, headache and rarely granulocytopenia.

Uses Hyperthyroidism—antithyroid drugs are used in hyperthyroidism.

a. *Graves' disease* or diffuse toxic goitre needs long term (1-15 yrs) treatment with antithyroid drugs.
b. *Toxic nodular goitre* As an alternative—when surgery cannot be done as in case of the elderly patients.
c. *Preoperatively*—hyperthyroid patients are made euthyroid with antithyroid drugs and then operated.

Iodides inhibit the release of thyroid hormones and in thyrotoxic patients the symptoms subside in 1-2 days. The gland becomes firm, less vascular and shrinks in size over a period of 10-14 days. These effects are transient and decrease after 15 days.

Adverse effects include allergic reactions like skin rashes, conjunctivitis, swelling of the lips and salivary glands, fever and lymphadenopathy. Chronic overdose can cause *iodism* with metallic taste, excessive salivation, lacrimation, running nose, sore throat, cough and rashes.

Uses

1. ***Preoperative preparation for thyroidectomy*** Iodine is started just 10 days prior to surgery to make the thyroid gland firm and less vascular.
2. ***Severe thyrotoxicosis*** Iodides act rapidly to reduce the release of thyroid hormones.
3. ***Prophylaxis*** Iodide or iodate is added to salt used in cooking to prevent endemic goitre.
4. ***Antiseptic***
5. ***Expectorant*** Used in cough.

Radioactive iodine ^{131}I given orally as a solution is rapidly absorbed and is concentrated by the thyroid in the follicles. It emits β rays which penetrate only 0.5 mm to 2 mm of the tissue so that it destroys only the thyroid tissue without damaging the surrounding structures.

It is used in the treatment of hyperthyroidism and in thyroid carcinoma. Small dose is also used for diagnostic purpose in thyroid function tests.

Advantages of ^{131}I are that administration is simple and convenient; surgery and its associated risks can be avoided. The disadvantages are (i) the long time (3 months) taken for maximum response, and (ii) the risk of hypothyroidism.

β-adrenergic blockers Many of the symptoms of hyperthyroidism are of sympathetic overactivity as there is increased tissue sensitivity to catecholamines in hyperthyroidism. β adrenergic blockers like propranolol relieve symptoms like palpitation, tremors, nervousness, sweating and myopathy. They only afford symptomatic relief and are used as adjuvants.

Ionic inhibitors interfere with the concentration of iodine by the thyroid gland. Thiocyanate and perchlorate inhibit the organification of iodine but are not used now due to the adverse effects. Food like cabbage; cigarette smoking and sodium nitroprusside increase the concentration of thiocyanate in the blood and may result in hypothyroidism.

❑ INSULIN AND ORAL HYPOGLYCAEMICS

Diabetes mellitus is a chronic metabolic disorder characterised by hyperglycaemia and altered metabolism of carbohydrates, lipids and proteins. It is a common condition affecting 1-2% of population and has a strong hereditary tendency.

Diabetes mellitus can be of 2 types.

Type I Insulin dependant diabetes mellitus (IDDM) is an autoimmune disorder where antibodies destroy the β cells of the islets of Langerhans. It usually occurs in young children and adolescents (hence called juvenile onset diabetes mellitus).

Type II Non-insulin dependant diabetes mellitus (NIDDM) is of maturity onset. Most patients are obese. There is both reduced sensitivity of tissues to insulin and impaired regulation of insulin secretion.

INSULIN

In 1921 Banting and Best obtained insulin in the form of pancreatic extract. In 1922 the extract containing insulin was first used on a 14 years old boy suffering from severe diabetes mellitus with excellent response. Insulin was then purified in a few years.

Chemistry, synthesis and secretion Natural insulin is a polypeptide synthesized from the precursor proinsulin. Human insulin differs from bovine insulin by 3 amino acids and from porcine insulin by 1 amino acid. Hence porcine insulin is closer to human insulin. It is stored in granules in the β islet cells of the pancreas. Normal pancreas releases about 50 units of insulin everyday. The secretion is regulated by factors like food, hormones and autonomic nervous system. The islets of Langerhans are composed of 4 types of cells—β cells secrete insulin, α(A) cells glucagon, δ(D) cells somatostatin and P cells secrete pancreatic polypeptide.

Insulin is metabolised in the liver, kidney and muscle.

Actions of Insulin

1. **Carbohydrate metabolism** Insulin stimulates the uptake and metabolism of glucose in the peripheral tissues especially skeletal muscles and fat.

   It inhibits glucose production in the liver by inhibiting gluconeogenesis and glycogenolysis.

   By the above actions, insulin lowers the blood glucose concentration.
2. **Lipid metabolism** Insulin inhibits lipolysis in adipose tissue and promotes the synthesis of triglycerides. In diabetes, large amounts of fat are broken down. The free fatty acids so formed are converted by the liver to acetyl CoA and then ketone bodies. This results in ketonaemia and ketonuria.

   Insulin indirectly enhances lipoprotein lipase activity resulting in increased clearance of VLDL and chylomicrons. In insulin deficiency, there is hypertriglyceridaemia.
3. **Protein metabolism** Insulin facilitates amino acid uptake and protein synthesis and inhibits protein break down—anabolic effect.

In diabetes, there is increased catabolic effect and negative nitrogen balance.

Mechanism of action Insulin binds to specific receptors present on the surface of the target cells and produces its effects.

Side effects

1. **Hypoglycaemia** is the most common complication of insulin therapy. It may be due to a large dose of insulin, inappropriate time of administration, unusually small meal or vigorous exercise. Symptoms—sweating, palpitation, tremors, blurred vision, weakness, hunger and confusion. Severe hypoglycaemia may result in convulsions and coma.

   Treatment Glucose or fruit juice like orange juice can be given orally or in severe cases IV glucose promptly reverses the symptoms.
2. **Allergy** This is due to the contaminating proteins in the insulin preparation. Urticaria, angioedema and rarely anaphylaxis can occur. It is rare with purified preparations and human insulin.
3. **Lipodystrophy** Atrophy of the subcutaneous fat at the site of injection may be due to immune response to contaminating proteins. It is rare with purified preparations. Insulin absorption may be irregular. Lipodystrophy can be prevented by using different sites for injection.
4. **Oedema** Some severe diabetics develop oedema which is self-limiting.

Preparations of Insulin

Insulin preparations differ in their source and duration of action. Conventional preparations are obtained from bovine (cattle) and porcine (pig) pancreas. They may be short, intermediate or long-acting (Table 12.3). All preparations are given SC. Only regular (plane) insulin can be given IV in emergencies. Insulins are destroyed when given orally. Doses are expressed as units.

Mixtures of short-acting and intermediate/long-acting preparations are given for a rapid onset and long duration of action.

TABLE 12.3: Preparations of insulin

Preparation	*Onset*	*Duration*
SHORT-ACTING	(hr)	(hr)
Regular (Plane, soluble)	0.5-1	8
Semilente (amorphous insulin zinc suspension)	1	14
INTERMEDIATE-ACTING		
Lente (Insulin zinc suspension)	2	24
NPH (Neutral protamine hagedorn) or Isophane insulin	2	24
LONG-ACTING		
Ultra lente (crystalline insulin zinc suspension)	6	36
PZI (Protamine zinc insulin)	6	36
Insulin analogs		
Insulin lispro	0.25	3-5
Insulin aspart	0.25	3-5
Insulin glargine	2-5	18-24
Highly purified insulin		
Human insulin		

Highly purified insulins and human insulin are also available as regular and lente preparations

Disadvantages of the conventional preparations are that:

i. They are allergenic because of the impurities (1%) and their animal source.
ii. They are not very stable.

Hence highly purified preparations are now made available which have advantages of being less antigenic, more stable, less chances of insulin resistance and lipodystrophy. But they are all expensive.

Highly purified insulins Insulin are purified by more developed purification techniques like gel filtration and ion-exchange chromatography. As a result the contaminating protein content is negligible. They have the following advantages:

— they are less allergenic
— more stable
— less chances of resistance
— less chances of lipodystrophy

Human insulins are produced by recombinant DNA technology. Human proinsulin gene is introduced into *E.coli*, cultured and proinsulin is extracted. This is modified to get human insulin. It can also be obtained by enzymatic treatment of porcine insulin. Human insulin is available as regular, NPH, lente and ultralente preparations.

Human insulin is less immunogenic and is absorbed more rapidly; dose needed is lesser (10%). It is more expensive.

Indications for highly purified/human insulins:
1. Allergy to conventional preparations
2. Insulin resistance
3. Lipodystrophy at the site of injection
4. Pregnancy.

Insulin analogs with favourable pharmacokinetic properties have been synthesized. ***Insulin lispro, aspart and glargine*** are insulin and analogs. They are absorbed 3 times faster than human insulin can be given subcutaneously 10 minutes before food; chances of hypoglycemia are less with insulin analogs.

Glargine is a long-acting analog which acts for 24 hours.

Insulin delivery devices have been designed which make insulin administration more convenient. Portable *pen injectors* are small pen-size devices containing multiple doses of insulin and retractable needles. They can be carried while travelling and to the place of work. Insulin pumps deliver appropriate doses of insulin on the basis of selfmonitored blood glucose results. The set is inserted subcutaneously.

Alternate routes of Insulin delivery have been tried—inhaled insulin and insulin nasal spray are being evaluated for use.

Drug interactions

1. β adrenergic blockers mask tachycardia, the important warning symptom of hypoglycaemia. They also prolong hypoglycaemia by inhibiting compensatory mechanisms acting through β_2 receptors.
2. Salicylates precipitate hypoglycaemia by enhancing insulin secretion and β cell sensitivity to glucose.

Uses of insulin
1. Diabetes mellitus
2. Myocardial infarction. Insulin, glucose and potassium chloride drip has shown to reduce mortality.

3. Schizophrenia—Insulin coma was first produced and after 20 minutes glucose was given. This treatment is not recommended now.
4. Burns—In patients with severe burns, insulin may be given with glucose to reduce the loss of nitrogen and potassium.
5. Hyperkalemia—Insulin glucose drip may be tried
6. Anorexia nervosa—Insulin increases the appetite in such patients.

Oral Hypoglycaemic Drugs

The main disadvantage of insulin is the need for injection. The advent of oral hypoglycaemics came as a boon to millions of NIDDM patients with early and mild diabetes. Sulfonylureas were the first oral antidiabetics (OAD) to be made available in 1950s. We now have many oral hypoglycaemics.

Classification

1. *Sulfonylureas*
   - *I generation* – Tolbutamide, Chlorpropamide, Acetohexamide, Tolazamide
   - *II generation* – Glibenclamide, Glipizide, Gliclazide
2. *Biguanides* – Phenformin, Metformin
3. *Meglitinides* – Repaglinide, Nateglinide
4. *Thiazolidinediones* – Troglitazone, Rosiglitazone, Pioglitazone
5. *Alpha glucosidase inhibitors* – Acarbose, Miglitol

Sulfonylureas

A sulfonamide derivative used for its antibacterial effects in typhoid patients produced hypoglycaemia. This observation led to the development of Sulfonylureas.

Mechanism of action Sulfonylureas reduce the blood glucose level by:

1. stimulating the release of insulin from the pancreatic β cells.
2. increasing the sensitivity of peripheral tissues to insulin.
3. increasing the number of insulin receptors.
4. suppressing hepatic gluconeogenesis.

Sulfonylureas bind to receptors on pancreatic β cells, cause depolarization and Ca^{++} influx leading to increased insulin secretion. Thus some functional β cells are essential for their action.

Pharmacokinetics Sulfonylureas are well-absorbed orally, extensively bound to plasma proteins, metabolised in the liver and some are excreted in the urine. Hence they should be avoided in patients with renal or liver dysfunction.

Adverse effects Second-generation agents have fewer adverse effects. Hypoglycaemia is the most common adverse effect, least with tolbutamide due to short t½ and low potency.

Nausea, vomiting, jaundice, and allergic reactions can occur. Patients on sulfonylureas may have an increase in the rate of cardiovascular death. However this is still controversial and sulfonylureas continue to be used.

Drug interactions

I. *Drugs that augment hypoglycaemic effect.*
   - NSAIDs, warfarin, sulfonamides—displace sulfonylureas from protein binding sites.
   - Alcohol, chloramphenicol, cimetidine—inhibit metabolism

II. *Drugs that decrease the action of sulfonylureas*
   - Diuretics and corticosteroids—↑ blood glucose levels.

Biguanides

Biguanides lower blood glucose level by insulin-like effects on the tissues. Mechanism of action is not clear. They

- Suppress hepatic gluconeogenesis.
- Inhibit glucose absorption from the intestines.
- Stimulate peripheral uptake of glucose in tissues in the presence of insulin.

Phenformin is not used therapeutically as it causes lactic acidosis. Metformin is safer with lower incidence of lactic acidosis. It does not cause hypoglycaemia since it is an euglycaemic agent.

Biguanides

- Have insulin-like effects
- Do not cause hypoglycaemia
- Weight reduction—due to anorexia
- Nausea, diarrhoea, metallic taste are transient
- Preferred in obese diabetics either alone or with sulfonylureas
- Contraindicated in renal, hepatic and cardiac diseases

Adverse effects Nausea, diarrhoea, and metallic taste are self-limiting. Rarely lactic acidosis can occur. Anorexia is advantageous as it helps in reducing body weight. Long term use may interfere with vitamin B_{12} absorption.

Meglitinides Repaglinide and nateglinide increase the release of insulin by acting on pancreatic β-cells. They are well tolerated with minor adverse effects like hypersensitivity reactions, hypoglycaemia and gastrointestinal disturbances. Meglitinides may be used either alone or with biguanides in NIDDM patients.

Thiazolidinediones (TZDs) increase glucose transport into muscle and adipose tissue and reduce hepatic glucose output. They may cause oedema, weight gain and anaemia. Liver function should be monitored. TZDs may be used with other antidiabetics.

α-glucosidase inhibitors—Acarbose and miglitol inhibit the enzyme α-glucosidase present in the intestines and reduce the absorption of carbohydrates. They also inhibit the digestion of carbohydrates. Adverse effects include diarrhoea, flatulence and abdominal distension. They can be used with other antidiabetics.

Treatment of Diabetes Mellitus

The aim of treatment is to keep the blood sugar within normal limits and prevent complications of diabetes. In IDDM, insulin is the only treatment.

Mild NIDDM may be controlled by diet, exercise and weight reduction. When not controlled, an oral hypoglycaemic should be given. Most NIDDM patients may require insulin sometime later in life.

Status of oral antidiabetics Uncomplicated NIDDM patients not controlled by diet and exercise are given OAD. Mild NIDDM patients with recent onset diabetes, age above 40 years at the onset of diabetes, obese with fasting blood sugar < 200 mg/dl are candidates for oral hypoglycaemics. They are convenient to use. Sulfonylureas are preferred but, when blood sugar is not adequately controlled, metformin can be added. Metformin has the advantages of reducing appetite and being euglycaemic. In conditions like stress, surgery or in any of the complications of diabetes, insulin should be used (Table 12.4). In some patients, insulin may be given along with sulphonylureas as the latter increase the tissue sensitivity to insulin.

TABLE 12.4: Preparations of some oral antidiabetics

Drug	*Dose*	*Duration of action*
Tolbutamide (RASTINON)	500 mg q 8-12 h	6-8 hr
Chlorpropamide (DIABINESE)	250-500 mg q24 h	36-48 hr
Glibenclamide (DAONIL, EUGLUCON)	5 mg q 12-24 h	18-24 hr
Metformin (GLYCIPHAGE)	500 mg q 12-24 h	6-8 hr

Insulin is effective in all types of diabetes mellitus. The dose should be adjusted as per the needs of each patient—guided by blood sugar levels.

Insulin resistance is said to be present when the insulin requirement is increased to > 200 U/day. It is due to the antibodies to insulin which partly neutralise it. This is rare with purified preparations and human insulin. Hence in presence of resistance, it is necessary to change over to highly purified/human insulin.

Treatment of diabetic ketoacidosis Ketoacidosis may be precipitated by infection, trauma or stress and is more common in IDDM patients. Acidosis, dehydration, electrolyte imbalance, impaired consciousness, and hyperventilation are the common features seen. Treatment is with regular (plane) insulin by continuous IV infusion. Fluid and electrolyte replacement are important.

Glucagon

Glucagon is synthesized in the alpha (α) cells of the pancreatic islets of Langerhans; like insulin, the secretion of glucagon is regulated by nutrients—chiefly glucose, paracrine hormones and autonomic nervous system. Fasting stimulates glucagon secretion. It is degraded in the liver, kidney and plasma.

Actions Glucagon increases blood glucose level by glycogenolysis and gluconeogenesis in the liver. It evokes insulin release. It mobilises stored fat and carbohydrates. Glucagon increases heart rate and force of contraction. It also relaxes the intestinal smooth muscles.

Uses

1. Severe hypoglycaemia—glucagon can be used in the emergency treatment of severe hypoglycaemia due to insulin.
2. Diagnostic uses—for diagnosis of IDDM.
3. Radiology of the bowel—as glucagon relaxes intestines.

❑ CORTICOSTEROIDS

Corticosteroids are hormones produced in the cortex of the adrenal gland. They are glucocorticoids, mineralocorticoids and a small amount of androgens. Cortisol is the major glucocorticoid while aldosterone is the major mineralocorticoid. The secretion of adrenal cortex is under the control of ACTH secreted by the anterior pituitary and this is in turn regulated by CRF (Fig. 12.1). This is termed hypothalamic-pituitary-adrenal axis.

STRUCTURE AND SYNTHESIS

The corticosteroids have a steroid (cyclopentanoperhydrophenanthrene) ring. They are synthesized in the adrenal cortex from cholesterol (Fig. 12.2) under the influence of ACTH.

Every day about 10-20 mg of hydrocortisone (maximum in the early morning) and 0.125 mg of aldosterone are secreted. They are also released in response to stress.

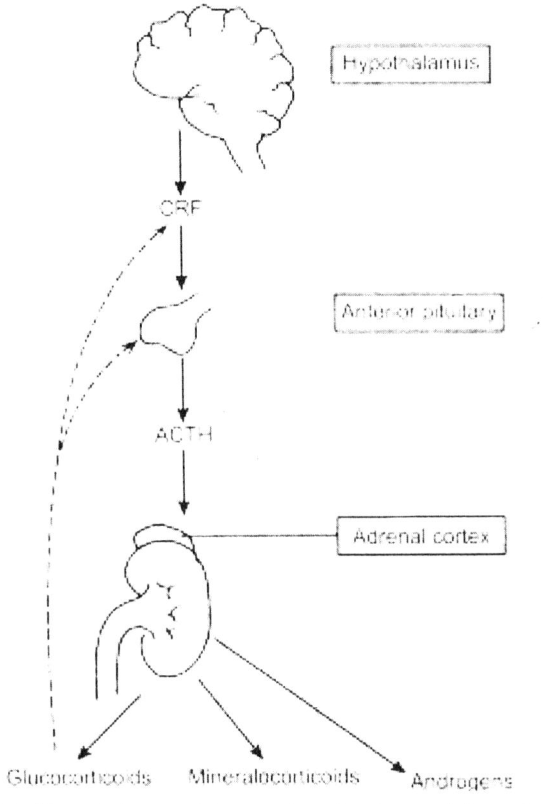

Fig. 12.1: Hypothalamo-pituitary-adrenal axis regulation of synthesis and secretion of adrenal corticosteroids

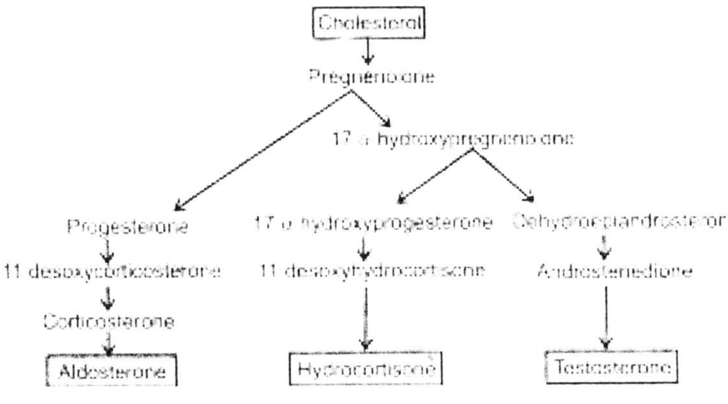

Fig. 12.2: Synthesis of adrenal steroids

ACTIONS

Glucocorticoid Actions

1. **Metabolic effects** *Carbohydrate, protein and fat metabolism*—Glucocorticoids promote gluconeogenesis and glycogen deposition in the liver and inhibit peripheral utilization of glucose resulting in increased blood glucose levels. They enhance protein breakdown and nitrogen is excreted leading to negative nitrogen balance. Glucocorticoids are catabolic hormones.

   They promote lipolysis and redistribution of fat takes place—fat is mobilised from extremities and deposited over the face, neck and shoulder and excess glucocorticoid activity results in moon face, fish mouth and buffalo hump.

2. **Anti-inflammatory and immunosuppressive effects** Glucocorticoids suppress the development of inflammatory response to all types of stimuli. They inhibit both early and late manifestations of inflammation. Inhibition of late response like capillary proliferation, collagen deposition, fibroblastic activity and scar formation may delay wound healing. They inhibit migration and depress the function of the leukocytes and macrophages including the release of chemical mediators. The ability of these cells to respond to antigens is decreased. In addition glucocorticoids also reduce the synthesis of prostaglandins and leukotrienes by inhibiting phospholipase A_2.

   Glucocorticoids thus suppress cell-mediated immunity, prevent manifestations of allergy and prevent homograft rejection. Large doses also inhibit antibody production.

3. **Other actions**
   - Glucocorticoids reduce capillary permeability, maintain the tone of arterioles and have a positive ionotropic effect. Prolonged use can cause hypertension.
   - They are essential for normal muscular activity.
   - They are required for normal functioning of the central nervous system. Deficiency results in apathy and depression while large doses result in restlessness, anxiety and sometimes psychosis.

- GIT—Glucocorticoids enhance the secretion of gastric acid and pepsin in the stomach.
- Calcium metabolism—Glucocorticoids inhibit absorption and enhance the renal excretion of calcium—they antagonise the effect of vitamin D on calcium absorption. Bone resorption takes place.
- Formed elements of blood—glucocorticoids have a lympholytic effect and this effect is very prominent in lymphomas. They also increase the number of platelets and RBCs.
- They are essential for maintaining normal GFR.

4. **Mineralocorticoid action** Glucocorticoids have a weak mineralocorticoid action—cause some salt and water retention and potassium excretion. Some synthetic glucocorticoids are devoid of this activity.

TABLE 12.5: Relative potency of some corticosteroids

Drug	*Glucocorticoid activity*	*Mineralocorticoid activity*	*Equivalent dose*
Short-acting (8-12 hr)			
Hydrocortisone	1	1	20 mg
Cortisone	0.8	0.8	25 mg
Intermediate-acting (18-36 hr)			
Prednisolone	4	0.8	5 mg
Methylprednisolone	5	0.5	4 mg
Triamcinolone	5	0	4 mg
Fludrocortisone	10	125	2 mg
Long-acting (36-54 hr)			
Paramethasone	10	0	2 mg
Dexamethasone	25	0	0.75 mg
Betamethasone	30	0	0.6 mg
Fludrocortisone	10	125	

MECHANISM OF ACTION

Corticosteroids bind to specific receptors in the cytoplasm, the drug- receptor complex is transported into the nucleus where it binds to specific sites on DNA and regulates the synthesis of new proteins that bring about the effects of glucocorticoids.

PHARMACOKINETICS

Most glucocorticoids are well-absorbed orally. Hydrocortisone undergoes high first pass metabolism. It is 95% bound to plasma proteins—transcortin. Glucocorticoids are metabolised by microsomal enzymes in the liver and are excreted by the kidneys. The t½ varies with each agent and we have short, intermediate and long-acting agents.

TABLE 12.6: Preparations and dose of some commonly used glucocorticoids

Glucocorticoid	*Trade name*	*Daily dose*
Hydrocortisone hemisuccinate	EFCORLIN	30-100 mg
Prednisolone	WYSOLONE	5-60 mg, 10-40 mg IM
Methylprednisolone acetate	SOLVMEDROL	4-32 mg
Triamcinolone	KENACORT	4-20 mg
Dexamethasone	DEXOMA	0.5-5 mg oral, 4-20 mg IV/IM
Betamethasone	BETNESOL	0.5-5 mg oral, 4-20 mg IM/IV

Topical Preparations

Several glucocorticoid preparations are available for topical use as creams, ointments, nasal and eye drops. Some of them also contain antibiotics (Table 12.7).

TABLE 12.7: Some topical glucocorticoid preparations

Hydrocortisone (LYCORTIN Oint)	1%
Triamcinolone (LEDERCORT ACETONIDE Oint)	0.1%
Dexamethasone (DECADRON Cream)	0.1%
Flucinolone acetamide (FLUCORT Oint)	0.025%
Betamethasone (BETNOVATE Oint, Cream)	0.025%
Beclomethasone dipropionate (BECLATE Cream)	0.025%
Clobetasol propionate (TENOVATE Cream)	0.05%

- Hydrocortisone, the chief natural glucocorticoid is used orally and parenterally; in emergencies it is used intravenously.
- Prednisolone has potent glucocorticoid with mild mineralocorticoid activity. It is the most commonly used preparation.
- Prednisone is a prodrug converted to prednisolone in the liver.
- Methylprednisolone is similar to prednisolone and is used as retention enema and for high dose pulse therapy.
- Triamcinolone, dexamethasone, betamethasone have no mineralocorticoid activity and have selective, potent glucocorticoid effects.

Inhalation steroids	
Beclomethasone (BECLATE INHALER)	50 μg, 100 μg 200 μg/metered dose
Budesonide (BUDECORT)	200 μg/metered dose
Fluticasone (FLOHALE)	25, 50, 150 μg/metered dose

Adverse effects of glucocorticoids Adverse effects of glucocorticoids (Fig. 12.3) are dependent on dose, duration of therapy and the relative potency of additional mineralocorticoid effects. Whenever possible, they should be used topically to avoid systemic effects. Single doses are harmless while short courses are well-tolerated. Prolonged use is associated with toxicity. Adverse effects include:

1. *Cushing's syndrome* with characteristic appearance of moon face, buffalo hump, truncal obesity, muscle wasting, thinning of the limbs and skin, easy bruising, purple striae and acne.
2. *Hyperglycaemia* and sometimes diabetes mellitus may be precipitated.
3. *Susceptibility to infection* is increased and the severity of any infection may be more because of immunosuppression. Opportunistic infections may occur. Previously dormant tuberculosis may become active.
4. *Osteoporosis* especially of the vertebrae is more common in the elderly.

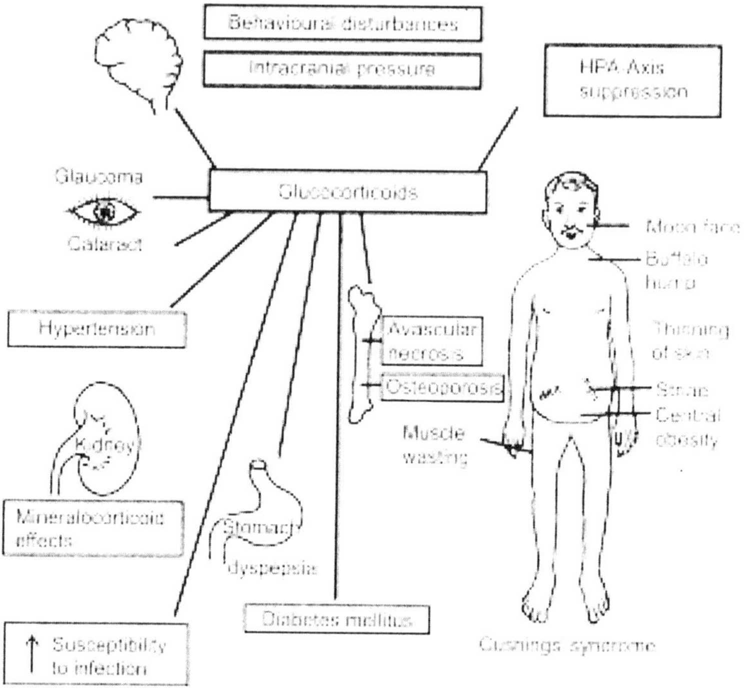

Fig. 12.3: Adverse effects of glucocorticoids

5. *Avascular necrosis* of the bone due to restriction of blood flow through bone capillaries may cause pain and restriction of movement. Growth in children may be suppressed.
6. *Peptic ulceration* may sometimes occur on prolonged therapy especially when other ulcergenic drugs (e.g. NSAIDs) are used concurrently.
7. *Mental disturbances* like euphoria, psychosis or depression can occur with high doses.
8. *Cataract* and glaucoma may follow long-term use of glucocorticoids even as eye drops.
9. *Delayed wound healing* Steroids may delay wound healing.
10. *Other effects* include raised intracranial pressure, convulsions, hypercoagulability of the blood and menstrual disorders.

11. *HPA axis suppression* depends on the dose, duration and time of administration. After prolonged steroid therapy, adrenal cortex gradually atrophies due to feedback inhibition. If steroid administration is suddenly stopped, acute adrenal insufficiency results. Hence after prolonged administration, steroids should be tapered before withdrawal to allow HPA axis to recover. Prior to surgery or general anaesthesia, it is advisable to elicit proper drug history. If the patient has received long-term steroids within previous six months, prophylactic hydrocortisone should be administered to avoid shock. Two weeks of use of > 20 mg hydrocortisone/day needs tapering of the dose.

    In order to minimize HPA axis suppression, (i) *lowest effective* dose of a glucocorticoid for the *shortest possible period* should be used, (ii) the drug should be given in a *single morning dose*, (iii) administration on *alternate days* is found to be associated with least/no HPA axis suppression and whenever possible this measure should be followed, especially when long-term steroids are needed.
12. *Mineralocorticoid effects* including salt and water retention, oedema, hypokalaemia and hypertension are rare with selective glucocorticoids.

Uses

I. Replacement therapy

A. *Acute adrenal insufficiency* is an emergency condition that could be precipitated by an infection or sudden withdrawal of steroids. Intravenous hydrocortisone hemisuccinate 100 mg bolus followed by infusion is given immediately. Correction of fluid and electrolyte balance are important.
B. *Chronic adrenal insufficiency* (Addison's disease). Oral hydrocortisone 20-40 mg daily is given. Some patients may need additional fludrocortisone (a mineralocorticoid)

II. Pharmacotherapy Glucocorticoids have been used in a variety of nonendocrine conditions where they may even be life saving.

1. *Rheumatoid arthritis* In progressive disease steroids are given with NSAIDs. If 1-2 joints are involved, intraarticular injections are preferred.

2. *Osteoarthritis* Steroids are given as intra-articular injections.
3. *Rheumatic carditis* Severely ill-patients with fever and carditis but not responding adequately to NSAIDs require glucocorticoids.
4. *Acute gout* When treatment with NSAIDs have not been successful, prednisolone is used as an adjuvant.
5. *Allergic conditions* like angioneurotic oedema, hay fever, serum sickness, contact dermatitis, urticaria, drug reactions and anaphylaxis—steroids are indicated. Steroids are slow acting and in less severe cases, antihistamines should be preferred.
6. *Bronchial asthma*
   - Acute exacerbations—a short course of prednisolone
   - Status asthmaticus—intravenous hydrocortisone hemisuccinate
   - Chronic asthma—steroids are used as supplement to bronchodilators. Inhalational steroids are used and in more severe cases low dose oral prednisolone is indicated.
7. *Collagen diseases* like polyarthritis nodosa, lupus erythematosus, polymyositis, Wegener's granulomatosis and other rheumatoid disorders respond to glucocorticoids.
8. *Eye diseases* Allergic conjunctivitis, uveitis, optic neuritis and other inflammatory conditions are treated with steroids. In ocular infections, steroids are contraindicated.
9. *Renal diseases* like nephrotic syndrome are treated with steroids.
10. *Skin diseases* Atopic dermatitis, seborrhoeic dermatitis, inflammatory dermatoses and other local skin conditions are treated with topical steroids. Systemic steroids are *life saving* in pemphigus.
11. *Gastrointestinal diseases* Mild inflammatory bowel diseases like ulcerative colitis are treated with steroid enema while severe cases need oral prednisolone.
12. *Liver diseases* Steroids are useful in conditions like chronic active hepatitis and alcoholic hepatitis.
13. *Haematologic disorders* like purpura and haemolytic anaemia having immunological aetiology respond to steroids.

14. *Cerebral oedema* Large doses of dexamethasone is given.
15. *Malignancies* Because of their lympholytic effects, steroids are used in the treatment of acute lymphocytic leukaemia and lymphomas—as a component of combination chemotherapy. Steroids are used for rapid symptomatic relief in other cancers like breast cancer.
16. *Lung diseases* Apart from bronchial asthma, steroids are used in other diseases like aspiration pneumonia and prevention of infant respiratory distress syndrome.
17. *Organ transplantation* For prevention and treatment of graft rejection, high doses of prednisolone are started at the time of surgery with immunosuppressive agents.

Contraindications to glucocorticoid therapy

Steroids should be used with caution in:

1. Peptic ulcer	6. Psychoses
2. Hypertension	7. Epilepsy
3. Infections	8. CCF
4. Diabetes mellitus	9. Glaucoma
5. Osteoporosis	10. Renal failure

MINERALOCORTICOIDS

The most important natural mineralocorticoid is aldosterone which is synthesized in zona glomerulosa of the adrenal cortex. Small amounts of desoxycorticosterone is also released.

Actions Mineralocorticoids promote sodium and water retention by distal renal tubules with loss of potassium. They act by binding to the mineralocorticoid receptor.

Adverse effects include weight gain, oedema, hypertension and hypokalaemia.

Fludrocortisone has predominantly mineralocorticoid properties and is used for replacement therapy in aldosterone deficiency as in Addison's disease. Although aldosterone is the principle natural mineralocorticoid, it is not used therapeutically since it is not effective orally.

Inhibitors of Adrenal Steroids Synthesis

Metyrapone, trilastane, aminoglutethimide and ketoconazole These drugs inhibit the synthesis of adrenal steroids by inhibiting certain enzymes involved in steroid synthesis. They are used in Cushing's syndrome and some prostatic and breast cancers.

❑ OESTROGENS, PROGESTINS AND ORAL CONTRACEPTIVES

PHYSIOLOGIC CONSIDERATION

At puberty, the ovary begins its cyclic function called menstrual cycle which stretches over 30-40 years characterised by regular episodes of uterine bleeding.

The hypothalamus releases the GnRH in pulses which stimulates the release of FSH and LH from the anterior pituitary. At the beginning of each cycle, a number of follicles in the ovary begins to enlarge in response to FSH. After 5-6 days, one of the follicles begins to develop more rapidly. The granulosa cells of this follicle multiply and under the influence of LH, synthesize oestrogens. This oestrogen inhibits FSH release, resulting in regression of the smaller follicles. Just before the midcycle, the oestrogen secretion reaches a peak, stimulating a brief surge in FSH and LH levels which results in **ovulation** by around the 14th day of the cycle (Fig. 12.4).

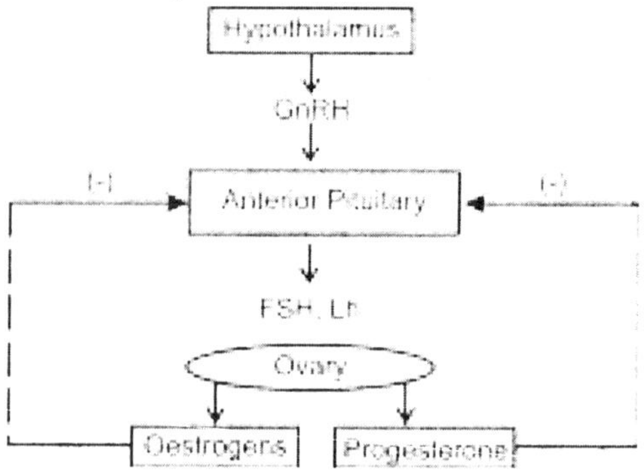

Fig. 12.4: Regulation of secretion of gonadal hormones

OESTROGENS

The oestrogens are produced by the ovaries, placenta and in small amounts by the adrenals and testes. During the first part of the menstrual cycle, oestrogens are produced by the theca cells in the ovarian follicle and after ovulation—by the granulosa cells of the corpus luteum. The major oestrogens are oestradiol, oestrone and oestriol. Oestradiol is converted to oestrone and oestriol by the liver and other tissues.

Natural oestrogens Oestrogens, Oestradiol, Oestrone, Oestriol.

Synthetic oestrogens Ethinyl oestradiol, Stilboestrol and Mestranol.

Actions Oestrogens are required for—

1. the normal maturation of the female reproductive tract.
2. development of secondary sexual characters in the female.
3. stimulation of preovulatory endometrium.
4. metabolic effects—oestrogens inhibit the resorption of bone and maintain the bone mass. They promote the fusion of epiphyses.
5. oestrogens are important for the maintenance of normal structure of the skin and blood vessels in women.
6. oestrogens decrease plasma LDL cholesterol and raise HDL cholesterol and triglycerides.
7. effect on blood coagulation—oestrogens enhance the coagulability of the blood.

Pharmacokinetics Natural oestrogens are metabolised rapidly in the gut—hence are not effective orally; they have a short t½. All oestrogens get absorbed through the skin and mucous membrane. They are largely bound to plasma proteins. Synthetic oestrogens are orally effective and are long-acting.

Adverse effects Nausea, breast tenderness, migraine headaches, hyperpigmentation, hypertension and cholestasis may be seen. In men gynaecomastia and feminization can occur. *Cancers* Increased incidence of endometrial and breast cancers are reported on long-term oestrogen therapy.

Teratogenic When given to a pregnant lady, oestrogens may cause:

- in female child—increased risk of vaginal and cervical cancers
- in male child—genital abnormalities.

Preparations Oestrogens are available for oral and parenteral use. A transdermal patch for cyclic oestrogen therapy is also available.

Uses

1. *Replacement therapy* In primary hypogonadism—oestrogen started at 11-13 years of age stimulates the development of secondary sexual characters and menstruation.
2. *Postmenopausal syndrome* Due to decreased oestrogen production at menopause, hot flushes, anxiety, fatigue, sweating, muscle and joints pain are common. Other longer-lasting changes including osteoporosis, genital atrophy, skin changes, increased risk of cardiovascular disease and psychological disturbances may be seen. Oestrogens given in low doses is highly effective in reversing most of the changes.
3. *Senile vaginitis* is common in elderly women due to oestrogen withdrawal from ovary. Oestrogen cream is used topically.
4. *Osteoporosis* In postmenopausal oesteoporosis, oestrogens restore calcium balance and need to be given for a long time.
5. *Oral contraceptives* Oestrogens are used (page 387).
6. *Dysmenorrhoea* Oestrogens combined with progestins suppress ovulation and such anovulatory cycles are painless. Oestrogens are used only in severe dysmenorrhoea.
7. *Dysfunctional uterine bleeding* Oestrogens are used along with progesterone.
8. *Carcinoma prostate* is an androgen dependent tumour. Oestrogens antagonise the action of androgens, suppress androgen production and are useful for palliative therapy.

Contraindications Oestrogen dependent tumours, liver disease, thromboembolic disorders.

ANTIOESTROGENS

Tamoxifen binds to the oestrogen receptors and competitively blocks the binding of oestrogens to its receptor. It is also a partial agonist at certain tissues. It is given orally.

Side effects include hot flushes, nausea, vomiting, vaginal bleeding and skin rashes.

Uses

Breast cancer Tamoxifen is used in advanced breast cancer in postmenopausal women with oestrogen receptor-positive tumours.

Clomiphene citrate binds to the oestrogen receptors and acts as a competitive inhibitor of endogenous oestrogens. Like tamoxifen, it is also a partial agonist. Clomiphene opposes the negative feedback of endogenous oestrogens on the hypothalamo pituitary axis resulting in increased gonadotrophin secretion and thereby induces ovulation.

Side effects include ovarian hyperstimulation resulting in multiple pregnancy, ovarian cysts, hot flushes, headache and skin rashes.

Uses

1. *Infertility* Clomiphene citrate is used to induce ovulation in infertility due to ovarian disorders.
2. *In vitro fertilization* Clomiphene induced ovulation is also useful in *in vitro* fertilization.

PROGESTINS

Progesterone is the natural progestin synthesized in the ovary and placenta. It is also synthesized by the testis and adrenals where it acts as a precursor of various steroid hormones (see under corticosteroids).

Progestins	
Natural	Progesterone
Synthetic	Medroxyprogesterone acetate Allylestrenol Megestrol Norethisterone acetate Lynestrenol Norgestimate

Actions

1. *Uterus* The secretory changes in the uterine endometrium like increased tortuosity of the glands are due to progesterone. In pregnancy, decidual changes in the endometrium take place under the influence of progesterone. Progesterone is very important for the maintenance of pregnancy (*Progestin* = favours pregnancy).
2. *Cervix* The watery secretion of the cervix is changed to a thick scanty secretion by progesterone.

3. *Vagina* Vaginal epithelium changes to that seen in pregnancy by the influence of progesterone.
4. *Breast* Along with oestrogen, progesterone is responsible for the development of the secretory apparatus in the breast and prepares the gland for lactation.
5. *Body temperature* Increase in the body temperature by 1°C that is seen during luteal phase which begins at ovulation is due to progesterone.

Adverse effects Headache, breast engorgement, rise in body temperature, oedema, acne and mood swings may be seen. Progesterone is teratogenic.

Uses

1. *Contraception* (see below).
2. *Hormone replacement therapy (HRT)* Progestins are combined with oestrogens in HRT of postmenopausal women. Oestrogen administration increases the risk of endometrial cancer—supplementing it with progestin counters this risk.
3. *Ovarian suppression* Progestins are used to suppress ovulation in dysmenorrhoea, endometriosis, dysfunctional uterine bleeding (DUB) and premenstrual syndrome.
4. *Threatened or habitual abortion* Efficacy in such patients is not proved.
5. *Endometrial carcinoma* Progestins are used as a palliative measure in cases with metastasis.

Therapeutic uses of oestrogens and progestins

Oestrogens	*Progestins*
1. HRT — Primary hypogonadism — Postmenopausal syndrome	1. HRT 2. Contraception
2. Contraceptive	3. Dysmenorrhoea
3. Senile vaginitis	4. DUB
4. Osteoporosis	5. Endometriosis
5. Carcinoma prostate	6. Premenstrual syndrome
6. DUB	7. Endometrial cancer
7. Dysmenorrhoea	

ANTIPROGESTINS

Mifepristone binds to the progesterone receptor and blocks the actions of progesterone. When given in early pregnancy—abortion occurs.

Mechanism Mifepristone blocks the progesterone receptors in the uterus and thereby causes decidual breakdown; blastocyst gets detached, HCG and progesterone secretions fall. This in turn increases prostaglandin levels and stimulates uterine contractions. It also softens the cervix and facilitates expulsion of the blastocyst. If given during the follicular phase—it also delays ovulation.

Mifepristone also binds to glucocorticoid receptors.

Uses

1. *Termination of pregnancy* Early pregnancy up to 9 weeks can be terminated with a single oral dose—600 mg of mifepristone followed 48 hr later by a prostaglandin to increase uterine contractions and facilitate expulsion of the blastocyst.

   Adverse effects include heavy bleeding, nausea and abdominal pain.
2. *Postcoital contraceptive* Mifepristone prevents implantation when given within 72 hr after coitus.

Regular use of mifepristone in late luteal phase acts as a contraceptive.

HORMONAL CONTRACEPTIVES

Millions of women around the world use hormonal contraceptives making them one of the most widely prescribed drugs. When properly used, they are the most effective spacing method of contraception. Hormonal contraceptives have greatly contributed to the control of population throughout the world.

Oral Pills

1. Combined-pill
2. Mini-pill
3. Postcoital pill

Depot preparations

1. Injectables
2. Subcutaneous implants

Combined pill contains low doses of an oestrogen and a progestin. They are highly efficacious (success rate 98%).

Ethinyloestradiol or mestranol are the oestrogens used. Newer progestins like desogestrel and norgestimate cause least side effects. The pill is started on 5th day of the menstrual cycle, taken daily for 21 days followed by a gap of 7 days during which bleeding occurs. This is monophasic regimen.

Oral contraceptives are also available as biphasic or triphasic preparations (Table 12.8). This reduces the amount of hormones needed and more closely mimics menstrual cycles.

If a woman misses a pill, she should take 2 pills the next day and continue the course. If more than 2 pills are missed, then that course should be withdrawn, should follow an alternate method of contraception for that particular cycle and restart the course of oral contraceptives on the 5th day of the next menstrual cycle. If the woman has conceived, the pregnancy should be terminated because these hormones are teratogenic.

TABLE 12.8: Oral contraceptive preparations

Regimen	*Oestrogen*	*Progestin*	*Trade name*
Monophasic	Ethinyl oestradiol 50 μg Ethinyl oestradiol 30 μg	Norgestrel 0.5 mg Levonorgestrel 0.15 mg	OVRAL-G OVRAL-L
Biphasic	Ethinyl oestradiol 35 μg	Norethindrone 0.5 mg (10 days) 1 mg (11 days)	—
Triphasic	6 days Ethinyl oestradiol 30 μg; next 5 days Ethinyl oestradiol 40 μg: next 10 days Ethinyl oestradiol 30 μg	Levonorgestrel 50 μg Levonorgestrel 75 μg Levonorgestrel 125 mg	TRIQUILAR
Mini-pill	Nil	Norgestrel 75 μg	OVRETTE
Postcoital pill	Diethyl stilboestrol (25 mg/day for 5 days) Or Combined pill (2 stat and 2 after 12 hr)	—	—

Mini-pill A low dose progestin is taken daily without a gap. As oestrogen is not used, its adverse effects are also eliminated. But efficacy is lower, menstrual cycles may be irregular and is therefore not popular and not preferred.

Postcoital contraceptives High dose of an oestrogen was used earlier. The combined pill is now preferred due to lower doses needed and lesser side effects reported. The pill should be started within 72 hours of coitus and has an efficacy of 90-98%. It is advocated as an emergency method in situations following rape or contraceptive failure.

Depot preparations are given as:

1. Intramuscular injections of progesterone at 3-6 months intervals, e.g. depot medroxyprogesterone acetate (DMPA) (150-400 mg) or Norethisterone enanthate (NET EN) (200 mg).
2. Implants—They are implanted under the skin.

> ***Contraindications* to combined pill:**
> - Thromboembolic and cerebrovascular disease
> - breast cancers
> - liver disease
> - OCs should be used with caution in diabetes, hypertension, convulsive disorders, oedema and CCF.

Norplant capsules implanted subcutaneously in the forearm or upper arm work for 5 years.

Disadvantages i. Amenorrhoea is frequent
ii. Permanent sterility may occur.

Mechanism of action of oral contraceptives The combined pill blocks the release of gonadotrophins from the pituitary and thereby inhibits ovulation.

Progestin only preparations make the cervical mucus thick and scanty and thereby inhibit sperm penetration. They also inhibit tubal motility and delay ovum and sperm transport.

Adverse effects Headache, nausea, vomiting, breast tenderness, amenorrhoea and irregular menstrual cycles may be commonly seen. Weight gain, acne, mood swings and hirsutism may occur. More severe side effects include—cardiovascular effects—in women >35 years there is an increased risk of MI and venous thromboembolism.

Cancers OCs may increase the incidence of cervical, breast and other cancers—but is controversial.

Cholestatic jaundice and gallstones Incidence may be higher.

Benefits of combined pills

1. Effective and convenient method of contraception.
2. Reduced risk of ovarian and endometrial cancers.
3. Reduced incidence of pelvic inflammatory disease and ectopic pregnancy.
4. Menstrual benefits—loss menstrual blood less, less iron-deficiency; premenstrual tension and dysmenorrhoea are less intense.

Centchroman a chroman derivative is a nonsteroidal oral contraceptive developed by research institute (CDRI), Lucknow. It has antioestrogenic and antiprogestogenic activity and may act by preventing implantation. Onset of action is quick (< 60 minutes) and duration of action is 7 days. Dosage (SAHELI, CENTRON) 30 mg twice a week for 3 months followed by once a week till contraception is desired (The tablet should be continued without withdrawing for menstruation).

Centchroman has the following advantages:

1. Success rate claimed is 97-99%
2. It is devoid of the side effects of hormonal contraceptives
3. Long t½ allows once a week administration
4. No teratogenicity, carcinogenicity or mutagenicity reported
5. It is well tolerated.

Centchroman may cause prolongation of menstrual cycles in 10% of women. It may cause ovarian enlargement and should be avoided in polycystic ovaries. It should also be avoided in renal and hepatic dysfunction, tuberculosis and in lactating mothers.

❑ ANDROGENS AND ANABOLIC STEROIDS

Androgens are produced chiefly in the testis and small amounts in the adrenal cortex. In the females, small amounts of androgens are produced in the ovary and adrenal cortex. Testosterone is the most important natural androgen. In the adult male, 8-10 mg of testosterone is produced daily. Secretion is regulated by gonadotrophins and GnRH.

Physiological actions In the male, testosterone is essential for the development of secondary sexual characters and sex organs. It is necessary for normal spermatogenesis and is important for maintaining sexual function in men. Testosterone promotes bone growth, enhances the muscle mass, protein synthesis and positive nitrogen balance—has anabolic actions.

Mechanism of action is similar to other steroids. Androgens bind to androgen receptors on the target cells, the complex moves to the nucleus where it stimulates protein synthesis.

Adverse effects Masculinization and acne in females, hepatotoxicity, increased libido and precocious puberty can occur in young boys. With large doses, salt and water retention, suppression of spermatogenesis resulting in infertility can be seen. Feminizing effects like gynaecomastia in men can occur as some androgens are converted to oestrogens.

Uses

1. *Testicular failure* Androgen replacement therapy in primary and secondary testicular failure.
2. *Other uses* Androgens may be used in senile osteoporosis and carcinoma of the breast in premenopausal women.

ANABOLIC STEROIDS

Anabolic steroids are synthetic androgens with higher anabolic and low androgenic activity. These are believed to enhance protein synthesis and increase muscle mass. But with higher doses, the relative anabolic activity is lost and these drugs act like other androgens.

Adverse effects are similar to those caused by androgens.

Preparations of anabolic steroids

Anabolic steroid	*Route*	*Dose*	*Trade name*
Methandienone	Oral	2-10 mg/day	PRONABOL
Nandrolone phenylpropionate	IM	10-50 mg/wks	DURABOLIN
Nandrolone decanoate	IM	25 -100 mg/3 wks	DECADURABOLIN
Ethylestrenol	Oral	2-4 mg/day	ORABOLIN
Oxandrolone	Oral	5-10 mg/day	ANAVAR
Stanozolol	Oral	2-10 mg/day	STROMBA

Uses

1. *Catabolic states* Anabolic steroids may benefit patients following surgery, trauma, prolonged illness and debilitating conditions. Given during convalescence, the negative nitrogen balance is corrected, appetite improves and there is a feeling of well being.
2. *Senile osteoporosis* seen in elderly males respond by formation of new bone tissue.
3. *Growth stimulation in children* Anabolic steroids promote linear growth in prepubertal boys. They may be used only for short periods—but actual benefit on final height is not established.
4. *Other uses* Anabolic steroids are tried in chronic renal failure to reduce nitrogen load on the kidneys. They may benefit in refractory anaemias with bone marrow failure.
5. *Abuse in athletes* Anabolic steroids enjoy a reputation for improving athletic performance. When combined with adequate exercise, the muscle mass increases. But the dose used by athletes is very high and is associated with serious adverse effects like testicular atrophy, sterility and gynaecomastia in men and virilizing effects in women; increased aggressiveness, psychotic symptoms and increased risk of coronary heart disease in both sexes. Moreover, there is no evidence that athletic performance improves. Hence the use of anabolic steroids by athletes has been banned and is medically not recommended.

Contraindications for the use of androgens.

1. Pregnancy
2. Carcinoma of prostate/breast in males
3. Infants and chlidren
4. Renal/cardiac/liver disease.

ANTIANDROGENS

Cyproterone acetate—a derivative of progesterone competitively binds to androgen receptors and thus blocks the action of androgens. It also has progestational activity.

Cyproterone is used to treat severe hypersexuality in males, in carcinoma prostate and in female hirsutism.

Flutamide is a potent competitive antagonist at androgen receptors. It is used in the treatment of carcinoma prostate.

Finasteride inhibits the enzyme 5-alpha reductase and thus inhibits the convertion of testosterone to its active metabolite dihydrotestosterone which acts mainly in the male urogenital tract. Fenasteride is used in benign prostatic hypertrophy to reduce the prostate size.

Inhibitors of androgen synthesis Gonadotrophin releasing hormone or its agonist like leuprolide when given continuously inhibit LH and testosterone secretion resulting in pharmacological castration—used in men with prostatic cancer (Table 12.9).

Antifungal agent *ketoconazole* also inhibits steroid hormone synthesis and thereby inhibits androgen synthesis.

TABLE 12.9: Antagonists of sex hormones and their uses

Hormone	*Receptor antagonist*	*Uses of antagonist*
Oestrogen	Tamoxifen	Breast cancer
	Clomiphene citrate	• Infertility • *In vitro* fertilization
Progesterone	Mifepristone	Termination of pregnancy
Androgen	Flutamide	Carcinoma prostate
	Cyproterone	• Carcinoma prostate • Hypersexuality in men • Female hirsutism

MALF CONTRACEPTIVES

The requirement of a safe and effective chemical contraceptive in men has not been fulfilled largely because it is difficult to totally suppress spermatogenesis. Various compounds including testosterone with progestin, oestrogens with progestins, antiandrogens like cyproterone acetate have been tried, but are neither reliable nor safe.

GnRH agonists and antagonists along with testosterone inhibit gonadotrophin secretion and is being studied.

Gossypol, a cotton seed derivative has shown to produce oligozoospermia and impair sperm motility in Chinese studies. This effect is reversible in a few months. Hypokalaemia is the major adverse effect.

DRUGS USED IN SEXUAL IMPOTENCE

Sexual impotence is the inability of a man to have satisfactory sexual intercourse due to inability to have and maintain an erection. Very often it is psychological while in some cases there could be an organic cause.

Several drugs have been tried including testosterone, yohimbine, papaverine and antidepressants. The recent introduction—Sildenafil (Viagra) has been a success in a large percentage of them.

Sildenafil (Viagra)

Sildenafil inhibits the enzyme phosphodiesterase in the penis and thus prolongs the life of cyclic GMP. This causes relaxation of smooth muscle in the corpus cavernosum and vasodilation—both resulting in cavernosal engorgement and penile erection.

Sildenafil is given orally (50-100 mg) 1 hour before sexual activity.

Adverse effects and precautions Due to vasodilation—headache, dizziness and nasal stuffiness can occur. Sildenafil potentiates the hypotensive action of nitrates and is contraindicated in patients on nitrates and in patients with coronary artery disease. Elderly men above 60 years need less dose (25 mg). Patients with liver disease, kidney disease, bleeding disorders and elderly people are at a higher risk of toxicity. Several deaths have been reported in such patients.

❑ AGENTS AFFECTING BONE MINERAL TURNOVER

Calcium and phosphorus are the most important minerals of the bone with 1-2 kg of calcium and 1 kg of phosphorus stored in it. Calcium and phosphorus metabolism are chiefly regulated by vitamin D and parathormone. Other hormones that also influence calcium and phosphorus metabolism are calcitonin, growth hormone, insulin, thyroid hormone, prolactin, glucocorticoids and sex hormones.

CALCIUM

Calcium is essential for tissue excitability, muscular excitation-contraction coupling, secretion from glands, myocardial contractility and formation of bone and teeth. It also maintains the integrity of mucous membranes and cell membrane. Calcium is essential for normal blood coagulation.

Calcium is absorbed from the small intestine by a carrier mediated active transport. Normally about 30% of the dietary calcium is absorbed, while in Ca^{++} deficiency, the absorption increases under the control of vitamin D (Fig. 12.5). The normal plasma calcium level is 9-11 mg/dl. It is excreted in faeces, urine and sweat.

Some preparations of calcium

Salt	*Formulation*	*Dose*
Calcium gluconate	10% inj—given IV 500 mg, 1 g tablets	10-20 ml
Calcium chloride	5-10% solution IV	5-10 ml

Adverse effects Oral calcium can produce constipation.

Uses

1. To prevent and treat calcium deficiency. Calcium supplements are given orally in children, pregnant and lactating women and in postmenopausal osteoporosis to prevent calcium deficiency.

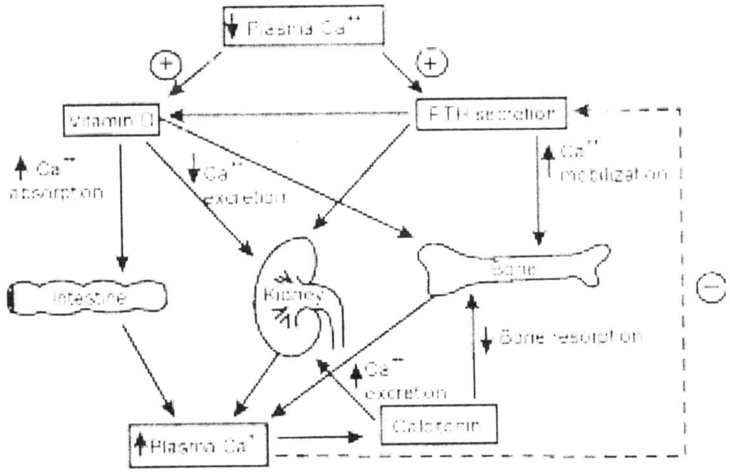

Fig. 12.5: Regulation of plasma calcium level

Tetany: 5-10 ml IV calcium gluconate followed by 50-100 ml slow IV infusion promptly reverses the muscular spasm. The injection produces a sense of warmth. This is followed by oral calcium 1.5 g daily for several weeks.

2. Vitamin D deficiency rickets—calcium is given along with vitamin D.
3. As an antacid—calcium carbonate is used.
4. For placebo effect—IV calcium is used in weakness, pruritus and some dermatoses. The feeling of warmth produced by the injection could afford psychological benefit.

PHOSPHATE

Phosphates play a vital role in various enzymatic reactions, are important for the structure and function of the cells and are important constituents of teeth and bone. Phosphorus is absorbed by the small intestine and excreted through kidneys under the influence of parathormone.

Hypophosphataemia results in muscle weakness and abnormal bone mineralization.

PARATHYROID HORMONE (Parathormone, PTH)

Parathormone is a peptide secreted by the parathyroid gland. Secretion of PTH is regulated by plasma Ca^{++} concentration—low plasma Ca^{++} stimulates PTH release, while high levels inhibit secretion (Fig. 12.5). Parathormone maintains plasma calcium concentration by mobilising calcium from the bone, promoting reabsorption of Ca^{++} from the kidneys and by stimulating the synthesis of calcitriol which in turn enhances calcium absorption from the intestines. PTH also promotes phosphate excretion.

Hypoparathyroidism is characterised by low plasma calcium levels with its associated manifestations. Hyperparathyroidism which is most commonly due to parathyroid tumour produces hypercalcaemia and deformities of the bone.

PTH is not therapeutically used. It is used for the diagnosis of pseudohypoparathyroidism.

Hormones that influence bone metabolism
• Vitamin D
• Paratharmone
• Calcitonin
• Glucocorticoids
• Estrogens

VITAMIN D

Vitamin D a fat-soluble vitamin, is a prehormone produced in the skin from 7-dehydrocholesterol under the influence of ultraviolet rays. It is converted to active metabolites in the body which regulate plasma calcium levels and various functions of the cells.

Source

- Diet—as ergocalciferol (vitamin D_2) from plants.
- Cholecalciferol (vitamin D_3) is synthesized in the skin from 7-dehydrocholesterol.

Cholecalciferol (vitamin D_3) is converted to 25-OHD_3 (calcifediol) in the liver (Fig. 12.6) which is in turn converted to 1,25-dihydroxycholecalciferol (calcitriol) in the kidneys.

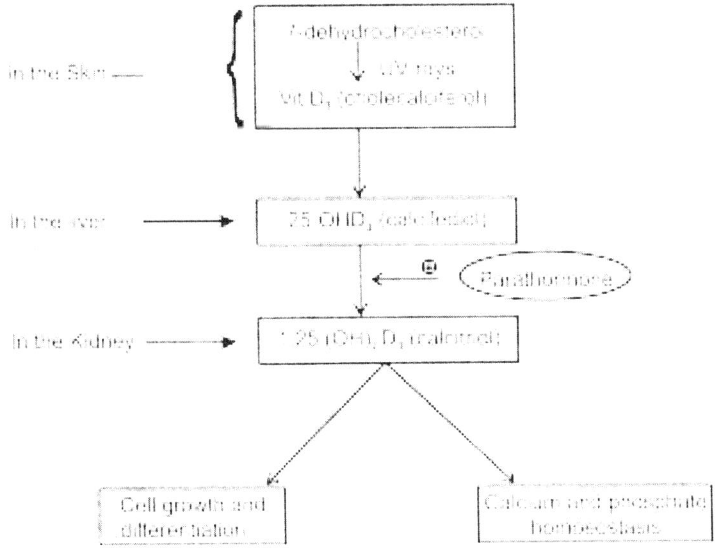

Fig. 12.6: Synthesis and functions of vitamin D

Calcitriol is the active form of vit D while calcifediol is the main metabolite in circulation. Convertion of calcifediol to calcitriol is influenced by PTH and plasma phosphate concentration.

Actions The chief actions of calcitriol are:

- it stimulates calcium and phosphate absorption in the intestine
- mobilises calcium from bone by promoting osteoclastic activity
- increases reabsorption of Ca^{++} from kidney tubules.

Calcitriol is essential for normal bone mineralization. It is essential for skeletal muscles as well as cellular growth and differentiation.

Vitamin D deficiency results in low plasma calcium and phosphate levels with abnormal mineralization of the bone; causes rickets in children and osteomalacia in adults.

Daily requirement—400 IU (10 mg).

Pharmacokinetics Given orally, vit D is well-absorbed from the small intestines in the presence of bile salts. It is converted to 25-OHD_3 in the liver and circulates in the plasma, bound to a protein and is stored in the adipose tissue. Vitamin D is also degraded in the liver and the metabolites are excreted in the bile.

Preparations

- Calciferol capsules 25000; 50,000 IU.
- Cholecalciferol granules—oral 60,000 IU in IG; 3,00,000 IU/ml; 6,00,000 IU/ml inj.
- Shark liver oil with vit D—1000 IU/ml, vit A—6000 IU/ml.

Adverse reactions High doses of vitamin D used for long periods result in hypervitaminosis D manifesting as generalised decalcification of the bones, hypercalcaemia, hyperphosphataemia resulting in weakness, drowsiness, nausea, abdominal pain, thirst, renal stones and hypertension. Hypervitaminosis D in children is most often due to unnecessary vit D supplementation by parents.

Uses

1. *Prophylaxis*—400 IU daily or 3,00,000 IU every 3-6 months IM prevents vit D deficiency. Adequate dietary calcium and phosphate intake is necessary. In the breastfed infants, from the first month onwards oral vit D supplements are needed. In obstructive jaundice, prophylactic 6,00,000 units vit D given IM prevents deficiency.
2. *Nutritional rickets and osteomalacia* 6,00,000 units IM repeated after 4-6 weeks is needed in rickets and osteomalacia along with calcium supplements.
3. *Vitamin D resistant rickets* is a hereditary disorder with abnormality in renal phosphate reabsorption. Phosphate with vitamin D is found to be useful.
4. *Vitamin D dependent rickets* is due to calcitriol deficiency (inability to convert calcifediol to calcitriol) and is treated with calcitriol.
5. *Senile osteoporosis* Oral vit D supplements with calcium may be tried.
6. *Hypoparathyroidism* Calcitriol with Ca^{++} supplements are beneficial.

CALCITONIN

Calcitonin is a peptide hormone secreted by the parafollicular 'C' cells of the thyroid gland. Secretion is regulated by plasma Ca^{++} concentration, i.e. high plasma Ca^{++} stimulates calcitonin release.

Actions The chief effects of calcitonin are to lower serum calcium and phosphate by its actions on the bone and kidney. It inhibits osteoclastic bone resorption and in the kidney, it reduces both calcium and phosphate reabsorption.

In general the effects are opposite to that of PTH. Calcitonin is used to control hypercalcaemia, Paget's disease, metastatic bone cancer and osteoporosis and to increase bone mineral density.

Other hormones that regulate bone turnover are glucocorticoids and oestrogens. Glucocorticoids antagonise vitamin D stimulated intestinal calcium absorption and enhance renal Ca^{++} excretion. Oestrogens reduce bone resorption by PTH and also enhance calcitriol levels. Oestrogen receptors are found in bone which suggests that they may also have a direct effect on bone remodeling.

BISPHOSPHONATES
(Etidronate, Pamidronate, Alendronate)

Bisphosphonates are analogs of pyrophosphate; they inhibit bone resorption. Bisphosphonates get incorporated into bone matrix, are imbibed by osteoclasts and then incapacitate the osteoclasts resulting in reduced bone resorption. They also slow the formation and dissolution of hydroxyapatite crystals.

Fever, gastritis and hypocalcaemia can occur. Long-term use can lead to osteomalacia due to inhibition of bone mineralization.

Uses Bisphosphonates are used in Paget's disease of the bone, hypercalcaemia and is tried in postmenopausal osteoporosis.

Index

A

B

D

E

F

G

H

M

N

T